# Sports Injury Prevention and Rehabilitation

World-class preparation and rehabilitation of the injured athlete integrates best practice in sports medicine and physical therapy with training and conditioning techniques based on cutting-edge sports science. In this ground-breaking new book, leading sports injury and rehabilitation professionals, strength and conditioning coaches, biomechanists and sport scientists show how this integrated model works in practice across the full spectrum of athlete care, from the prevention of sports injury to the assessment and treatment of injuries, and the design and implementation of effective rehabilitation programmes. Crucially, in every chapter, there is a sharp focus on return to performance, rather than just a return to play.

The book introduces evidence-based best practice in all the core functional and professional areas of sports injury prevention and management, including:

- the performance framework for rehabilitation;
- end-stage rehabilitation, testing and training for a return to performance;
- performance frameworks for medical and injury screening;
- the psychology of injury and rehabilitation;
- developing core stability and flexibility;
- assessment of training and rehabilitation loads;
- performance retraining of muscle, tendon and bone injuries;
- recovery from training and rehabilitation;
- the influence of pain on performance;
- running, throwing and landing mechanics and their contribution to injury and performance.

Every chapter is set up as a masterclass from world-leading practitioners from a range of elite sports teams and is written to have real-world application. Chapters contain best practice protocols, procedures and specimen programmes designed for high performance, with examples drawn from a wide range of individual and team sports.

No other book examines rehabilitation in such detail from a high-performance standpoint, and therefore *Sports Injury Prevention and Rehabilitation* is essential reading for any course in sports injury, sports therapy or sports medicine, and for any clinician, physical therapist, coach or sport scientist working to prevent or rehabilitate sports injuries.

**David Joyce** is an athletic performance and rehabilitation specialist who has worked at the highest levels of world sport and with multiple national, world and Olympic champions. He holds masters degrees in both sports physiotherapy and strength and conditioning and has worked at two Olympic Games as a physiotherapist and performance coach (with Team Great Britain at the 2008 Olympics in Beijing and with Team China at the 2012 Olympics in London). He has also worked in elite rugby (Western Force, Hull FC and Saracens) and football (Blackburn Rovers and Galatasaray SK). He is the co-editor and key contributor of *High Performance Training for Sports*, presents internationally on high-performance management and injury rehabilitation, and lectures on the Masters of Strength and Conditioning course at Edith Cowan University in Perth, Western Australia. David is currently the Head of Athletic Performance at the Greater Western Sydney Giants in the Australian Football League and lives in Sydney, Australia.

**Dan Lewindon** graduated with a BSc (Hons) in physiotherapy from Nottingham University in 2000. He spent three years working in the National Health Service, gaining experience in all aspects of physiotherapy, before seeking expertise in his chosen field of sports medicine. Dan joined Northampton Saints RFC in 2003, working full time with the Senior Team and progressing to the Lead role in 2008. He completed an MSc in sports medicine at Queen Mary's University of London in 2007 and a second MSc in exercise science (strength and conditioning) at Edith Cowan University in Australia in 2011. Dan was appointed Physiotherapist for the England Senior Rugby Team in 2009 and now works with them full time. Dan is the co-editor of and key contributor of *High Performance Training for Sports* and through his work has developed particular interest and expertise in lower limb and soft tissue injury and rehabilitation. Dan has lectured internationally in injury screening, rehabilitation and prevention strategies and lives in Market Harborough, England.

# Sports Injury Prevention and Rehabilitation

Integrating medicine and science
for performance solutions

Edited by David Joyce
and Daniel Lewindon

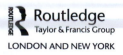

Routledge
Taylor & Francis Group

LONDON AND NEW YORK

First published 2016
by Routledge
2 Park Square, Milton Park, Abingdon, Oxon OX14 4RN

and by Routledge
711 Third Avenue, New York, NY 10017

*Routledge is an imprint of the Taylor & Francis Group, an informa business*

© 2016 D. Joyce & D. Lewindon

*British Library Cataloguing in Publication Data*
A catalogue record for this book is available from the British Library

*Library of Congress Cataloging-in-Publication Data*
Sports injury prevention and rehabilitation : integrating medicine and
   science for performance solutions / edited by David Joyce and Daniel
   Lewindon.
      pages cm
   Includes bibliographical references and index.
   1. Sports injuries—Prevention.   2. Sports injuries—Patients—
Rehabilitation.   I. Joyce, David, 1976– editor.   II. Lewindon, Daniel, editor.
   RD97.S658 2016
   617.1′027—dc23
   2015024428

ISBN: 978-0-415-81505-5 (hbk)
ISBN: 978-0-415-81506-2 (pbk)
ISBN: 978-0-203-06648-5 (ebk)

Typeset in Baskerville
by Apex CoVantage, LLC

# Contents

*List of contributors*                                                      ix

**PART I**
**The performance team**                                                     1

1  Reconditioning: A performance-based response to
   an injury (*Bill Knowles*)                                                3

2  Strength and conditioning in injury prevention
   and rehabilitation (*Ben Rosenblatt*)                                    11

3  Psychology in injury prevention and rehabilitation (*Tig Calvert*)       22

4  Nutrition in injury prevention and rehabilitation (*Matt Lovell*)        31

**PART 2**
**Athletic competencies**                                                   43

5  Medical assessment and pre-participation screening
   (*Mike Bundy and Lisa Hodgson*)                                          45

6  The injury risk profiling process (*David Joyce and Dan Lewindon*)       62

7  Assessing and developing the kinetic chain (*Ian Prangley*)              77

8  Assessing athletic qualities (*Nick Winkelman*)                          95

9  Running mechanics in injury prevention and performance
   (*Frans Bosch and John IJzerman*)                                       106

10 Landing mechanics in injury prevention and performance
   rehabilitation (*Julie Steele and Jeremy Sheppard*)                     121

11 Throwing mechanics in injury prevention and performance
   rehabilitation (*Steve McCaig and Mark Young*)                          139

12  Core stability in injury prevention and performance
    (*Lee Burton and Gray Cook*)                                              153

13  Flexibility in injury prevention and performance (*Anthony Blazevich*)    169


**PART 3**
**Injury processes, prevention and return to performance**                   179

14  Muscle injuries (*Dan Lewindon and Justin Lee*)                          181

15  Tendon injuries (*Craig Ranson, David Joyce and Polly McGuiggan*)        199

16  Bone injuries (*Henry Wajswelner and Sophia Nimphius*)                   212

17  Pain and performance (*David Joyce and David Butler*)                    223

18  Determining return to play (*Calvin Morriss and Phil Pask*)             232


**PART 4**
**Managing the injured athlete**                                             243

19  The athletic neck (*Kay Robinson*)                                       245

20  The athletic shoulder (*Ian Horsley and Ben Ashworth*)                   259

21  The athletic elbow (*Adam Olsen and Mike Reinold*)                       274

22  The athletic spine (*Tim Mitchell, Angus Burnett and Peter O'Sullivan*) 289

23  The athletic hip and groin (*Enda King*)                                 307

24  The athletic knee (*Chris Mallac and David Joyce*)                       322

25  The athletic shin (*Andy Franklyn-Miller*)                               337

26  The athletic foot and ankle (*Dan Lewindon and David Joyce*)            346


**PART 5**
**Managing the training athlete**                                            371

27  Managing pre-season and in-season training (*Raphael Brandon*)           373

28  Monitoring training load (*Stuart Cormack and Aaron Coutts*)             380

29  Optimizing athlete recovery (*Christian Cook, Liam Kilduff
    and Blair Crowther*)                                                      392

30  Environmental stress – heat and altitude (*Chris R. Abbiss*)             401

**PART 6**
**Special considerations**                                              413

31  The developing athlete (*Ian Jeffreys*)                             415

32  The female athlete (*N. Travis Triplett and Margaret Stone*)        429

33  The travelling athlete (*Shona Halson and Emidio Pacecca*)          436


    *Index*                                                             445

# Contributors

**Chris R. Abbiss,** Associate Professor – Physiology, and Postgraduate Course Coordinator, Exercise and Health Science, Edith Cowan University, Australia

**Ben Ashworth,** First Team Physiotherapist, Arsenal Football Club, UK

**Anthony Blazevich,** Associate Professor in Biomechanics, Director of Centre for Exercise and Sports Science Research, Edith Cowan University, Australia

**Frans Bosch,** International Sports Performance consultant and lecturer, Fontys University, Netherlands

**Raphael Brandon,** Head of Science and Medicine, England and Wales Cricket Board, UK

**Mike Bundy,** Consultant in Sports and Exercise Medicine, Pure Sports Medicine, UK

**Angus Burnett,** Project Manager, Sports Spine Centre, Aspertar, Qatar Orthopaedic and Sports Medicine Hospital, Qatar

**Lee Burton,** President, Functional Movement Systems, USA

**David Butler,** Director, Neuro Orthopaedic Institute, Australia; Adjunct Senior Lecturer, University of South Australia, Australia

**Tig Calvert,** Independent Sports Psychologist, UK

**Christian Cook,** Professor, Sports Science, Bangor University, UK; Technical Advisor, Rugby Football Union, UK

**Gray Cook,** Founder, Functional Movement Systems, USA

**Stuart Cormack,** Senior Lecturer, School of Exercise Science, Australian Catholic University, Australia

**Aaron Coutts,** Professor of Sport and Exercise Science, University of Technology Sydney, Australia

**Blair Crowther,** Research Associate, Hamlyn Centre, Imperial College London, UK

**Andy Franklyn-Miller,** Consultant in Sports and Exercise Medicine, Sports Surgery Clinic, Dublin, Ireland

**Shona Halson,** Senior Physiologist, Australian Institute of Sport, Australia

**Lisa Hodgson,** Assistant Professor in Sport and Exercise Medicine, University of Nottingham, UK; Managing Director, Corobeus Sports Consultancy, UK

**Ian Horsley,** Regional Lead Physiotherapist (NW), English Institute of Sport, UK; Associate Lecturer, University of Salford, UK

**John IJzerman,** Sports Physician, Dutch Olympic Committee, Netherlands

**Ian Jeffreys,** Reader in Strength and Conditioning, University of South Wales, UK; Proprietor, All-Pro Performance, UK

**Liam Kilduff,** Professor of Elite Performance, A-STEM, College of Engineering, Swansea University, UK

**Enda King,** Head of Performance Rehabilitation, Sports Surgery Clinic, Dublin, Ireland

**Bill Knowles,** Director of Reconditioning and Athletic Development, HP Sports, USA

**Matt Lovell,** Sports Nutritionist, Perform and Function Ltd, UK

**Chris Mallac,** International Course Presenter, Rehab Trainer International; former Head of Performance, London Irish Rugby, UK

**Steve McCaig,** Senior Physiotherapist, England and Wales Cricket Board, UK

**Polly McGuiggan,** Lecturer in Biomechanics and Director of Studies, MSc Sport and Exercise Medicine, University of Bath, UK

**Tim Mitchell,** Specialist Musculoskeletal Physiotherapist, Senior Lecturer, School of Physiotherapy and Exercise Science, Curtin University, Australia

**Calvin Morriss,** Head of Performance Support, British Cycling, UK

**Sophia Nimphius,** Senior Lecturer, Edith Cowan University, Australia

**Adam Olsen,** Athletic Trainer and Physical Therapist, St. Louis Cardinals, USA

**Peter O'Sullivan,** Professor, School of Physiotherapy and Exercise Science, Curtin University, Australia

**Emidio Pacecca,** Senior Physiotherapist, Western Force Rugby, Australia

**Phil Pask,** Senior National Team Physiotherapist, England Rugby Team (RFU), British and Irish Lions (2005, 2009, 2013)

**Ian Prangley,** Consultant Physiotherapist and Physical Performance Coach in professional tennis, London, UK; former National Physiotherapy Manager, Tennis Australia

**Craig Ranson,** Programme Director of Sports and Exercise Medicine, Cardiff Metropolitan University, UK; National Team Physiotherapist, Welsh Rugby Union, UK

**Mike Reinold,** President and Founder, Champion Physical Therapy and Performance, Boston, MA, USA

**Kay Robinson,** Sports Physiotherapist, Balmain Sports Medicine, Australia; former Lead Physiotherapist, British Skeleton, Team GB and English Institute of Sport, UK

**Ben Rosenblatt,** Senior Strength and Conditioning Coach, Great Britain Hockey and English Institute of Sport, UK

**Jeremy Sheppard,** Head of Strength and Conditioning /Sports Science Manager, Surfing Australia; Senior Lecturer, Edith Cowan University, Australia

**Julie Steele,** Director, Biomechanics Research Laboratory, University of Wollongong, Australia

**Margaret Stone,** Director, Centre of Excellence for Sport Science and Coach Education/ Olympic Training Site, East Tennessee State University, USA

**N. Travis Triplett,** Professor and Chair, Health and Exercise Science Department, Appalachian State University, Boone, NC, USA

**Henry Wajswelner,** Course Coordinator, Master of Sports Physiotherapy Programme, La Trobe University, Australia

**Nick Winkelman,** Director of Movement (Performance Innovation Team), EXOS, USA

**Mark Young,** Physiotherapist, Geelong Football Club, Australia

# Part I

# The performance team

# Chapter 1

# Reconditioning

## A performance-based response to an injury

*Bill Knowles*

## Introduction

For the past 25 years, I have been working with professional, world-class and Olympic-level athletes in the field of Sports Reconditioning and Performance Training. This journey continues to explore the relationship between evidence-based medicine and experience-based evidence. Even today, there continues to be a blend of the "art" and the "science" when working with athletes.

The purpose of this chapter is to explore the cornerstones of a performance rehabilitation model by considering the definitions and concepts we must consider when preparing our athletes for a return to the highest level of function following injury.

## Definitions

Throughout my career I have seen many medically led rehabilitation protocols designed for elite athletes striving to return to the highest level of competition. We do need to understand, however, that there is a big difference between protecting and restoring tissue health and preparing the athlete for a return to competition.

> If you are not qualified or experienced enough to design a performance training program for a professional or world-class athlete pre-injury, how are you able to design a performance training program or Return to Competition (RtC) strategy post-injury?

*Rehabilitation* is a *medical or clinical model* for treating individuals who *may or may not* be athletes. Often, a surgeon will design and/or direct this protocol. With operations, the focus of the protocol is on the surgery, wound healing and early stages of rehabilitation. They usually emphasize protecting the peripheral lesion first, and then promote slow controlled motion and activities of daily living. This continues for many months with the aim on "doing no harm" to the repair. Eventually, basic athletic preparation is typically encouraged to begin once biological healing time of the graft has advanced.

> Just because biological healing has occurred, it does not mean the athlete is prepared for performance.

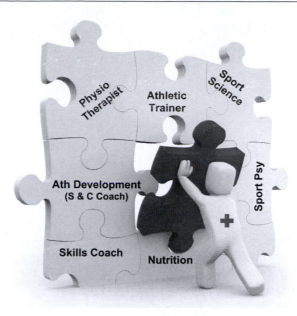

*Figure 1.1*  Reconditioning – Performance-based and medically supported

*Reconditioning* is a *performance-based model* for training athletes following injury or surgery. It is directed by the performance team and is medically supported. The program design begins with the end goal in mind, which is a *Return to Competition*. We then design a progression backward to the surgery/injury date. This process allows the performance team to address all aspects of athletic development immediately post-injury or surgery to best prepare the individual for the true demands of competition that lay ahead.

Returning to competition is easy; continuing to compete is more difficult.

## Training around the injury

Reconditioning follows a functional path immediately post-injury and continues this progression until the athlete has returned to competition. We recognize that a serious injury should be looked upon as a neurophysiologic dysfunction, not just a common peripheral musculoskeletal injury. It is a peripheral injury, but with a central consequence. With this in mind we must train the brain through movements, not just muscles, during all stages of post-injury care. Most protocols that restrict active motion, like brace joints, assist motion via continuous passive motion (CPM) machines or prevent loading are affecting the normal patterning that an athlete needs in order to best prepare for higher quality training in the weeks and months to come. For joint injuries, the best brace is neuromuscular control and coordinated movement patterns. These *can* be developed early and often if the protocol encourages doing so.

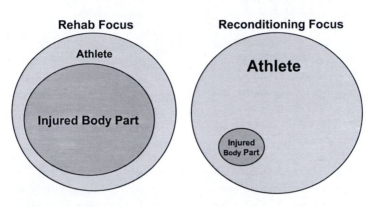

Figure 1.2 Training around the injury

Often, rehabilitation protocols are centred on what an athlete *cannot* do, as opposed to what an athlete *can* do. While this is often a consequence of protecting the repair/injury, these limitations can compromise the short- and long-term movement qualities of the athlete. Unfortunately, rest is often the chosen form of protection, yet the short- and long-term neuromuscular inhibition that accompanies this approach may actually put the repair at greater risk as the athlete progresses.

The reconditioning model also respects protecting the repair and maintaining joint homeostasis but encourages more athletic ways to train the individual. Because reconditioning is performance-based, we prepare the athlete – we don't just treat the injury. This is done through coaching movements that occur in daily training for the athlete, albeit at the correct intensity and load. This strategy maintains and/or restores coordinated movement patterns that are essential for athletic success in the future. Whether the response is physiological, psychological or both, the outcomes are excellent. The traditional medical model of rehabilitation, which focuses more on the injury, underestimates the total body healing response that training familiar movements has on athletes.

## The load compromised athlete

When an athlete injures a joint surface, ligament, muscle or tendon it is, to some degree, forever compromised. With increased severity comes an increased challenge to keep the tissue healthy over an athlete's career. There is clear evidence that an anterior cruciate ligament (ACL) injury leads to early onset osteoarthritis (OA) 5–15 years after injury, 'aging' the knee roughly 30 years.[1] These degenerative changes can often exact a toll later in an athlete's career. For knee injuries, these changes are attributed in part to quadriceps weakness as a result of arthrogenic muscle inhibition (AMI). AMI is an ongoing neural inhibition that prevents the quadriceps from fully activating and is believed to result from pain, swelling, inflammation, joint laxity and structural damage. Altered afferent information from the damaged knee joint is believed to have both spinal and supraspinal pathways.[2] This 'central consequence' may alter dynamic neuromuscular activation patterns that affect lower extremity kinematics and kinetics leading to a negative change in load distribution across the knee joint.[1]

> Arthrogenic muscle inhibition occurs bilaterally after unilateral knee injury.[1]

For example a grade III medial collateral ligament injury can permanently retain laxity in the absence of pain, swelling or decreased performance. Yet this new 'biomechanical set-up' (altered kinetics) with laxity on one side of a joint is not normal and may predispose the athlete to other concerns down the line; especially in high-intensity multidirectional sports. These bilateral concerns are OA, meniscal tears, ACL injury and poor power output via AMI.

Whilst research into AMI has traditionally been centred on the sequelae from knee injuries, there is increasing interest in similar neuromuscular 'depowering' following muscle injuries. Such acute neural responses can reduce muscle strength and endurance and alter agonist/antagonist activity and coordination in both static and dynamic motor tasks.[3]

Being 'load compromised' means questioning whether the musculoskeletal injury *and* the neurophysiological function of the athlete can successfully sustain the mechanical loads of high-intensity training and competing over time. In the *reconditioning model*, once an LCA (load compromised athlete), forever an LCA. Regardless of whether the tissue is considered biologically 'healed' and functionally restored, accepting the athlete's LCA status should be a catalyst for designing the best Return to Competition and injury prevention program possible. In high-performance sport, the reality is it is often easier to get an athlete back to competition than it is to sustain them at this level. With this in mind, developing an athlete sustainability program (ASP) is a critical part of reconditioning because it is a performance-based model. On the contrary, most rehabilitation protocols dedicate very little time in this area, as they are more interested in restoring general function often at the neglect of true high-performance training.

Given that significant levels of AMI may still be present 18–33 months following knee joint injuries,[2] the central tenet of an ASP is that an athlete's reconditioning must continue well after they return to competition. The reality is, after long-term injuries, we must continue to implement strength, power and coordination training throughout the season, the year and their career. In addition, LCAs cannot take more than two weeks off from strength training or they risk a neuromuscular 'switching-off' that can predispose them to re-injury.

## Athletic development

As a performance-based model, reconditioning is identified more closely with the field of Athletic Development than Sports Therapy. As an Athletic Development professional, I am a part of a performance team whose goal is to train all components of athleticism to the level required by the sport in which the athlete participates. The performance team is comprised of the team physician, therapists, athletic development coaches, nutritionists, sport scientists, performance psychologists and technical sport coaches.

In reconditioning, we need to appreciate that our job is to enhance athleticism, which is the ability to perform athletic movements at optimal speed with precision, and efficiency.[4] This means that reconditioning follows that same functional path immediately post injury or following surgery until the athlete returns to competition. It is a path that explores what an athlete *can do* as they begin their preparation for more advanced training. In order to prepare for quality movements with precision and style, all treatment decisions following injury greatly matter. If you brace a knee, for example, for 12 weeks following surgery, you can expect a conflict with achieving optimal speed with grace when it matters most. This happens due to the altered mechanics that a brace inflicts on the athlete. But if you were to progressively re-establish neuromuscular control to stabilise the knee (utilizing the body's own intrinsic 'bracing') with properly loaded sport-specific movement patterns, you may actually improve the quality of speed in competition.

Following the progressive path that reconditioning advocates requires knowledge and experience to understand the movements that transfer to sport performance. The specialist involved in the reconditioning process must have the personality to 'coach' the athlete consistently towards improved movement proficiency. The adage that 'practice does not make perfect; practice makes permanent,' should be apparent here. You must coach consistently well or be prepared for compromised performance or potential re-injury in the future.

Injury should never interfere with an opportunity to train an athlete. We need to look at ways to train *around* the injury. Unfortunately, most early and middle-stage rehabilitation protocols are designed to protect the injury by preventing or limiting normal movement patterns. Reconditioning takes an Athletic Development approach during this same stage by encouraging normal movement patterns as soon as possible. This is done in creative ways that protect the injury but always contribute towards re-establishing proper athletic patterns. The brain is extremely plastic; thus every movement pattern that is imparted on the athlete during a post-op period may affect performance. For example allowing an athlete to squat in waist-to-chest-deep water following hip surgery offers a low load functional movement pattern at the ankle, knee and hip that the brain recognizes as segmentally correct movements without pain. This movement on land is often discouraged for many weeks for fear of harming the healing structures; thus it becomes about what you *cannot do* (as water is not discussed as an option). I feel the less we move correctly, the more harm we may be doing – at many different levels.

## Preparation

In a performance-based retraining model, we view post-injury care as a *preparation period* rather than a rehabilitation phase. This is a subtle but critical paradigm shift as we are preparing the athlete for a return to competition, not just repairing the injury. The goal of the preparation period is to return the athlete to the highest level of training within the shortest period of time while respecting homeostasis, and then staying there for a significant period of time to demonstrate sustainability. These qualities must be planned starting immediately after injury or surgery to achieve high performance upon their return. Adaptive qualities take time to develop and are dependent on fundamentally sound movement patterns. Too often athletes have 'adapted' to the physician's/therapist's protocol over months; yet this protocol often underestimates the true demands that team training or competition requires. This is an example where the athlete is *not* 'adaptable' based on the program design and thus cannot sustain high intensity efforts over time.

## Return to competition phases

The end-stage goal of rehabilitation is commonly referred to as Return to Play (RTP). Yet in performance training, that term is rarely used to describe a phase of preparation or training in an annual plan. Most commonly we discuss *training, rest-recovery, competition-competing* and *performance-performing*. The medical community has used the term Return to Play to broadly describe a final rehabilitation phase that represents skill training, team training, scrimmages, games and/or competition. The RTP stage of a typical rehabilitation protocol usually designs a less structured, under-developed plan to prepare the athlete for high-intensity competitive training or games. This is not surprising, as it is not an area of expertise for traditionally trained medically minded professionals.

The reconditioning model uses the term Return to Competition as it represents a more realistic understanding of the demands that are about to be placed on the athlete. Competition is usually more intense and more demanding on the body than team training or play. In most sports, injury and re-injury happen more often in competition than in training/ practice. Therefore, to earn the right to compete you must have progressed successfully through a high-intensity preparation period over time to show your ability to sustain that stress. An experienced athletic development coach who truly understands performance and the demands a particular sport requires must develop this level of program design.

**Build backwards**: A performance team looks carefully at how the athlete physically needs to look to be competitive and to reduce the risk of injury. It then strategically builds backwards to address the post-injury and post-operative plan. This plan is developed *with* the Medical Team, but not owned by one particular profession. For example there should be significant contact time with the athletic development staff during all RtC stages. All professions need to work in an interdisciplinary manner to ensure that the athlete is kept safe and healing structures are protected, and that they are skilfully trained in all aspects of athletic competency.

Reconditioning programs are criteria-based, not protocol-driven. There should be no steadfast timeline that controls the progression an athlete moves towards a return to training and, ultimately, return to competition. Guidelines should be created to monitor homeostatic responses to the weekly/monthly training, and biological healing should be respected and monitored as indicated. Movement quality training, strength, coordination, speed and power will address the neurophysiologic dysfunctions that occur with injury, *but* they must be developed early and often throughout the program. Ultimately, consistent Performance Team reviews will determine an athlete's preparedness for the next level of reconditioning. This is very important to avoid detrimental phases (down-time) in a program where athletes are not allowed to progress at a rate necessary to keep them safe and promote performance.

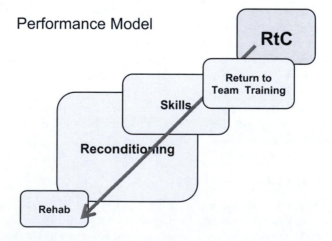

*Figure 1.3* Build backwards from Return to Competition to injury

### Case example: Limitations of the 'traditional' model in ACL rehabilitation

Traditional rehabilitation protocols do not satisfactorily develop the lower extremity strength required to effectively protect the knee and enhance performance. For multidirectional sports, athletes must sufficiently develop their fast-twitch, Type II muscles. These are responsible for high-intensity force production, stabilization and force reduction.

Knee joint injuries negatively affect neuromuscular control (AMI) of the lower extremity and specifically affect Type II fast-twitch muscle. The exercises used to best develop this Type II neurophysiological profile are often contra-indicated for 3–5 months to protect the healing graft (such as heavy resistance training, plyometrics, sprinting, fast-eccentric and concentric training). While strength training is encouraged during this time (0–5 months), it is still underestimating what will be required to best protect the knee in competition. Moderate intensity functional exercises (targeting Type I muscle) often predominate the rehabilitation protocol.

High-intensity 'sport-specific' training is usually indicated by months 5–6 post-op. This usually involves sprinting, cutting, technical sport skills and other plyometric training. Following this, athletes are typically cleared to 'Return to Play' at 6 months post-op after spending the least amount of time training the muscle fibre types (Type II) that contribute the most to protecting the knee under high stress. The Return to Competition program would not allow an athlete to return to team training following ACL surgery without multiple months of progressive Type II activation training as part of an overall plan of reconditioning. A qualified athletic development professional makes decisions from a preparation and performance perspective, not a timeline based on biological healing.

## Multidimensional speed and agility

Another very generic rehabilitation term is the return to running program. From a Reconditioning perspective for multidirectional athletes, we tend to avoid the use of the terms 'running' or 'jogging'. It is preferable to speak in terms of acceleration, deceleration, stabilization and change of direction. This approach is called multidimensional speed and agility, or MDSA.[4] Most rehabilitation protocols use return to running as an indicator of functional restoration midway through a return to sport progression. This imparts a false sense of security for the athlete, as basic linear running requires very little strength and coordinative abilities. Yet the athlete feels a connection to function that clouds their vision of the essential athletic qualities that are still required to perform at a high level. Typically, this quickly leads towards sport-specific physical and technical skills that continue in the absence of the necessary strength and coordination required for deceleration and change of direction actions, thus potentially predisposing the athlete to re-injury or poor performance.

A performance-based model understands that injury most often occurs during deceleration actions. Thus the Performance Team should focus on the complex movements of MDSA. Since perception, decision-making and speed in change of direction are critical factors in the performance of agility tasks, it is helpful to think of agility as having both motor and cognitive components.[4] This must be trained at progressive levels throughout the entire Reconditioning Program. It cannot wait until the often-prescribed final phase of the 'rehabilitation program'.

## If you can't slow it down, don't speed it up

This is a basic message to stress the importance of delaying running until the athlete establishes significant strength to support change of direction and stopping. My experience is that, after injury, acceleration and other forms of force production are much easier to express than deceleration. This is why I support MDSA versus the Return to Running Program for most athletes. MDSA can be implemented early and often in the Reconditioning Program at low intensity where it represents technical training only. In fact, the early post-operative phase is a perfect time to introduce basic running mechanics as static or slow images of the whole movement that is coming in the very near future. These static images become dynamic over time but require a foundation of coordination and strength to protect the athlete.

## Summary

If a professional athlete is following the same post-injury program for the first three months that an average adult would follow for the same injury, then the concept of 'sports rehabilitation' is greatly misunderstood by the practitioner designing and/or implementing such protocol. We must continue to advance the quality of post-injury protocols for athletes by having discussions and sharing experiences with the orthopaedic community as they can significantly influence the path reconditioning can follow. By ensuring we operate as an interdisciplinary team, whereby performance coaches are involved in the decision making processes, along with medical professionals, we may further understand that full athletic preparedness is not a given just because the peripheral musculoskeletal injury was repaired.

## Notes

1 Palmieri-Smith, R. M., and Thomas, A. C. (2009). A neuromuscular mechanism of posttraumatic osteoarthritis associated with ACL injury. *Exercise and Sport Science Review, 37*(3), 147–53.
2 Rice, D. A., and McNair, P. J. (2010). Quadriceps arthrogenic muscle inhibition: Neural mechanisms and treatment perspectives. *Seminars in Arthritis and Rheumatism, 40*(3), 250–266.
3 Fyfe, J. J., Opar, D., Williams, M. J., and Shield, A. J. (2013). The role of neuromuscular inhibition in hamstring strain injury recurrence. *Journal of Electromyography and Kinesiology, 23*(3), 523–30.
4 Gambetta, V. (2007). *Athletic development: The art and science of functional sports conditioning.* Champaign, IL: Human Kinetics.

Chapter 2

# Strength and conditioning in injury prevention and rehabilitation

*Ben Rosenblatt*

## Introduction

Injuries occur as a consequence of fatigue, previous trauma, lack of physical preparation and occasionally, bad luck. The strength and conditioning (S&C) coach not only has the knowledge and insight to physically prepare athletes for competition, but also has the unique position within an interdisciplinary team (IDT) to characterise the stress of training and an athlete's response to it. This has probably been best demonstrated by the work of Cormack et al.,[2] who developed valid and reliable tools to quantify the stress of and the athlete's response to training.

The purpose of this chapter is to detail the specific role an S&C coach can play in the prevention and rehabilitation of sports injuries. This will be achieved by introducing the concept of injury risk and illustrating the role of the S&C coach by using examples from elite athletes.

## Injury prevention

Injuries cannot be totally prevented, but the risk of injuries occurring can certainly be reduced. Musculoskeletal trauma occurs as a consequence of tissue being placed under greater stress that it can tolerate. Subsequently, the purpose of injury prevention is to:

1    Find methods of reducing the acute or chronic stress placed through a tissue; and/or
2    Increase the stress a tissue can tolerate prior to failure.

It is clear that certain tissues are more plastic in nature than others and can adapt to stress placed through them. For example ligaments are far less plastic than muscle tissue. To reduce the risk of injury to a ligament, one must reduce the stress placed through it. Equally, to reduce the risk of injury to a muscle, we should seek to increase the stress it could tolerate by increasing its cross sectional area and force production/absorption qualities.

### Reducing biomechanical stress on non-plastic structures

There are two methods of reducing the stress placed through the musculoskeletal system. The first is to ensure that the movement patterns that the athlete is undertaking do not place excessive force through structures that cannot tolerate it or are not particularly plastic in nature. In order to achieve this, the S&C coach must have a thorough understanding of both functional anatomy and clinical biomechanics. Whilst these two topics are not typical of the education of an S&C coach, they can certainly seek this knowledge from the medical team supporting the athlete. For example, anterior cruciate ligament (ACL) injuries occur as a consequence of excessive or rapid knee valgus. In order to reduce the risk of ACL injuries, the S&C coach must prioritise exercises that reduce frontal or transverse plane forces through the knee joint. Examples include stiff-leg kettle bell swings and single-leg landing drills with no frontal or transverse plane motion of the pelvis, knee or foot.

## Fatigue management

The second method of reducing stress in the musculoskeletal system is to manage the fatigue an athlete is experiencing. Fatigue can reduce a muscle's capacity to generate large, rapid forces and reduce reaction times, concentration and joint proprioception. All of these factors can reduce an athlete's capacity to tolerate stress through specific structures in the musculo-skeletal system. Subsequently, managing fatigue is a vital component of reducing injury risk. As the S&C coach has the knowledge, insight and position within an IDT to modulate and prescribe training volume and intensity, they are the best placed person to undertake this vital role.

Planned variation of training load on a daily, weekly and monthly basis reduces the monot-ony of training, which reduces the risk of injury and illness in athletes.[3] Probably more important is to monitor each athlete's psychological and physical response to training in order to make sure that they are not competing in a fatigued state, and if they are training in a fatigued state, they have appropriate periods of recovery to adapt to the overall training stress. This is discussed in detail in chapter 31.

Fatigue is an important part of the training process, but it also increases the risk of injury. The S&C coach must characterise the response to and load of training in order to determine how fatigued an athlete is, the importance of this to the training process and what training has taken place to achieve this state. Fatigue management will certainly reduce the stress placed through the body and reduce injury risk.

## Increasing tolerance

Whilst reducing stress going through the MSK system is one approach to injury risk reduc-tion, it is important to realise that too great a reduction will result in insufficient adaptive stress and decreased opportunity for technical improvement. As a consequence, we should look to couple this approach with strategies to increase tissue tolerance. Tissue failure occurs when the stress/strain placed through the structure exceeds its plastic region (exceeds its capacity to adapt).

It is possible to alter the amount of stress/strain a structure can tolerate by changing the length of the tissue or its capacity to generate force. The nature of the change required is determined by the most likely mechanism of injury. For example increasing stress tolerance by increasing hamstring length may reduce hamstring injury risk in gymnasts who are required to operate through large ranges of hip flexion with an extended knee. By the same token, increasing strain tolerance by increasing hamstring strength may reduce hamstring injury risk in sprinters who are not required to operate through extreme ranges of motion but do have to take high levels of force through their hamstrings. As such, the interventions required that reduce the risk of ham-string injury would differ between a sprinter and a gymnast, as they have different stress/strain requirements of the hamstring and the likely mechanisms of injury are unique.

There are several ways the S&C coach can reduce the risk of athletes getting injured. Through movement-based training, the biomechanical load going through structures which cannot tolerate them can be reduced. Fatigue can also be managed to reduce the biomechanical stress going through the MSK system. Finally, the amount of stress the MSK system can tolerate can be increased with appropriate training.

## Injury risk model

In order to reduce the risk of injury to athletes, it is possible to establish injury risk models and identify the interventions the S&C coach can put in place as part of a regular training programme. The process is one of establishing the most common and severe injuries in the athlete's sport, identify the risk factors, determine appropriate measurement tools to represent the risk, identify criteria for athletes to meet and put interventions in place which are representative of reducing the risk that each particular athlete faces.

### Identifying risk factors

In order to identify risk factors, the mechanisms of injury must be fully understood. ACL sprains occur as a consequence of the magnitude and rate of knee valgus whilst landing or turning. Posterior shoulder impingements occur as a consequence of a decreased capacity to decelerate the internal rotation of the humeral head whilst throwing or pushing. Lateral ankle sprains occur due to the magnitude and rate of inversion during landing and turning. To understand the risk of injury, the S&C coach must understand the mechanism. Once the mechanism is understood, the risk can be identified. To reduce knee valgus during landing or cutting activities, the medial hamstrings are required to rapidly and forcefully contract. To decelerate the internal rotation of the humeral head whilst throwing, the external rotators of the shoulder must rapidly and forcefully contract. To prevent the ankle inverting whilst landing or turning, the ankle evertors must rapidly and forcefully contract at the appropriate time.

### Establishing assessments

Assessments should directly reflect the physical characteristics which underpin the risk of injury. Assessments must be used to determine which interventions each athlete requires. One injury may have several risk factors, of which only one may be relevant to an athlete. For example isokinetic assessment of eccentric external rotation could be used to determine whether an athlete has the strength to decelerate the internal rotation of the humerus.

### Identify criteria

Criteria should be developed based on either published data or sound reasoning. Foster[3] identified that >6,000 AU of training and a monotony of >2.0 increases risk of injury and illness. However, some athletes may regularly exceed the training volume. As such, in order to manage fatigue to reduce injury risk, S&C coaches could ensure that training monotony does not exceed 2.0 on a weekly basis. Equally, there is strong evidence to suggest that an eccentric hamstring to concentric quadriceps ratio (during isokinetic knee flexion and extension) of less than 0.9 places an athlete at a high risk of ACL injury.[1] As such, one may choose to use this criterion to determine whether an athlete requires greater eccentric hamstring strength. Ultimately, athlete-, sport- and injury-specific criteria must be identified in order to appropriately determine who needs what.

## Training interventions

Once the needs of an athlete have been established, the role of the S&C coach is to use their knowledge of functional anatomy, the principles of training and their coaching skills to coach training programmes which reduce an athlete's risk of injury. As with any training programme, after a sufficient period of time, the assessments should be re-taken to determine the success of the training interventions.

### Case study 1: Reducing risk of lower back pain in an elite female hockey team as part of a strength and conditioning performance programme

Due to prolonged periods in spinal flexion, large rotational forces through the spine, a high running demand and a dense competition schedule (7 international matches in 11 days), female hockey players are at risk of developing lower back pain. To improve physical performance in hockey, activities should focus on absorbing and generating power through the lower body, developing a large aerobic capacity and improving context-specific change of direction and sprint performance. The challenge is to include activities to reduce risk of lower back pain without reducing the volume of activities to improve hockey performance.

Lack of anti-extension capacity, anti-lateral flexion capacity and rotation control were considered as risk factors, and assessments and criteria were established to measure these risk factors within the athlete group (Table 2.1). For the capacity assessments, athletes were timed in the testing positions until technical failure. During the control assessment, a qualitative assessment was employed. The athlete was instructed to maintain a neutral posture and raise one arm above her head. If a technical error was observed (e.g. thoracic flexion or a weight shift), a score was given to the athlete. A score of zero represented no technical errors.

None of the squad reached the criteria, so a 10-station circuit of trunk exercises to reduce the risk factors were employed. The circuit was employed twice per week at the end of a gym session, and the numbers of sets and time per exercise were manipulated on a daily basis to increase the total work duration over a four-week period (Figure 2.1).

Table 2.1 The risk factors, assessments and criteria utilised to determine whether an athlete was at risk of lower back pain

| Risk Factor | Assessment | Criteria |
| --- | --- | --- |
| Anti-extension capacity | Flexion hold | Greater than 2.5min |
| Anti-lateral flexion capacity | Side hold | Greater than 2min |
| Rotation control | Plank with arm raise | Qualitative score of 0 |

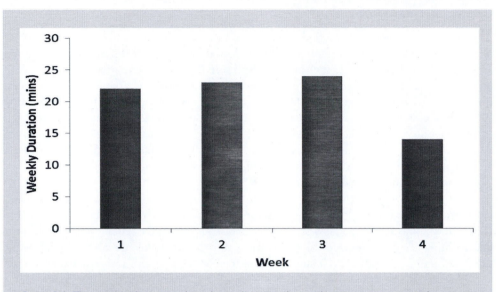

*Figure 2.1* The weekly duration of trunk conditioning during the intervention period

*Table 2.2* The results of the assessments pre- and post-training intervention. An effect size of greater than 1.2 represents a large change

| Assessment | Pre (n=20) | Post (n=20) | Effect size |
|---|---|---|---|
| Flexion hold (s) | 130 | 140 | 0.22 |
| Side hold (average of left and right) (s) | 85 | 113 | 0.95 |
| Plank with arm raise (compensations) | 1.4 | 0.4 | 1.2 |

This took no longer than 12 minutes to deliver. To improve motor control, exercises were utilised which required a knowledge of result with an external focus of attention[7] (e.g. in a forward crawling plank with a foam roller across the back, if the foam roller fell off, it indicated to the athlete that she had lost rotational control).

Table 2.2 clearly demonstrates that the short training intervention resulted in a large improvement in rotation control and moderate improvement in capacity to resist lateral flexion. The advantage of this training approach was that an intervention which reduced risk of lower back pain was able to be utilised without encroaching on any other time to be committed to improving physical performance.

## Rehabilitation

When an athlete gets injured, the S&C coach has an essential role to play. Not only does the S&C coach have the skill sets to change physical characteristics that reduce injury risk, but they can also prepare an athlete for the increasing task demands of subsequent phases of rehabilitation and use the time as an opportunity to make gains in physical performance in other areas.

## Criteria-driven approach

As with any other period of training, rehabilitation should begin with the end in mind. What physical demands will be placed on the athlete when they return to training and competition and what physical qualities do they need to display in order to tolerate those demands? With these questions in mind, it is possible to put in place a bespoke rehabilitation strategy that is driven by increasing task demands. The progression of activities through rehabilitation should be determined by achievement of clear clinical or functional criteria. As discussed earlier, the criteria should be driven by the risk factors of the specific injury. A criteria-driven approach to rehabilitation has been shown to produce favourable outcomes and provide a framework for the S&C coach to operate within during rehabilitation.[5]

Having a clear understanding of both the biomechanical and physiological demands of the sport the athlete is returning to, and the mechanism of injury provides an end point for a rehabilitation programme. In order for an athlete to return to competition or training they must be able to tolerate the biomechanical and physiological stress placed through the system. As detailed above, this can be achieved by both increasing the capacity of structures to tolerate stress or reducing the stress placed through a structure. Thus, the role of the S&C coach during rehabilitation is to train an athlete to improve their ability to tolerate the physical demands of training and competition.

As detailed in the section on reducing injury risk, a sport-specific activity which has previously caused trauma will have several different risks associated with it. In a rehabilitation paradigm, these risks can be described as fundamental competencies for an athlete to achieve. Each fundamental competency is determined by key physical characteristics. For example inability to decelerate the internal rotation of the humerus whilst throwing may be a risk factor for shoulder injuries. Subsequently, this is a fundamental competency for an athlete to achieve prior to returning to throwing. The physical characteristics that underpin this competence include eccentric strength of the external rotators, rate of force development of the external rotators, maintenance of scapula-thoracic position and timing of external rotation eccentric contraction. These characteristics can be independently assessed in order to determine which training interventions are required to rehabilitate an injured athlete's shoulder.

A hierarchy of needs exists based on the biomechanical stress of the training interventions on the injured structure. For example it would be inappropriate to start placing high forces through a shoulder joint in order to improve strength if the athlete had inappropriate control of their scapula. This would place greater stress through injured structures than it could tolerate and be detrimental to rehabilitation process. Thus, the stages of rehabilitation are determined by increasing biomechanical demand and specificity and the healing of the injured structure. It is important that assessments are put in place that represent the underpinning physical characteristics required to support a fundamental competence. Also, clear criteria should be established within the assessments to determine whether the athlete has achieved the competence to reduce that aspect of injury risk.

A hierarchical, criterion-driven approach to rehabilitation ensures that athletes can achieve fundamental competencies which allow them to undertake activities of increasing biomechanical demand and specificity. This approach is particularly appealing, as it provides goals for athletes to strive for and ensures that athletes are capable of tolerating the biomechanical demand placed through their injured structure prior to returning to training and competition. This also provides the S&C coach with a framework to apply their knowledge of functional anatomy and the principles of training to put in place bespoke training interventions, which will increase an athlete's ability to tolerate the increased biomechanical demand of returning to sport-specific activities and accelerate their rehabilitation.

**Case study 2: *Increasing hamstring capacity, strength and rate of force development during the rehabilitation of an ACL injury***

A male handball player ruptured his hamstring 18 weeks prior to the Olympic Games. To increase the chance of him competing, he decided to adopt a conservative strategy instead of reconstructive surgery. As co-activation of the medial hamstrings reduces the ACL stress by providing a posterior drawer on the tibia, it was decided that this muscle function would be one of the targets of his rehabilitation. In order to determine which exercises and loading regimes he required, a hierarchical assessment strategy was utilised (Table 2.3). To determine whether he had the capacity to tolerate high forces through this muscle group, a single leg hamstring bridge (knee flexed to 20°) was used. To determine whether he was capable of tolerating large eccentric forces through this muscle to protect the knee, an isokinetic assessment was undertaken. Finally, to determine whether he had the pre-activation strategy and rate of force development to protect his knee, the activation of his medial hamstring was recorded (using EMG) 20ms pre contact, on ground contact and at peak force during an unpredicted land and cut onto a force plate. The assessments were hierarchical and he was not allowed to undertake each assessment until he had passed the first one.

He initially held the hamstring bridge for only 35s. A continuous muscle conditioning circuit (Table 2.4) was utilised for three weeks, and the volume of work was manipulated by changing the number of sets used per session (Figure 2.2). By week four he was capable of holding the bridge for over two minutes.

*Table 2.3* The risk factors, assessments and criteria utilised to determine which type of activities the athlete should use to help him rehabilitate his ACL injury

| Risk Factor | Assessment | Criteria |
| --- | --- | --- |
| Load tolerance | Single-leg hamstring bridge | 2min |
| Eccentric strength | Isokinetic | Eccentric peak torque 30% > concentric peak torque |
| Rate of force development | EMG functional analysis | Early activation of medial hamstrings |

*Table 2.4* The hamstring conditioning circuit

| Exercise | Time |
| --- | --- |
| Single-leg bridge hold (short) (left) | 30s |
| Single-leg bridge hold (short) (right) | 30s |
| Single-leg bridge hold (long) (left) | 30s |
| Single-leg bridge hold (long) (right) | 30s |
| Bridge walkouts | 30s |
| Single-leg Swiss ball hamstring curl (left) | 30s |
| Single-leg Swiss ball hamstring curl (right) | 30s |

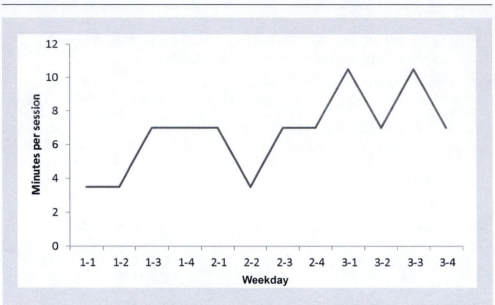

*Figure 2.2* The daily and weekly duration of hamstring muscle conditioning to improve medial hamstring load tolerance

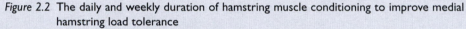

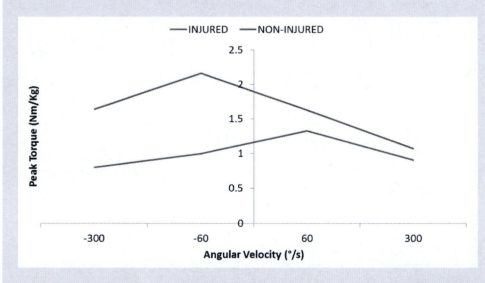

*Figure 2.3* The eccentric and concentric isokinetic torque velocity curve of the hamstrings of the injured and non-injured legs

The isokinetic assessment was then undertaken and revealed that he was not capable of producing enough torque eccentrically to protect his knee (Figure 2.3). Subsequently, heavy strength training was utilised to induce muscle hypertrophy and reduce the post-synaptic inhibition which had resulted in the eccentric strength deficit. Sumo stance deadlifts, stiff-leg kettlebell swings and single-leg prone hamstring curls were all utilised to target the deficit. In order to ensure full motor unit recruitment to stimulate the adaptive process,[6] heavy loads and lower reps were utilised with the deadlifts and moderate loads to failure were used for the swings and single-leg curls. The athlete utilised this strength regime three times per week for three weeks. The sets and reps were manipulated within the week to facilitate training variety and to allow the athlete to express maximal intent during each session. A week's training is detailed in Table 2.5.

After three weeks of training, the athlete had reduced their strength deficit and the functional assessment of rate of force development was undertaken. The graph in Figure 2.3 demonstrates that the athlete was not capable of recruiting his medial hamstring on his injured side early enough or to the same magnitude as the non-injured side. In order to reduce this deficit, work had to be done to increase the medial hamstrings' rate force development and early activation. Small amplitude multidirectional hopping was utilised to develop pre-activity.[3] A hamstring bridge with foot on a box (knee flexed to 20°) with rapid swinging of the opposite leg was utilised to develop the rate of force development of the medial hamstrings. Although the volume of work appeared greater, due to the speed of activity, the muscles were under tension for shorter periods of time but had to produce more force more rapidly (Table 2.6). Only two weeks of training was required to increase the magnitude of muscle activity 20ms pre-impact during an unanticipated cut (see Figure 2.4).

Table 2.5 The weekly strength training regime to increase muscle hypertrophy and reduce the eccentric strength deficit

| Day | Exercise | Notes | Sets | Reps | Recovery |
| --- | --- | --- | --- | --- | --- |
| 1 | Sumo Deadlift | Superset (max load) | 4 | 6 | 30s |
| | Kettlebell swing | | 4 | Max | 3min |
| | Prone hammy curl | Injured only | 4 | Max | 30s |
| 2 | Sumo Deadlift | Superset | 3 | 8 | 30s |
| | Kettlebell swing | | 3 | Max | 3min |
| | Prone hammy curl | Injured only | 3 | Max | 30s |
| 3 | Sumo Deadlift | Superset – use Day 1 load | 5 | 4 | 30s |
| | Kettlebell swing | | 5 | Max | 3min |
| | Prone hammy curl | Injured only | 4 | Max | 30s |

Table 2.6 The weekly training regime to increase medial hamstring pre-activity and rate of force development

| Day | Exercise | Notes | Sets | Reps | Recovery |
| --- | --- | --- | --- | --- | --- |
| 1 | Single-leg hopping | Random surfaces and obstacles, minimise contact times | 4 | 12 | 2min |
| | Box bridge swings | Heel on box, rapid swings | 4 | 10 | 2min |
| 2 | Single-leg hopping | Random surfaces and obstacles, minimise contact times | 3 | 8 | 2min |
| | Box bridge swings | Heel on box, rapid swings | 3 | 8 | 2min |
| 3 | Single-leg hopping | Random surfaces and obstacles, minimise contact times | 5 | 10 | 2min |
| | Box bridge swings | Heel on box, rapid swings | 5 | 10 | 2min |

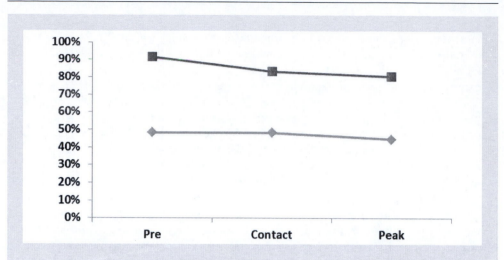

*Figure 2.4* The magnitude of medial hamstring activity recorded 20ms pre contact (pre), at contact (contact) and at peak force (peak) during an unpredicted cut from a 30cm landing on the injured (gray) and non-injured (black) legs. Medial hamstring activity was normalised to maximum recorded during a bilateral countermovement jump

## Opportunity to develop competition performance

When an athlete gets injured, the S&C coach must have performance in mind. It is imperative that athletes maintain whatever sport-specific training they can physically perform, and other training modalities can be used to maintain physical qualities. Tools such as session RPE to monitor training load can be utilised to ensure that athletes maintain total training load and there is a stepwise progression back to sport-specific training to ensure they are not over-reaching. Due to busy competition schedules and conflicting demands and pressures of training, sometimes athletes never have an opportunity to truly develop physical qualities that limit their performance.

The S&C coach can contribute to rehabilitation by working with the rest of the support team to establish clear criteria for progression based on the biomechanical demand of the activities the athlete needs to return to. They can then work with the team to put in appropriate training interventions to ensure that the athlete meets these criteria. Rehabilitation is also an excellent opportunity for the S&C coach to coach an athlete to improve their physical performance.

## Summary

The S&C coach is a vital member of the multidisciplinary team (MDT) for both reducing risk of injury and rehabilitating an athlete to return to training and competition. Through the identification of an injury risk model, S&C coaches can apply the principles of training to target interventions which will both reduce the stress placed through the MSK system or increase its capacity to tolerate stress. Finally, rehabilitation provides the S&C coach with an exciting opportunity to help athletes make gains that are not possible throughout the rest of the competition calendar.

## Notes

1 Aagaard, P., Simonsen, E. B., Magnusson, S. P., Larsson, B., & Dyhre-Poulsen, P. (1998). A new concept for isokinetic hamstring: quadriceps muscle strength ratio. *American Journal of Sports Medicine, 26*(2), 231–37.
2 Cormack, S. J., Newton, R. U., McGuigan, M. R., & Cormie, P. (2008). Neuromuscular and endocrine responses of elite players during an Australian rules football season. *International Journal of Sports Physiology and Performance, 3*(4), 439–53.
3 Foster, C. (1998). Monitoring training in athletes with reference to overtraining syndrome. *Medicine and Science in Sports & Exercise, 30*(7), 1164–68.
4 Moritz, C. T., & Farley, C. T. (2004). Passive dynamics change leg mechanics for an unexpected surface during human hopping. *Journal of Applied Physiology, 97*, 1313–22.
5 Myer, G. D., Paterno, M. V., Ford, K. R., Quatman, C. E., & Hewett, T. E. (2006). Rehabilitation after anterior cruciate ligament reconstruction: Criteria-based progression through the return-to-sport phase. *Journal of Orthopaedic & Sports Physical Therapy, 36*(6), 385–402.
6 Spiering, B. A., Kraemer, W. J., Anderson, M. J., Armstrong, L. E., Nindl, B. C., Volek, J. S., & Maresh, C. M. (2008). Resistance exercise biology: Manipulation of resistance exercise programme variables determines the responses of cellular and molecular signalling pathway. *Sports Medicine, 38*(7), 527–540.
7 Wulf, G., McConnel, N., Gärtner, M., & Schwarz, A. (2002). Enhancing the learning of sport skills through external-focus feedback. *Journal of Motor Behavior, 34*(2), 171–182.

Chapter 3

# Psychology in injury prevention and rehabilitation

*Tig Calvert*

## Introduction

Psychology has a central role to play in successful rehabilitation and, indeed, has value in the prevention of injury. Rather than the mind being separate from the body as was once thought, modern science has shown a very different and much more interesting picture. The psychology of the athlete is crucial in rehabilitation, as their emotions, beliefs and thoughts all affect how their body responds to injury. The mind and body interact. It is because of this intrinsic connection between the body and the mind that psychological techniques can be used to support rehabilitation and can also be useful in helping athletes to be more robust psychologically to reduce the risk of injury.

In relation to rehabilitation, sport psychology has traditionally focused on helping the athlete adjust to injury, in adherence to rehabilitation, and in preparation for return to sport, but without the specific remit to aid physical rehabilitation. Now, within a new paradigm, rehabilitation psychology specifically aims to aid the physical healing and repair of the body through psychological means, via the biological interaction between the mind and body.

The role of the rehabilitation psychologist is to help the athlete to develop and use their psychological resources to aid effective healing and successful rehabilitation with the aim of producing robust physical and psychological health in the athlete. This chapter describes the scientific evidence showing the link between the psychology and the physiology of the athlete in relation to rehabilitation following sport-related injury and presents a framework for the psychologist within the rehabilitation team.

In practice there are various opportunities for psychological intervention to assist rehabilitation. However, it is important to recognise that psychology is not only the remit of the psychologist but forms part of the natural relationship an athlete has with many members of the team. How an athlete interacts and the attitude and relationships between coaches, athletes, physiotherapists, doctors, strength and conditioning coaches, massage therapists and nutritionists can help or hinder the psychological health of the athlete, as well as affecting the athlete's belief system which, as we see, is fundamental to successful rehabilitation.

## Theoretical basis of rehabilitation psychology

Based on the theoretical knowledge from psychoneuroimmunology (PNI), the investigation of the pathways connecting the mind and the body, we have a greater understanding of how both positive and negative states of mind can affect immune system responses and repair of tissues. One of the ways the body and mind communicate is through the central nervous system, and this has particular relevance to how negative emotions and stress can inhibit rehabilitation.

In the 1970s, Robert Ader, a psychologist and immunologist, showed that the mind and body communicate with each other in a bidirectional flow of hormones, neurotransmitters and cytokines (cells of the immune system).[1] The brain and immune system represent a single, interactive system of defence. Thoughts, beliefs and emotions have neurochemical consequences and have a direct effect on both the immune system and individual cells in the body. Emotions and health interact. This interaction between crucial areas of the brain and the immune responses of the body is governed by the hypothalamus. The hypothalamus, an almond-shaped area deep within the brain, controls many of our everyday functions. It regulates body temperature, hunger, thirst, sleep and libido, and has a role to play in emotions.

Through a feedback system called the hypothalamic-pituitary-adrenal (HPA) axis the hypothalamus also controls the body's response to stress. The HPA axis is extremely effective in situations of acute stress. However, in chronic, long-term stress it can fail to regulate itself leading to an over-production of cortisol. This weakens the functioning of the immune system. In chronic stress, pro-inflammatory cytokines are over-expressed and their anti-inflammatory counterparts are down-regulated.[2]

The immune system does not just search and destroy pathogens; it also has a major role in tissue regeneration and aiding recovery from injury. The immune system recognises and eliminates cells or tissues damaged by injury, and therefore any weakness can inhibit rehabilitation. Marucha et al. showed that the healing of a mouth biopsy in dental students took 40 per cent longer during exams than during the summer break.[3] Critically, the production of IL-1 mRNA, a mediator of the inflammatory response, altered by 68 per cent in the same interval.

Clearly, stress can hinder the body's ability to heal. In the case of athletes, the injury itself is often a source of stress. Due to the detrimental physical result of stress on the immune response, we could argue that psychological intervention during long-term rehabilitation could be useful for all athletes. Identifying and assessing the levels of anxiety surrounding injury is important.

> Often, athletes who appear on the surface to be coping well may have underlying issues. All members of the team should therefore be aware of the importance of early identification of anxiety and stress symptoms.

As well as producing 'stress' hormones the hypothalamus also produces calming hormones, such as oxytocin, to promote healing of the body. This leads us to examine whether positive psychological states can mitigate some of the negative consequences of stress and, in addition, help the body to produce hormones that promote healing. Oxytocin is generally associated with nurturing in females. However, it is produced in both males and females and has a major role to play in successful rehabilitation. The main role of oxytocin in the body is to effect growth and repair.[4]

Oxytocin creates a feeling of well-being, reduces experiences of pain and decreases anxiety. Oxytocin levels increase when we do pleasurable things, have physical contact and are sociable. If an athlete is isolated during rehabilitation, this can reduce the production of oxytocin and inhibit the ability of their body to heal. Oxytocin can be increased with psychological therapies, such as deep relaxation or hypnotherapy, and is one of the biological consequences of sports massage. Oxytocin levels are also affected by the social environment. During rehabilitation it is important to create an environment for the athlete that not only decreases the stress response but also enhances the likelihood of healing hormones such as oxytocin.

> Social support has been shown to be pivotal and low levels of oxytocin have been shown in people with little social support.[5,6] It is therefore important to recognise that the social environment that the athlete experiences is crucial to successful rehabilitation.

Suggestions to improve the social environment of the athlete include:

- Arrange regular interaction with the medical and rehabilitation team even at times when no active therapy is appropriate;
- Assign a non-injured teammate to liaise with the injured athlete to ensure that they still feel included in the team and to keep up to date with day to day activities;
- Encourage team activities that the injured athlete can still attend, including social activities;
- Encourage contact with other injured athletes in the same or different sports to provide support and encouragement.

## Thoughts and beliefs in rehabilitation

It is not only emotions that have a corresponding biological effect; other cognitions are important too. Thoughts and, in particular, beliefs can have a physical effect on the body. This has been studied extensively observing the placebo effect. The placebo effect, in which an inert substance has a measurable effect on the physical body, is not only a good example of how the mind and body interact, but also allows us to examine specific beliefs. Examination of the placebo effect reveals that biological changes occur in the body that mimic the actions of the actual medication, and actual biological changes thus occur based on beliefs.[7] The placebo effect is particularly strong in relation to pain relief, as pain signals are intrinsically linked to areas of the brain that also respond to emotions. This is discussed in detail in chapter 17.

The nocebo effect, on the other hand, occurs when a patient who believes that a treatment will cause harm experiences an adverse effect.[8] This is particularly relevant to rehabilitation. It is important for athletes to hold positive beliefs regarding their treatment and the outcome. The nocebo effect seems to stem from the hippocampus, and as a consequence, memory is important.[9] So too, therefore, is an athlete's prior experience of injury treatment. If an athlete is identified as having negative beliefs regarding recovery or treatment, psychological intervention is especially warranted.

Examining how the placebo and nocebo effects occur highlights the psychological traits that are relevant. Placebo effects depend on the functioning and efficiency of the reward system, and individuals' responses to placebos differ. Expectation, conditioning and beliefs are important. Branded pills work better than generic. Because of previous experience affecting expectations, placebo prescribed four-times-a-day is more potent than twice-a-day, and injections are more effective than tablets.[7] The stronger the expectation, the stronger the effect. Athletes base their beliefs on prior experience and from interaction with the rehabilitation team.

The language we use is important. For example referring to an injured leg as 'the bad leg' can instil negative beliefs in the athlete unintentionally and affect the healing process and the athlete's perception of the injured area and levels of pain. Ensuring that the athlete receives consistent, positive communication from all members of the team is important.

## Application of theory in practice

Using the scientific basis of PNI and knowledge from placebo research we can develop therapeutic techniques with the intention of helping athletes influence their own natural healing processes to enhance their rehabilitation.

Ideally, the psychologist would have the opportunity to assess the athlete as soon as possible post injury and work with the rehabilitation team throughout the rehabilitation process regarding the needs and support requirements for the athlete depending on expected length of rehabilitation.

The psychologist has a role to play in the acute stage post injury and prior to treatment. The earlier the athlete can have help managing their anxiety post injury the better. Early intervention can ensure that any psychological trauma encountered at the time of injury can be alleviated before it creates biological effects that can hinder fast and efficient healing. Psychological intervention prior to surgery has also been shown to be effective in reducing post-operative pain, level of pain medication required and length of hospital stay.[10] One study using a brief relaxation intervention reduced patient stress and improved collagen deposition in surgical wounds leading to faster healing.[11] This is particularly relevant in relation to highly anxious athletes.

### *Reducing anxiety in the injured athlete*

Reducing anxiety, mediating the stress response and helping the athlete produce beneficial physical responses during rehabilitation are the cornerstones of rehabilitation psychology. Techniques such as deep relaxation or clinical hypnotherapy are particularly useful in helping an athlete to achieve a state of parasympathetic dominance of their central nervous system. This reduces the level of cortisol in the body and increases serotonin and oxytocin, thereby providing the body with the optimum state for repair. In conjunction, helping the athlete to produce healthy cognitions and expectations can support a robust psychological basis for successful rehabilitation.

Psychological responses to injury include devastation, isolation, feeling cheated and restlessness.[12] In addition, many athletes experience an array of emotional responses, including anger, regret, lack of control, which can lead to helplessness, and disappointment, which can lead to despair. During the process of rehabilitation, athletes can also experience feelings of isolation and loneliness. Rehabilitation can also be hindered through lack of motivation, feelings of apathy and, in some cases, denial.

These emotional states may result from the injury or may not. Some athletes fare well and respond well to injury. Developing healthy expectations and a positive belief system can act as a psychological buffer to stress and protect against the physical consequences of stress. As well as reducing stress, positive psychology interventions (PPIs) such as learned optimism[13] can have psychological and physical benefits.[14] Research has shown a relationship between positive psychological well-being and health, even to the extent of longevity of life.[15] Importantly, these attributes can be learned and developed.

### The ABCDE method

The ABCDE method can help the athlete reassess their beliefs surrounding injury and rehabilitation.[16] ABCDE (which refers to *adversity, belief* and *consequence* leading to *disputation* and finally *energisation*) forms a way of helping the athlete re-evaluate their beliefs surrounding the injury and enables the athlete to develop more optimistic coping strategies. Pessimistic athletes tend to view their injury as more personal to them; they blame themselves and often feel they are unlikely to recover and that there is little they can do about it. Helping athletes develop a more optimistic coping style helps them to see that injuries are not personal, recovery is possible and they can be proactive in their recovery.

### Maintaining motivation

Lack of motivation is a common psychological sequela of injury, which can impact on rehabilitation. Motivation is governed by the neurotransmitter dopamine. Levels of dopamine are dependent upon a feedback system, which may be disrupted through injury. Athletes are often used to a strenuous training programme and an active lifestyle. The consequences of a sudden halt to these activities can have a rebound effect on the normal production of dopamine and serotonin, leading to low mood and lack of motivation. Dopamine levels can be rebalanced through having goals which are positive and achievable, enabling the athlete to build belief that they can recover.[17] Rehabilitation can be a time of frustration for an athlete concerned about losing their skills, fitness and confidence. Maintaining a positive, optimistic outlook has biological and psychological effects that can help the process of rehabilitation. Encourage the athlete to partake in other activities that increase dopamine levels, for example competitive non-active pastimes or hobbies.

## Identification of psychological ill health

Athletes can experience grief and symptoms of depression following career-threatening injury. Indeed, in some instances, levels of depression following injury can be so severe[18] that athletes can become suicidal. Identifying symptoms of possible psychological disorders requiring medical consultation is essential. Eating disorders may become more apparent during periods of rehabilitation, and injury can also cause symptoms of post-traumatic stress disorder (PTSD). Any concerns about clinical disorders should be discussed with the medical team.

All members of the rehabilitation team should be aware of the following symptoms that may be indicative of a clinical disorder.

Symptoms of depression include:

- early morning wakefulness, insomnia or excessive sleepiness
- appetite disturbances
- mood changes
- anhedonia, where the athlete no longer finds pleasure in activities that were once pleasurable.

Symptoms of eating disorders include:

- mood changes
- nail, hair and skin changes
- weight changes
- secretive eating
- vomiting or use of laxatives
- over-concern about weight
- inaccurate self-perceptions.

Symptoms of PTSD include:

- flashbacks
- nightmares
- anxiety.

Psychological intervention to support the medical team and, if appropriate, the nutritionist is recommended.

However many issues are of a non-clinical level. An athlete may not show symptoms that require clinical intervention but may have emotions that are preventing their body from healing effectively. During rehabilitation, psychological issues can hinder progress. It is important for the psychologist to address these non-clinical issues and be trained in techniques to assist non-clinical emotional disorders.

Two techniques which have been shown to be particularly helpful in clinical settings are Eye Movement and Desensitisation and Reprocessing (EMDR[19]) and Emotional Freedom Technique (EFT[20]). These techniques are easy to learn and safe to use and can offer immediate and permanent relief from emotional issues that could hinder rehabilitation. EMDR has a wealth of supporting research demonstrating its benefits in treating psychological trauma and, in particular, PTSD. EFT is particularly useful during rehabilitation, as studies have shown a decrease in cortisol levels following EFT with corresponding decrease in stress symptoms,[21] implying that the technique has a generic effect on the central nervous system in a similar way to meditation, deep relaxation or hypnosis. EFT can be useful in rehabilitation psychology as a means of mitigating the effects of stress on the immune system, as well as being effective at relieving immediate emotional issues.

## Returning to sport

A review of concerns that athletes have about returning to sport following injury shows a number of areas of anxiety concerning the ability to perform to pre-injury standards or the standards of their teammates.[22] Athletes can lose their identity as an athlete while injured and face anxieties about suffering a subsequent injury when returning to sport. Fears and anxieties lead to poor outcome and if identified can be reduced with psychological techniques. Psychology throughout the rehabilitation process can aid a successful return to sport and the prevention of further injury. During the period when an athlete is preparing to return to sport, it is important to be innovative when designing activities, so that the returning athlete can compete along with their teammates. Injured athletes often report learning a great deal about themselves and their bodies through the process of rehabilitation. Encourage the athlete to share this knowledge with teammates and allow their development and growth through rehabilitation to be of benefit to all.

## Prevention of injury

The mechanisms discussed in this chapter are not only applicable to an athlete once they are injured, but are also important to the prevention of injury. Educating and assisting athletes to control and regulate their own physiological response to stress is useful in the prevention of injury, as well as giving them tools to aid with rehabilitation. Teaching deep relaxation techniques to all athletes to enable their bodies to naturally produce a state conducive to healing can prevent minor injuries from becoming more serious and make them less susceptible to injury. One role of the psychologist is to help their athletes to become psychologically robust to prevent injury. Research has demonstrated that athletes high in hardiness are less prone to injury, and that hardiness can facilitate the rate and quality of their recovery from injury.[23] What athletes experience prior to injury is important, and there is a good level of evidence to support the argument that an athlete can have a psychological vulnerability to injury.[24]

Hardiness refers to the athlete's ability to withstand difficulties and adversity and is a concept well known in performance psychology. The aspects of hardiness that seem to affect successful rehabilitation are confidence and optimism. Using techniques such as the ABCDE technique and other PPI interventions can help athletes to develop a robust defence against the psychological effects that can lead to a vulnerability to injury.

## Psychological health

Below is a suggested programme designed to help athletes attain a psychological state conducive to good psychological health and in the prevention of injury. The programme can be conducted as a two-day workshop or as a weekly session over a 6-week period. The programme can be used to include all members of the team including support staff and coaches and could be conducted across sports or within a team.

The three cornerstones of the programme are education in how the body and mind interact, relaxation and positive psychology tasks. Participants are encouraged to keep a positive psychology diary where they can record the completion of their tasks. These are personal reflections and should remain confidential. Positive psychology tasks have been shown to help produce positive emotions and develop optimism.

These include:

- designing a vision board to express desires and goals;
- expressing gratitude, recording three things they are grateful for in their daily diary;
- practising kindness, such as opening doors, smiling and chatting with people they meet, going out of their way to be helpful if a situation arises;
- increasing and becoming aware of 'flow', where the athlete is fully emerged in an activity;
- challenge negative beliefs with the ABCDE method.

Through our knowledge of psychoneuroimmunology and the development of positive psychology interventions we can ensure that athletes develop strong psychological health and corresponding physical well-being. It is important that we use this knowledge in an area like sport where the health of the athlete is paramount to sporting success.

## Summary

Recognising the links between the mind and the body has enabled research to ascertain that negative states – i.e. anger, hostility, anxiety and stress – can hinder physical recovery, and that positive psychological states can encourage physical recovery. In addition, specific beliefs, expectations and conditioning are also important. This knowledge can help rehabilitation psychologists to focus on helping athletes to form psychologically healthy emotional states, beliefs and cognitions to aid rather than hinder their rehabilitation.

Rehabilitation psychology, based on the theoretical basis of psychoneuroimmunology, uses psychological techniques to enhance the athlete's ability to repair following injury. Each athlete has facets to their psychological make-up that can be harnessed to benefit their recovery. Utilising these aspects can also be beneficial in preventing injury, by decreasing the risk, and in successful rehabilitation following injury. Sport is leading the way in integrating new scientific knowledge into practical application to the benefit of athletes.

The five key things every injury specialist should consider:

- Maintaining a positive, trusting environment is beneficial in prevention of injury and successful rehabilitation following injury.
- If an athlete is psychologically stressed, their body is more vulnerable to injury – keep an eye on their mental as well as physical health.
- Sleep and nutrition are essential to injury prevention and successful rehabilitation. They are both intrinsically linked to the immune system through the hypothalamus and are excellent markers of good physical and psychological health.
- Isolation and loneliness are common during rehabilitation. Active engagement with the athlete whenever possible and encouraging them to remain part of the team during rehabilitation are recommended.
- Injury can be a turning point in an athlete's career, for better or worse. Successful rehabilitation can ensure the athlete returns to sport a more robust and confident athlete.

## Notes

1 Ader, R., & Cohen, N. (1993). Psychoneuroimmunology: Conditioning and stress. *Annual Review of Psychology, 44*, 53–85.
2 Maes, M., Songa, C., Lina, A., De Jongha, R., Van Gastela, A., et al. (1998). The effects of psychological stress on humans: increased production of pro-inflammatory cytokines and th1-like response in stress-induced anxiety. *Cytokine, 10*(4), 313–18.
3 Marucha, P. T., Kiecolt-Glaser, J. K., & Favagehi, M. (1998). Mucosal wound healing is impaired by examination stress. *Psychosomatic Medicine, 60*(3), 362–65.
4 Moberg, K. (2003). The oxytocin factor. Cambridge, MA: Da Capo Press Inc.
5 Antoni, M. H. (2006). The influence of bio-behavioural factors on tumour biology: pathways and mechanisms. *Nature Reviews Cancer, 6*, 240–48.
6 Gidron, Y., & Ronson, A. (2008). Psychosocial factors, biological mediators, and cancer prognosis: a new look at an old story. *Current Opinion in Oncology, 20*(4), 386–92.
7 Benedetti, F. (2009). Placebo effects: Understanding the mechanisms in health and disease. New York: Oxford University Press.

8  Data-Franco, J., & Berk, M. (2013). The nocebo effect: A clinician's guide. *Australian and New Zealand Journal of Psychiatry, 47*(7), 617–23.
9  Kaptchuk, T. J., et al. (2010). Placebos without deception: A randomized controlled trial in irritable bowel syndrome. *PLoS ONE 5*(12), e15591.oi:10.1371/journal.pone.0015591
10 Sullivan, M. (2009). Psychological determinants of problematic outcomes following total knee arthroplasty. *Pain, 143*(1), 123–29.
11 Broadbent, E., Kahokehr, A., Booth, R. J., Thomas, J., et al. (2012). A brief relaxation intervention reduces stress and improves surgical wound healing response: A randomised trial. *Brain, Behavior, and Immunity, 26*(2), 212–17.
12 Evans, L., Hardy, L., Mitchell, I., & Rees, T. (2008). The development of a measure of psychological responses to injury. *Journal of Sport Rehabilitation,17*(1), 21.
13 Seligman, M.E.P., & Csikszentmihalyi, M. (2000). Positive psychology: An introduction. *American Psychologist, 55*(1), 5–14.
14 Cohn, M.A., & Fredrickson, B.L. (2010). In search of durable positive psychology interventions: Predictors and consequences of long-term positive behaviour change. *Journal of Positive Psychology, 5*, 355–66.
15 Chida, Y., & Steptoe, A. (2008). Positive psychological well-being and mortality: A quantitative review of prospective observational studies. *Psychosomatic Medicine, 70*(7), 741–56.
16 Seligman, M.E.P. (2002). Positive psychology, positive prevention, and positive therapy. *Handbook of Positive Psychology 2*, 3–12.
17 Scheier, M. F., & Carver, C. S. (1992). Effects of optimism on psychological and physical well-being: Theoretical overview and empirical update. *Cognitive Therapy and Research, 16*(2), 201–28.
18 Appaneal, R. N., Levine, B.R., Perna, F.M., & Roh, J.L. (2009). Measuring postinjury depression among male and female competitive athletes. *Journal of Sport & Exercise Psychology, 31*(1), 60–76.
19 Shapiro, F. (2002). *EMDR as an integrative psychotherapy approach: Experts of diverse orientations explore the paradigm prism.* Washington, DC: American Psychological Association.
20 Craig, G. (2010). EFT for Sports Performance. Fulton, CA: Elite Books.
21 Church, D. (2013). Clinical EFT as an evidence-based practice for the treatment of psychological and physiological conditions. *Psychology, 4*(8), 645–54.
22 Podloga, L., Dimmock, J., and Miller, J. (2011). Strategies for enhancing recovery outcomes. *Physical Therapy in Sport, 12*, 36–42.
23 Wadey, R., Evans, L., Hanton, S., & Neil, R. (2012). An examination of hardiness throughout the sport injury process. *British Journal of Health Psychology, 17*, 103–28.
24 Arvinen-Barrow, M., & Walker, N. (Eds). (2013). The psychology of sport injury and rehabilitation. London: Routledge.

# Chapter 4

# Nutrition in injury prevention and rehabilitation

*Matt Lovell*

## Introduction

Nutrition plays a critical role in the training and rehabilitation processes, and it is no wonder that the well-nourished athlete recovers faster and with better body-component structure repair than his undernourished cousin. And yet, the importance of the diet during rehabilitation is often overlooked.

This chapter outlines the considerations that impact eating for injury recovery. It uses a systems-based approach to highlight the areas of nutrition that must be factored into an athlete's strategy. As knowledge and practice continues to develop, or as the needs of your own athletes diverge from the examples given, these principles can be used to guide a methodical, safe and effective nutritional approach to injury rehabilitation.

## Strategic nutrition

A sound nutritional strategy is required for the optimization of the regeneration environment. This involves limiting the primary damage incurred from injury (or training) and ensuring the tissues surrounding the affected area are free from metabolites or chemical messengers that may subsequently retard the regenerative process.

Parts of this nutritional foundation include eating to balance the acid/alkaline balance within the body, as well as to help the body regulate inflammation. Of primary importance is consuming the appropriate amount of energy (calories) and macronutrients (protein, carbohydrates and fats), balancing the altered requirements arising from the athlete's reduced training load (and increased risk of harming body composition) with the requirements of rehabilitation.

Additionally, we must provide the body with the relevant building blocks for repair and rebuilding. Initial strategies should focus on forming robust nutritional habits with an athlete that encourages consumption of adequate micronutrients and macronutrients to aid rehabilitation. Specific strategies to address particular injuries will then further guide food choices and supplementation.

This process is outlined in Figure 4.1 and then discussed in the following sections.

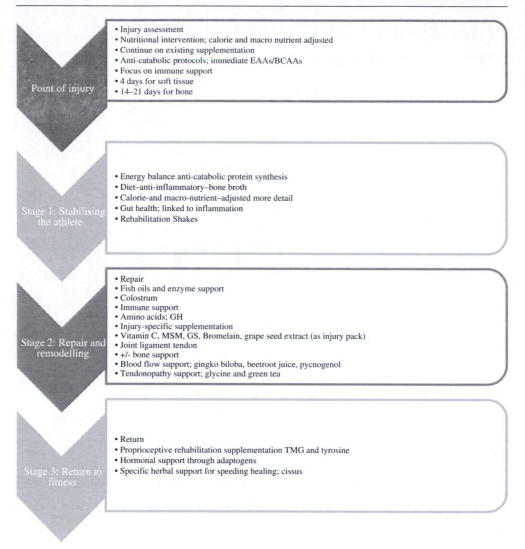

*Figure 4.1* Nutritional strategies to support the phases of injury rehabilitation

## Stage 1: Stabilising the athlete

The stages of injury need to be considered when deciding which dietary protocols to apply, and with which nutrients to intervene. The healing process needs to be supported by nutrient-dense foods, and this needs to be coupled by the need to maintain the body's acid/alkaline balance. Complicating this is the fact that over-consumption of energy during this period of reduced energy expenditure will lead to increased body fat and negatively impact on the athlete's fitness.

The other key consideration in this stage is the paradox of the inflammatory response. Inflammation is fundamental to the healing process following injury; it must be regulated to prevent it becoming a problem in its own right. Therefore, a balance needs to be struck between limiting damage and allowing the body's own immune system to function as it is designed.

## Energy balance

Following injury, energy expenditure is lowered due to reduced training load, necessitating calorific adjustments to preserve the athlete's physique and fitness. To do this, pre- and post-training carbohydrate intake should be adjusted based on basal metabolic rate (BMR) plus activity-factor calculations. Special emphasis should be placed on branched chain/essential amino acids (BCAAs/EAAs), which are the limiting factors for protein synthesis and can also be catabolized for energy. These high-quality protein precursors can be found in high concentrations in whey, dairy and meats and reflect a basic first step to recovery. Emerging evidence on 'adaptogenic' herbs such as *cissus quadrangularis* (cissus) is revealing a role for these enigmatic ingredients, but this level of nutritional support should be done alongside a trained herbalist and/or a sound drug testing protocol.

Energy balance and macronutrient provision depends entirely on the type of injury, the individual athlete and their physical exertion throughout rehabilitation. As a basic first step, we should look to increase intake of polyphenol-rich herbs, spices and vegetables, using these as a base for most meals. This results in a higher nutrient density and lower energy intake to reflect the reduction in activity and increased nutrient requirement for repair. Also, home-made stock/bone broth will not only add flavour when sugars and fats are being limited, but provide micronutrients to impact on processes of repair and inflammation. Table 4.1 highlights the critical building blocks for nutrition to support adaptation and rehabilitation during both rehabilitation and heavy training.

*Table 4.1* Template for building meals to support the healing process

| Food Class | Food Example | Benefit for healing |
| --- | --- | --- |
| Quality functional protein | Grass-fed beef | Building blocks for tissue repair |
| High polyphenol carbohydrate Brassica vegetables | Kale Broccoli Cabbage | Concentrated source of micro-nutrients and anti-inflammatory flavanoids |
| Starchy carbohydrate with additional flavanoid | Camargue 'red' rice or Thai 'black' rice | Nutrient-dense with inflammation regulation properties |
| Herb (culinary) | Oregano Basil | Facilitates digestion, high antioxidant potential |
| Spice | Turmeric Cinnamon | Anti-catabolic and anti-inflammatory |
| Tea | Green tea | Anti-inflammatory, antioxidant, thermogenic and calming properties |
| Functional sweetener | Glycine | Important component of collagen |

## Acid/base balance

The body's acid/base balance (pH) is tightly controlled to ensure the maintenance of the optimal environment for enzyme function. This can easily be disrupted, by a mismatch in the consumption between acid-forming foods (excessive meat and grain consumption) and alkali-forming foods (fruits and vegetables), increasing the body's workload to maintain the appropriate pH level. Calcium can be leached from the bones, which not only affects bone health but also the equilibrium and movement of many minerals in the body. This can make conditions for protein synthesis and rehabilitation sub-optimal. Hence, a good intake of vegetables is doubly important for recovery, hormonal output and acid/alkaline balance.

## Eating to support and regulate the inflammatory response

Inflammation is a necessary response to illness and injury, as it helps direct nutrients and immune factors (via blood and lymph) to an affected area, facilitating repair. As such, care should be taken with substances that may suppress it. Eating an appropriate balance of essential fatty acids, as well as micronutrients, provides the body with the precursors to efficiently and naturally *regulate* inflammation.

It is possible, however, for the inflammatory response to be excessive in both volume and chronicity. Whilst it aids energy provision for the immune response/repair by increasing breakdown of the body's stores, muscle is often sacrificed to provide fuel for this response, and there is a risk that chronic, poorly regulated inflammation can lead to catabolism.

## Step-by-step guide to addressing inflammation

From a nutritional perspective, we should not look to intervene to directly influence the inflammatory process in the acute period 72 hours for soft tissue injuries and 14–21 days for bone injuries. This will allow for a normal inflammatory response to occur.

As micronutrient status as well as omega-3:6 ratio can affect healing and inflammation on a number of levels, taking a selective panel of bloods can enable the practitioner to titrate dosages of essential micronutrient support and guard against deficiencies, optimizing the nourishment status of the athlete.

Good reference points to consider when interpreting red blood cell counts can be found in Table 4.2.

## Addressing deficiencies

If blood work reveals micronutrient deficiencies, a multi-nutrient containing a balanced complex of vitamins, minerals and co-factors should be taken daily. However, care must be taken to avoid 'mega-dosing' on certain anti-inflammatory nutrients and quenching the inflammatory response. *Concentrated flavonoid extracts* are an example of such a group of nutracueticals. By mopping up free radicals and exerting an antioxidant effect, they may interfere with cell signalling needed to mediate the inflammatory response. When in doubt, go to the (natural) source. The meals template above should be expanded to include brightly coloured foods like berries (particularly blueberries) and green tea (great natural sources of flavonoids). In general, brighter spices, herbs and vegetation will be higher in these antioxidants.

*Table 4.2* Red blood cell analysis

| Nutrient | Optimal range | Relevance |
| --- | --- | --- |
| Magnesium (RBC levels) | >35mg/L | Immune function/rehabilitation. Multiple benefits for human health. |
| Vit D D3 (25[OH]D) | >100 nmol/L | Immune function, protein synthesis, bone formation, calcium metabolism and anti-cancer effects. |
| Vit K (pertinent to Vit D function) undercarboxylated osteocalcin (ucOC) | Mid-range plus 20% | |
| Vit A (pertinent to Vit D function) Serum | Average of 125 mic/DL | |
| Iron profile | | Immune function, nutrient delivery, B12 for brain and nervous system function and the normal production of healthy blood. Folate is essential to proper DNA repair, red blood cell formation and methylation. |
| Ferritin | >75 <150 | |
| Total iron binding capacity | 20–55 mid-range + 20% | |
| Active Vit B12 RBC levels | >95pmol/L | |
| RBC Folate | Mid range +20% | |
| Omega-3:6 RBC levels | <1:3 >1:2 | Inflammation, multiple benefits to cellular function and immune regulation. |

---

**Rehab shakes**

One excellent way to achieve high levels of the valuable nutrients needed when injured is through a smoothie. The key is to understand the value each nutrient has in the healing process and to blend them in a way that is palatable and easy to digest. Taking too many of some aminos has caused GI distress, but this recipe is tried, tested and delicious when blended with ice:

    400 ml water
    5g BCAAs
    5g EAAs

Heaping teaspoon each of: Glycine, glutamine, arginine, OAKG, citrulline, creatine, HMB, and leucine.

Add in another heaping teaspoon each of: Blueberry extract, raw cacao nibs, manuka honey and flavouring.

Sip gradually over 30–45 minutes.

---

## Fatty acids

Obtaining an optimal balance of essential fatty acids within the body is vital for regulating inflammation. Omega-3 and omega-6 fatty acids provide precursors to inflammatory compounds, which interact to regulate inflammation.

• Athletes falling far below the optimal 3:6 ratio should be subject to dietary analysis, and if increased oily fish intake is not possible, supplement according to body weight up to three grams EPA per day.

- High dose supplementation also needs to include certain omega-6 fatty acids to help regulate the inflammatory response:

  - GLA: best taken as borage oil to ensure a pure source without excessive levels of other omega-6 fatty acids;
  - AA: supplements and foods such as eggs and prawns can be considered.

### The 'guts' of the inflammatory problem

Inflammation is a reaction of the immune system. The immune system must defend the body from foreign invaders, so it makes sense that much of these front-line ('innate') immune defences are in the gut. A compromised gut impacts on general immune function,[1] with knock-on effects that may impair mental well-being.[2]

   To regulate inflammation via the gut, three main factors should be considered:

1   Pro- and prebiotic strategies (eating 'good bacteria' or foods that support their growth in the gut). Yogurt and fermented foods such as sauerkraut are ideal additions to support the gut's growth of probiotics and should be included in the diets of all injured athletes. Aim for 30 billion live cultures each day, something that can be found in most probiotic formulations available in health food stores. Look for heat-stable non-competitive strains of bacteria. These will be manufactured in order to be stable outside of the fridge, below 25 degrees.
2   A sensible approach to anti-inflammatory medications formulated alongside a physician, because, whilst they may have their place, they may also obstruct probiotic gut health strategies.[3]
3   A dietary intake or supplement strategy that aims to tighten up the permeability or 'leakiness' of the gut. Certain nutrients can reduce gut permeability. Bovine colostrum has such an effect in athletes,[4] whilst the daily consumption of a simple homemade stock/bone broth to the food plan may also assist gut function and healing.

## Stage 2: Repair and remodelling – rebuilding the athlete

Once the injured athlete has been stabilized, we need to shift our focus to the process of rebuilding. This is a multi-pronged approach that must consider:

- Nutrient delivery and waste removal (supporting healthy circulation)
- The regeneration of damaged structures
- The central coordinating role of the immune system

### Circulation and vasodilation

Many circulatory strategies revolve around enhancing vasodilation to optimise blood flow. This occurs in response to the release of nitric oxide (NO). Eating foods rich in nitrates ($NO_3$) and nitrites ($NO_2$) can support NO production in the body. Again, basing the diet on organically grown fruits and vegetables will meet most requirements,[5] whilst herbs and spices will also add salicylates, blood-thinning agents to aid circulation.[6]

Other novel ingredients may also help blood flow. *Gingko biloba* potentiates blood-flow, although care should be taken with anti-coagulant medication and the use of this herb,[7] whilst *L-arginine and citrulline* are also NO precursors that may aid circulation.[8] Two–three grams of arginine and citrulline with 120 mg of standardized gingko extract twice daily is a good starting dosage. These are generally available in health food shops or online (see note below about World Anti-Doping Agency [WADA]–approved substances).

## Regeneration: Promoting protein synthesis and anti-catabolic strategies

Protein synthesis lies at the heart of any adaptation, rehabilitation or recovery process. The main factors increasing protein synthesis are resistance exercise and the intake of dietary protein (particularly 'high-quality' proteins rich in EAAs or leucine), and impairment of any of these following an injury slows healing rates. Our injury-eating template (Table 4.1) will provide sufficient nutrients and protein-induced stimulus to maintain protein balance, whilst energy intake can be manipulated via the carbohydrate and fat content. Hydration should continue to be monitored and promoted.

### Beyond protein . . . the added extras once the basics are covered

Whilst most of the amino acid requirements can be taken care of in strategies above, some research suggests additional benefit may be gained through using specific AAs. *Secretagogues* stimulate the release of growth hormone, stimulating anabolism. Taken before bedtime and pre training, these AAs may work with the body's natural circadian rhythms of hormone release to aid rehabilitation.

*Ornithine alpha ketoglutarate* (OAKG) has been shown to be effective in an oral bolus.[9] It has potential benefit for muscle protein synthesis[10] and can be added to juices (not other protein-containing foods) and taken before bed in a dosage of 250 mg/kg each day. They are not found in wholefoods in significant amounts, and the single aminos supplement appears to elicit a better response than when they are found in complexes within protein-containing foods like chicken.

## Immune action: Support and stimulate immune function

Immune-regulating protocols will support and optimize the speed and efficiency of the healing process, influencing anabolic and catabolic processes. This can be done effectively by addressing any nutrient deficiency relevant to the immune system that has been uncovered by screening (Table 4.2). In addition, Echinacea shows immune-modulating and wound-healing properties,[11] whilst colostrum provides immune factors that may stimulate the body's own production of immune-boosting proteins.[12,13] Initial dosing protocols would start with 20–60 grams of colostrum, along with 1 gram of Echinacea every three hours. Low lactose is a preferred source of colostrum if consuming above 5 grams in a single serving.

Anti-catabolic substances, through their role in reducing excess stress hormone production, may also be beneficial to the immune system, with colostrum providing direct immune benefits,[14] as well as athletic advantages.[12] *Pycogenol*, a bark extract with antioxidant properties, also accelerates healing.[15] A summary of these substances is provided in Table 4.3.

*Table 4.3* Anti-catabolic agents to aid healing

| Substance/Factor | Mechanism | Dosage |
|---|---|---|
| Sufficient calories | Under-eating means energy needs will be met through catabolism of fat and body proteins. | Determine BMR and then add in activity factor. Use macro split to control body composition, e.g. 'zone' type split 30–40% protein, 30% fat 30–40% carbs. |
| Adequate protein | Protein is required for healing, whilst deficient consumption can retard the regenerative process. | 2.2 g/kg LBM divided into equal servings across 4–6 meals to avoid fasting. For the purposes of injury recovery, larger protein intake can be sandwiched around training /rehab sessions. |
| Leucine | More anabolic than anti-catabolic but an essential part of switching on muscle protein synthesis. | Use 0.3 g/kg in 3 divided dosages on waking, before bed and after training/rehab sessions. |
| HMB | Shown to slow catabolism in disease state and may be helpful for combatting the catabolic effects of overtraining syndrome. | Use 3–5grams earlier in the day or before training. |
| BCAAs | Provides building blocks for tissue reformation and mental acuity support for rehabilitation sessions. | Use 0.3 g/kg throughout the training/ rehab period, e.g. as part of pre-intra and post-training shake. |
| Turmeric/Curcumin | Anti-inflammatory, prevents breakdown of protein, enhances glucose uptake into muscle. | Use 1 gram of curcumin 3x/day or 5–7grams of turmeric in cooking throughout the day. |
| Omega-3 fat | Regulates inflammation and promotes muscle protein synthesis; effects greater in elderly and states of inflammation. | Use 2–3.5 g EPA/DHA blended minus amounts that occur from dietary sources. |
| Creatine | Protects muscle mass during inactivity/immobilization. | Use 1/16 body weight in grams/kg, e.g. 80kg = 5grams daily in PW shake |
| OAKG | Precursor for NO, aids tissue repair and healing. | Use 0.2 g in divided dosages PW and before bed. |
| Glutamine | Improves healing in experimental studies, supports gut health and integrity, offers some benefit for growth hormone release. | Use 0.2 g/kg spread throughout day as per BCAAs. |
| Arginine/citrulline | Immune system support, growth hormone secretion, conditionally essential during periods of growth. | 3–6 grams pre-training and again at night as part of sectretagoue amino blend. |

## Injury-specific supplementation

Bone broth probably surpasses most available supplementation as the 'go-to' food-based healing strategy, as it contains multiple substrates for tissue remodelling and gut health support. As well as eating to *systemically* aid healing, individualised supplementation can support rehabilitation in a more specific fashion. It is beyond the scope of this chapter to cover all possible injuries, but guidelines for bone, muscle and tendon injuries are as follows:

### Bone injuries

- Commence the anti-catabolic strategies outlined in Table 4.3 within the first 48 hours;
- Run the panel of bloods in Table 4.2 and supply the necessary nutrients in suitable amounts based on the results;
- Adjust the energy balance of the diet;
- Emphasize alkaline, pigment-rich food sources as per the meal matrix (Table 4.1);
- Consider secondary damage support through ergogenic supplements, e.g. vitamin C, MSM, bromelain, grape-seed extract and glycine;
- The repair and remodelling phase would then begin with additional protein building and anti-catabolic strategies, blood-flow nutrients like citrulline, gingko and arginine and further inflammatory and oxidative regulation through the use of green tea;
- Use a bone supporting formula with sufficient vitamin K2, magnesium, calcium in a 2:1 ratio along with trace minerals from strontium and boron.

### Soft-tissue injuries

- Immediately commence anti-catabolic strategies (see Table 4.3); increase protein and amino acid intake;
- Adjust the energy balance of the diet;
- Glycine and green tea have particular relevance for tendinopathy and ongoing tendon support. Around five cups per day are necessary for sufficient flavonoid intake; extracts provide concentrated and measured dosages and may be preferred in the clinical setting. *Matcha* green tea is the most concentrated form of green tea extract and is the best form of commercially available green teas.

> For the athlete, sourcing supplements can be a minefield. Make sure all your supplements are drug-screened at a suitable lab and pass for the contaminants related to WADA and your sport's governing body. It's your responsibility to do this. If in doubt, do not take it!

## Stage 3: The finish line – return to competition

The final stage of rehabilitation is characterised by re-integration into full training and competition loads, and so our nutrition strategy needs to reflect these increased physical and technical demands. Eating to provide the nutritional building blocks and support the hormonal environment is vital, as is supporting an athlete's energy levels for performance and to reduce injury risk.

*Table 4.4* Possible cortisol-modifying agents

| Cortisol-moderating agent | Mechanism |
| --- | --- |
| Carbohydrate | Opposes the catabolic/starved-state triggering of cortisol release. |
| Glutamine | Lowers cortisol levels. |
| Phosphatidlyserin | 600 mg shown to reduce cortisol levels when taken after exercise.[16] |
| Vitamin C | 1–1.5 g shown to reduce cortisol levels when taken after endurance exercise.[17] |
| Antioxidants | Antioxidants such as *quercetin* and polyphenols may help lower cortisol levels, reduce the levels of free radicals and prevent the cell/tissue damage caused by physical stress. |
| L-Lysine and L-Arginine | Normalizes the cortisol stress response in those with high trait anxiety.[18] |

Continuing the anti-inflammatory and anti-catabolic strategies previously described is important. The food choices will aid the insulin/cortisol balance, and secretagogue aminos such as arginine may also assist with normalizing the growth hormone (GH) response to training. GH is critical for tissue healing and the adaptation from the training loads necessary during the final stages of rehabilitation.

A key nutritional aim during the recovery processes is to optimise normal physiology and maintain hormonal homeostasis in the face of the stress and fatigue imparted by training. Cycled use of adaptogenic herbs, such as *holy basil, schizandra* and *rhodioloa rosea*, show some promise in aiding this process.

Another key factor that we can seek to manipulate through diet is the insulin/cortisol ratio. Insulin is the most anabolic hormone, as it acts to stimulate the muscular uptake of aminos and increases testosterone production. It is most commonly triggered by a rise of blood glucose, but AAs such as glutamine and leucine found in dairy can stimulate *muscle-specific* insulin action independent of carbohydrate.

Keeping insulin levels high is usually done in the post-training window when we eat food that is high in sugars. However, a recovering athlete must exercise caution with excess energy intake in order to avoid increasing body fat.

Cortisol is released when carbohydrates are scarce and in response to stress. Initially, acute elevations in cortisol switch off inflammation, cause fat oxidation and stimulate the body to synthesise blood sugar, but a chronic increase in cortisol can lead to muscle catabolism and prevent glucose uptake by muscles.

It is essential, therefore, to strike an anabolic and catabolic balance, and possible cortisol-moderating agents are shown in Table 4.4.

Finally, creating an environment where the individual is better able to handle the adverse circumstances related to injury may be aided through anti-fatigue AAs like tyrosine[19] and amino complexes like creatine.[20]

Body composition assessment is an essential part of athlete management, and a thorough, regular anthropometry forms part of the core management plan around returning players to full match fitness, regulating the rebuilding of cross-sectional areas of injured tissue and limiting catabolism in immobilized limbs.

# Summary

Injury is an inevitable part of athletic endeavour and all too often a routine part of an athlete's training. Injury protocols are really an extension (and concentration) of existing recovery protocols for normal day-to-day training.

An understanding of inflammation and catabolism and nutritional strategies to limit these sources of damage are an essential part of returning to full fitness. Having clear strategies to adjust calorie intake to match changes in energy expenditure and knowing which nutrients are key to avoiding catabolism will arm the savvy athlete with the skills to heal faster. More specific dietary and supplement-focused approaches can then be individualized with an athlete in a process of constant refining, adjustment and strengthening a working relationship.

# Notes

1 Mengheri, E. (2008). Health, probiotics, and inflammation. *Journal of Clinical Gastroenterology*, *42*, S177–78.

2 Fehér, J., Kovács, I., & Balacco Gabrieli, C. (2011). Role of gastrointestinal inflammations in the development and treatment of depression. *Orvosi Hetilap 152*(37), 1477–85.

3 Espinoza, L. R., & García-Valladares, I. (2013). Of bugs and joints: the relationship between infection and joints. *Reumatología Clínica 9*(4), 229–38.

4 Playford, R. J., MacDonald, C. E., Calnan, D. P., Floyd, D. N., Podas, T., Johnson, W., . . . & Marchbank, T. (2001). Co-administration of the health food supplement, bovine colostrum, reduces the acute non-steroidal anti-inflammatory drug-induced increase in intestinal permeability. *Clinical Science 100*(6), 627–33.

5 Baxter, G. J., Graham, A. B., Lawrence, J. R., Wiles, D., & Paterson, J. R. (2001). Salicylic acid in soups prepared from organically and non-organically grown vegetables. *European Journal of Nutrition*, *40*(6), 289–92.

6 Paterson, J. R., Srivastava, R., Baxter, G. J., Graham, A. B., & Lawrence, J. R. (2006). Salicylic acid content of spices and its implications. *Journal of Agricultural and Food Chemistry*, *54*(8), 2891–96.

7 Diamond, B. J., & Bailey, M. R. (2013). Ginkgo biloba: Indications, mechanisms, and safety. *Psychiatric Clinics of North America*, *36*(1), 73–83. doi: 10.1016/j.psc.2012.12.006.

8 Bescós, R., Sureda, A., Tur, J. A., & Pons, A. (2012). The effect of nitric-oxide–related supplements on human performance. *Sports Medicine*, *42*(2), 99–117.

9 Le Bricon, T., Coudray-Lucas, C., Lioret, N., Lim, S. K., Plassart, F., Schlegel, L., De Bandt, J. P., . . . & Cynober, L. (1997). Ornithine alpha-ketoglutarate metabolism after enteral administration in burn patients: Bolus compared with continuous infusion. *American Journal of Clinical Nutrition*, *65*(2), 512–18.

10 Walrand, S. (2010). Ornithine alpha-ketoglutarate: Could it be a new therapeutic option for sarcopenia? *Journal of Nutrition Health and Aging*, *14*(7), 570–77.

11 Zhai, Z., Haney, D. M., Wu, L., Solco, A. K., Murphy, P. A., Wurtele, E. S., Kohut, M. L., & Cunnick, J. E. (2009). Alcohol extract of Echinacea pallida reverses stress-delayed wound healing in mice. *Phytomedicine*, *16*(6–7), 669–78. doi: 10.1016/j.phymed.2009.02.010.

12 Davison, G. (2012). Bovine colostrum and immune function after exercise. *Medicine and Sport Science*, *59*, 62–9. doi: 10.1159/000341966.

13 Gleeson, M. (2013). Nutritional support to maintain proper immune status during intense training. *Nestlé Nutrition Institute Workshop Series*, *75*, 85–97.

14 Zimecki, M., & Artym, J. (2005). Therapeutic properties of proteins and peptides from colostrum and milk. *Postepy Hig Med Dosw*, *59*, 309–23.

15 Blazsó, G., Gábor, M., Schönlau, F., & Rohdewald, P. (2004). Pycnogenol accelerates wound healing and reduces scar formation. *Phytotherapy Research*, *18*(7), 579–81.

16  Starks, M. A., Starks, S. L., Kingsley, M., Purpura, M., & Jäger, R. (2008). The effects of phosphatidylserine on endocrine response to moderate intensity exercise. *Journal of the International Society of Sports Nutrition, 5*, 11.

17  Peters, E. M., Anderson, R., Nieman, D. C., Fickl, H., & Jogessar, V. (2001). Vitamin C supplementation attenuates the increases in circulating cortisol, adrenaline and anti-inflammatory polypeptides following ultramarathon running. *International Journal of Sports Medicine, 22*(7), 537–43.

18  Jezova, D., Makatsori, A., Smriga, M., Morinaga, Y., & Duncko, R. (2005). Subchronic treatment with amino acid mixture of L-lysine and L-arginine modifies neuroendocrine activation during psychosocial stress in subjects with high trait anxiety. *Nutritional Neuroscience, 8*(3),155–60.

19  O'Brien, C., Mahoney, C., Tharion, W. J., Sils, I. V., & Castellani, J. W. (2007). Dietary tyrosine benefits cognitive and psychomotor performance during body cooling. *Physiology & Behavior, 90*(2–3), 301–7.

20  Cook, C., Crewther, B., Kilduff, L., Drawer, S., & Gaviglio, C. (2011). Skill execution and sleep deprivation: effects of acute caffeine or creatine supplementation – a randomized placebo-controlled trial. *Journal of the International Society of Sports Nutrition 8*, 2.

# Part 2

# Athletic competencies

# Medical assessment and pre-participation screening

*Mike Bundy and Lisa Hodgson*

## Introduction

Pre-participation screening (PPS) has become a routine tool in the assessment of players at the beginning of a new season, or when a new player or athlete is introduced to a new training group. The spectrum of what is screened during this process, however, can vary tremendously, ranging from the all-encompassing pre-signing medical examination of a multimillion-pound footballer to a brief examination to fulfil legal requirements when competing in a single event. Equally, different sporting bodies and governments have differing criteria for what needs to be assessed during a screening. For example in Italy, every person wishing to participate in sport is required to have a cardiac screening assessment, with a view to reducing the incidence of sudden death.

Not all pre-participation medicals should therefore follow the same format, but should instead be tailored to the needs of the medical team, the organisation and the athlete. These can be divided into those aimed at detecting cardiovascular disease and those that assess other aspects of the athlete's history.

The aim of this chapter is to explain the principles, benefits and process of screening. As part of this, we will delve in detail into the process of cardiac screening.

## Principles of screening

The overarching aim of any screening process is to assess the welfare of the athlete involved. It should be based on sound scientific criteria and be performed by a physician trained and experienced in sports medicine as well as in the screening process. Clearly, preparation and planning in such a process is vital. In order to make a meaningful assessment, the athlete should be examined in a suitable environment, with the right equipment, privacy and notes available, including reports and scans from previous medical attendants.

Everyone involved in the screening process needs to understand that if a problem is identified, then important discussions need to be taken about the consequences of these findings, and it should not just be ignored. As such, it is vital that consent for this PPS is given prior to the commencement of the process. On rare occasions, the findings have serious consequences and impact on the athlete's ability to pursue their career. The athlete is always given a chance to withdraw from the rest of the screening process if a serious medical problem is identified, but they need full counselling regarding the decisions they are making. Written advice and a certificate following the process need to be given to all parties, with full consent.

The results of a PPS can have dramatic consequences and these need to be appreciated. For example as a result of this process, some athletes may either be totally or temporarily precluded from participation in sport whilst further assessment or treatment is conducted. In a study of 733 adolescent pupils, it was noted that 0.4 per cent were excluded from the sport totally, and 5.5 per cent were temporarily excluded whilst they had further assessment.[1]

A screening process obviously needs to be validated, and if we are targeting a specific abnormality, it is important that this condition is recognised as having a significant impact on the performance or health of the athlete. With any screening process, it is vital that abnormalities can be detected at an early stage and that early treatment is of benefit. In elite sport, there are several tests that would not be used in treating the general public, but these too have to show reliability, sensitivity, specificity and affordability. Such an example would be detecting iron deficiency anaemia in female endurance athletes with screening blood tests.

## Benefits of screening

As we have listed, there are many points that will come out of the screening process, but in the realms of sport, probably the most important is identifying musculoskeletal abnormalities that put the athlete at risk of injury. It is not always practical to give the whole squad a list of preventative pre-habilitation exercises in the hope that you will reduce the incidence of injuries to a minimum, but rather, tailor-make the preventative programme to each player, once you have identified their particular risk.[2,3] This is where the PPS programme can be so beneficial. This is discussed in greater detail in chapter 6.

## Elite pre-participation screening

The main reasons for performing a PPS in sport are to:

1   Identify conditions that might adversely affect the sport's participation and identify injury risk, need for pre-habilitation or rehabilitation;
2   Establish baselines of athlete health, from an orthopaedic/musculoskeletal and general medical (including cardiovascular) perspective;
3   Allow the medical team an opportunity to uncover and discuss high-risk behaviours, such as infections, alcohol use, drug use and smoking;
4   Meet the legal and insurance requirements of the sport and the laws of the game;
5   Discuss consent for the process and also discuss confidentiality regarding any of their medical problems – this needs to be clearly excluded and rules outlined as to what the medical team can discuss with coaches, and whether athletes want to be present during these discussions or whether there is consent to discuss their medical issues in their absence;
6   Discuss contractual conclusions, as a medical report often needs to be submitted as part of this negotiation;
7   Provide an opportunity to discuss with the athlete how the medical team and the club function.

## The PPS process

A suggested format for a PPS programme forms a part of this chapter. It is not necessarily complete, but it is comprehensive, identifies the process and points out important issues that need to be raised or assessed. These can be divided into the following sections:

1  **Patient details**

This is a good opportunity to find out as much as you can about the personal life of your athlete – not only their address and contact details, but more importantly, home and family life. Athletes spend a lot of time involved in their sport, and the family around them can be supportive but also demanding and distracting, thus affecting the athlete's performance.

2  **Past medical history**

(a)  Medical and social history

It is routine to go through the past medical history of all of your athletes. Mostly, they will be fit and well, but occasionally we may find an athlete who has had some birth defect or childhood illness, or has a genetic trait, such as sickle cell disease, that will impact upon their sporting performance. It may well be that the athlete wants to keep this confidential, but the medical team should be aware of the consequences of these findings on performance. It is important in female athletes to identify any past history of eating disorders, menstrual disorders or osteopenia as part of the triad that predisposes to bone stress and osteoporosis. Issues that are commonly ignored in the young, such as dental health, vaccination history, sexual health and lifestyle issues such as alcohol, smoking and drug use, need to be explored.

It is also vital to understand as well the prescribed medications and nutritional supplements that the athlete may consume. It is important at this stage not to miss the need for a Therapeutic Use Exemption (TUE) form for athletes who are on medication that requires notification.

(b)  Musculoskeletal history

A list of previous injuries and their management is vital, not only because they may have biomechanical consequences for the athlete, but also because they may not have been fully rehabilitated, and should be a focus for the examination part of the screening. Details of scans, surgical reports and previous rehabilitation need to be obtained.[4]

(c)  Sport-specific history

This includes details of the athlete's background within the sport, such as:

- playing history
- runs of games and fitness levels
- protective clothing and equipment used, as well as strapping needed
- concussion history (frequency and threshold)
- the type of footwear or orthoses used.

In addition, previous strength training programmes need to be identified, as do pre-habilitation or rehabilitation regimes. It is also useful to obtain Global Positioning System (GPS) data, to know what their normal load is throughout a week and to compare that to training load expected moving forward. This can help identify whether they need modifications to training load to avoid sudden spikes.

Often missed, but vitally important, is the need to know what nutritional input that they get in terms of supplementation, allergy medication or any special diet, and whether they have any particular sponsorships that mean that they have to wear certain footwear or equipment that may make it difficult to comply with medical needs.

In certain sports, there are injuries that are more likely, such as spondylolisthesis in cricket, stress fractures in endurance athletes and osteoporosis in female endurance athletes. All of these issues need to be explored, and it needs to be determined whether any baseline investigations such as MRI, DEXA scan or blood tests have previously been performed.

(d) Family history

It is important to be aware of an athlete's family history of either cardiovascular or respiratory disease, as well as any family members who have inflammatory disorders or spondyloarthropathy, or any conditions that may be associated with these, such as inflammatory bowel disease, iritis or psoriasis. Obviously, sudden death has a significant impact in the cardiovascular screening, but so do diabetes, dental illness and osteoporosis.

## Medical examination

It is possible to get carried away with the breadth of the examination that may be required. Most examination processes are tailored to the needs of the athlete and the medical team, but it is important to use this to obtain baseline readings on the general medical status of your athlete. Height, weight, BMI and other anthropometric measures such as skinfold thickness can be recorded, as can the hyperflexibilty of the athlete through a Beighton score. Visual acuity and colour recognition may be relevant to the sport, as may hearing. A dental assessment may be appropriate, and importantly, assessing cardiorespiratory, abdominal, pelvic and baseline neurological function. Musculoskeletal examination is discussed in greater detail in chapter 6.

### Respiratory disease screening

Exercise-induced asthma is highly prevalent in elite athletes (present in up to half of elite-level athletes,[7,8] yet usually remains inadequately diagnosed and treated, and can be associated with severe health implications.[4,5] It is estimated that 20 per cent of any squad will have some degree of exercise-induced asthma.[6] Therefore, screening for this is of undoubted benefit, and respiratory function tests, including spirometry or the more detailed eucapnic voluntary hyperventilation (EVH) test, may be more appropriate.[9]

### Neurological screening

In a sport where concussion occurs, baseline neuropsychological tests, such as CogState Sport and SCAT3, as well as balance tests performed pre-season are essential. The diagnosis of concussion has been controversial, and obtaining objective markers to diagnose, monitor progress of and recover from concussion is something we all strive for. Assessing cognitive function compared to a 'normal' baseline state is one way to determine whether recovery has occurred. It is therefore extremely important to have reliable 'normal' baseline test results with which to compare the concussed athlete to enable doctors to diagnose and assess recovery status. These baseline tests can be written scores, such as a SCAT3 test, or more elaborate computer-based neuropsychological tests, such as CogSport, and should be performed each pre-season together with a neurological examination set as a baseline with which to compare later on in the season.

### General health screening

Further investigations may be dependent upon what is found at the history and examination, but a series of blood tests, including full blood count, urea and electrolytes, liver function, thyroid function, calcium, vitamin D, iron studies, lipids, B12 and folate, coeliac screen and hepatitis screen may be relevant. In those athletes who have frequent bone stress or bone fractures, parathyroid hormone (PTH) levels may also provide useful information. It is important to note that in many instances, 'normal' values for an athlete may differ from 'normal' values for the general population, and this needs to be considered when interpreting results.

### Imaging studies

Imaging with x-rays, MRI, CT or ultrasound is commonly used in some professional teams' medicals. The use of these has to be guided by the knowledge that not all of the findings are symptomatic or relevant, and images should be carefully interpreted with a consultant radiologist to determine the importance of such findings. Having said that, the identification of a spondylolisthesis in a fast bowler in cricket may have consequences for whether his bowling action should be reassessed or altered. Likewise, a DEXA scan identifying osteoporosis in a female endurance athlete will have consequences for her predisposition to stress fractures or stress reactions.

As can be seen, the range of assessment available to perform on a player is vast, and this may well be prioritised over the past medical history gleaned from the athlete. Rather than performing a standard range of radiological scans, it may be better to target certain images for certain situations, e.g. the DEXA scan in an athlete with a history of stress fractures, a knee MRI in a footballer with previous ACL reconstruction and frequent knee effusions, or a shoulder MRI in an athlete with previously undiagnosed shoulder instability found on the screening examination.

## Consequences of the PPS process

It is important to have an action plan following the PPS. This can be divided according to contractual requirements, where the medical team may be required to report to the coach or club director as to whether there are any limitations or consequences that can impact upon the contractual negotiations. In simple terms, these can be divided into the following categories:

1   Athlete cleared without limitations
2   Athlete cleared but further analysis is required
3   Athlete cleared but with limitations and precautions
4   Athlete not cleared to be fit to train/compete.

From a medical point of view, there are certain decisions to be made following the assessment, and these can be defined as follows:

1 **Investigation or referral**

   If the medical team identifies any issue that needs further investigation, such as imaging or referral to a specialist, then this needs to be enacted to allow the severity of the condition/injury to be fully assessed.

2 **Pre-habilitation needs**

   During the assessment, it is possible that certain biomechanical, strength or structural abnormalities that will put the player at injury risk may be identified. These need to be corrected or minimised through a pre-habilitation programme.

3 **Rehabilitation needs**

   If the athlete is returning from injury it is important that rehabilitation needs are addressed and that a proper reintegration back into sport is monitored.

4 **Review time**

   Finally, it needs to be decided when this process is going to be reviewed and reassessed. Some issues such as cardiac screening can be reviewed annually, whilst others, such as reviewing the impact of vitamin D replacement therapy or assessing shoulder strength and stability following a surgical reconstruction, require more frequent reviews.

## Cardiac screening

Arguably the most contentious aspect of medical screening in sport surrounds cardiac screening. Whilst it is true that cardiac screening cannot identify every possible fault, this is no different from any other aspect of screening the medical profession advocates. It does, however, have the potential to reveal 'silent' conditions that if left uncovered can be fatal. As such, cardiac screening is aimed at identifying those athletes, between the ages of 14 and 35 years old, who may have underlying conditions that may lead to sudden cardiac arrest (SCA) or death.

Sudden cardiac death (SCD) is defined as an 'unexpected death occurring as a result of natural causes in which loss of all functions occurred instantaneously or within 6 hrs of onset of symptoms'.[10] It is not the purpose of this section to discuss the various causes that can lead to a SCA or death, nor to argue the pros and cons of cardiac screening and what to do with the information once it is identified. That will be the decision of the individual sport or national governing body. Equally, the 'if to exclude' question will not be addressed, as this will always be a sportsperson's own decision taking into account the cardiologist's recommendations and the by-laws of that sport.

Cardiac screening will continue to be a controversial topic, particularly given the infrequent number of deaths that occur in relation to the number of young people who participate in sport. The prevalence of cardiovascular disorders known to cause SCD in young athletes is approximately three athletes in 1,000,[11,12] but the death of a young and apparently healthy individual is catastrophic. It is estimated that 80 per cent of all non-traumatic deaths in young competitive athletes are due to inherited congenital structural or functional abnormalities, most of which can be identified during life.[10,13,14] Male athletes appear to be at a greater risk of exercise-related SCA, and a particularly vulnerable cohort is adolescent males below 18 years of age.[15] Race is also an influencing risk factor, with black athletes being at higher risk than white athletes, particularly concerning hypertrophic cardiomyopathy (HCM).[16]

> Most deaths (90 per cent) occur during or shortly after exercise, and athletes are twice as likely to stress their heart and therefore have an increased vulnerability to SCA.[15] Whilst it is true that exercise itself is not a direct cause, it is a trigger, as the stressed heart is more vulnerable.

## Who should be screened?

In 2005, European recommendations were established endorsing a screening protocol that prior to participation in organised sport any fit and healthy young person should have cardiac screening that includes a resting 12-lead Echocardiogram (ECG).[17] This recommendation was informed by the Italian experience of mandatory cardiac screening and has since been supported by such bodies as the International Olympic Committee (IOC), International Federation of Football Association (FIFA) and an institutional review board (IRB).[11,18]

> During 2012, the 'Advances in Sports Cardiology' meeting in Seattle, Washington, USA, provided further reading to support the education regarding these issues for those working in sport.[19] A themed journal was published in 2013 to aid ECG interpretation by physicians for athletes to improve cardiac care with international consensus collaboration.[20]

Whilst the concept of cardiac screening remains controversial, the knowledge that 70–80 per cent of all young athletes with congenital abnormalities, whether structural or electrical in origin, are asymptomatic prior to the event[10] provides the stimulus to do everything possible to uncover underlying cardiac abnormalities. Indeed, the athlete that displays 'red flag' warning symptoms, such as syncope, shortness of breath on exertion, chest pain and palpitations, could be considered 'lucky', as they are given clear clues to an underlying problem. This is why a structured screening process of *all* athletes, not just the symptomatic ones, is critical.

Whilst there are acquired traumatic events, such as commotio cordis or viral conditions such as myocarditis, that can lead to SCA but cannot be identified prior, nor be accounted for in a prophylactic program, evidence exists as to the overall effectiveness of a cardiac screening process, and this should be the end of the debate. The only question left should be *how do we conduct this screening?*

## Medical history and physical examination

To establish a family history, common questions (see below) can be incorporated as part of the screening protocol.[21] For younger athletes, it is best to include parents or guardians in this process to ensure accuracy of the family history.

- Do you have a family history of SCD or has anyone died suddenly in your family below the age of 35?

- Have you ever suffered an episode of syncope?
- Do you suffer from palpitations?
- Do you ever suffer from shortness of breath that is disproportionate to the activity you are performing?
- Have you ever been diagnosed as having a heart murmur?

Physical examination is a part of the process but not stand-alone. Auscultation using a stethoscope may help to identify structural disease. For example the presence of a heart murmur may indicate a valve leakage or an obstruction to flow caused by obstructive hypertrophic cardiomyopathy.[21]

The above procedures may indicate an urgent referral for future testing, especially if one of the questions is positive and if there is a family history, or if a heart murmur is identified. But a negative questionnaire and/or physical examination is not enough to clear an athlete. Further screening is still required to ensure a full cardiac screen.

## 12-lead echocardiogram (ECG)

The goal of screening is to classify the heart as either 'normal', requiring no further testing, or 'abnormal', requiring further evaluation. At times, this can be difficult in sport, as it is generally accepted that, following years of intense training, athletes have physiological changes related to their heart that in a non-athlete would be suggestive of an underlying pathological condition. Nonetheless, an ECG should detect 95 per cent of those with an underlying HCM, and 80 per cent of those with arrhythmogenic right ventricular cardiomyopathy (ARVC).[18] As such, a 12-lead ECG is recommended by the European Society of Cardiology and the IOC.[17,4] The false positive ECG rate is still widely discussed, but London's St George's Hospital has reduced the false positive rate to 4 per cent,[15] and ECG is still the most cost-effective cardiovascular PPS tool.[22]

To ensure that ECGs in athletes are correctly interpreted to avoid missing potentially dangerous cardiovascular conditions or ordering unnecessary follow-up testing, it is best that a clinician experienced with the athletic heart conducts the process. Also important is having a direct referral pathway to a specialist centre that can assist with further interpretation and follow-up testing.

Even with expert interpretation, however, the ECG will not detect all conditions at risk of SCD. Further diagnostic testing may be required as a result of family history or symptoms, or if a positive ECG is found. Briefly, the follow-up tests that may be employed are:

## Echocardiogram (ECHO)

ECHO uses ultrasound waves to look at the structure of the heart and is used in those with ECG changes. Some sports will employ both an ECG and an ECHO as basic screening tools, whilst others will opt for an ECG screening with the ability to obtain an ECHO immediately should the ECG identify an abnormality.

## Exercise stress test/ECG test

This is an ECG-evaluated test conducted before, during and after exercise on either a treadmill or bike using a set protocol. The cardiologist will interpret the electrical changes and patterns that occur within the heart during exercise. These are particularly useful in detecting some of the features that are apparent in ARVC or Long QT syndrome (LQTS).

## 24-hour Holter test

This is either a 3-lead or 12-lead ECG taped to the athlete's chest for a period of 24 hours to record the cardiac electrical activity. This is ideal in looking for arrhythmias that may be present in some conditions such as LQTS or Brugada syndrome.

## Cardiac MRI

Cardiac MRIs can detect 5–10 per cent of conditions that present with a normal ECG.[21] They are chosen when there is an abnormal pattern of test results or a mismatch between signs and symptoms. It is primarily concerned with the structure of the heart and can detect subtle cardiomyopathies that often mimic channelopathies. It can also detect congenital coronary anomalies, myocarditis or signs of coronary artery disease.

Once abnormalities are detected we are duty-bound to ensure a speedy follow-up and further investigation to prevent unnecessary psychological worries in our athletes. Whilst any positive screening is going to have a psychological impact and anti-screening arguments are often based on the false-positive impact factor, the negatives of this are far outweighed by the negatives of a SCD.

Despite the financial implications, best practice dictates the mandatory offer of cardiac screening to athletes. The athletes can then make an informed decision whether or not to opt in to the process. It is possible to conduct the medical history taking, physical examination and ECG testing and then use an online interpretation tool, but this should only be considered if a referral pathway is in place to allow for follow-up testing and appropriate management by sports cardiologists if necessary.

## Summary

There is no doubt that PPS can be a very involved process. It can expose the athlete's vulnerabilities, and the process is not without its risk of identifying a condition that may have career- and life-changing consequences. The purpose of the screening process needs to be clear from the outset, as should the consequences and expectations of all involved. Ideally, the process should be comprehensive but can be targeted towards the specific needs of the athlete, the team, the sport, the position and the skill of the athlete. Below is a template that you are welcome to use as part of your screening process.

Table 5.1  Pre-participation screening questionnaire

Name :                        Sex :              DoB :
Address :                                        Age :
Next of Kin :                                    Tel :
Regular Physician :
Sport :                       Position :         Level :

R or L footed / handed :

No Games in last 12 months :

## Medical History :   If answer yes then give details

Do you have an on-going chronic illness ?
Have you ever had surgery ?

### Cardiac

Have you ever passed out during or after exercise ?
have you ever been dizzy during or after exercise ?
Have you ever had chest pain during or after exercise ?
Have you ever had palpitations, racing or irregular heart rate during or after surgery ?
Are you ever excessively short of breath or tired during exercise ?
has any family member died of heart problems or sudden deaht before the age of 50?
Do you have high blood pressure or cholesterol ?

### Respiratory

Do you have asthma or any respiratory illness ?
Do you cough, wheeze or have breathing difficulty during or after exercise ?
Do you use an inhaler (even episodically) ?

### Abdominal

Do you have any digestive, kidney or liver problems ?
Ever had a spleen injury or surgery ?
Ever had a hernia ?

### Neurological

Ever had any fits ?
Do you have frequent or severe headaches or migraines ?
Ever been concussed or significant head injury ?

Do you suffer from Diabetes ?
Do you wear glasses or contact lenses ?
Any other eye disorders ?
Any hearing problems ?
Any other problems with your ears, nose or thoat ?
Ever had any skin disorders esp Psoriasis, eczema, infection ?
Ever had a sexually transmitted disease ?
Do you have any dental problems / false teeth ?
Do you visit a dentist regularly ?
Do you wear a gumshield / mouthguard ?

### Infection

Ever had Glandular fever, Hepatitis, Rheumatic fever or TB ?

### Males

Ever had any testicular problems ?
Ever had any prostate problems ?

### Females

Do you have regular periods ?
Are you on the contraceptive pill ?
Date of last period :
Date of last cervical smear ?
Date of last mammogram ?

Do you get Stingers / burners ?

Do you get numbness or tingling in your feet / hands ?

**Psychological**

Ever had any depression ?

Ever had any stress or anxiety illness ?

Ever had an eating disorder ?


Any birth defects :

Any Sickle cell disease :

Smoker ?

Alcohol :

Do you wear Orthotics :


**Significant past surgical / Injury history** (inc any time lost playingin the last 12 months)

Neck :

Thoracic :

Lumbar :

Sacral :


Give details :


**Allergies**

Are you allergic to any drugs, foods, contacts ?

Do you use an epipen ?

**Medications**

Are you on any regular medication ?

Do you take episodic medication including pre-match ?

Specific TUEs :

Do you take any supplements ?

**Date of last vaccinations :**

Tetanus :                    Measles / MMR :

Hepatitis :                  Influenza :

**Family History**

Any familiy history of :

Blood pressure, Cardiac, respiratory disease

Inflammatory bowel disease, Coeliac disease,Diabetes, Mental illness

Sudden death


Groin :

Hips :

Thighs / Quads :

Knees :

Shins :

Ankles :

Feet :


Shoulder :

Elbow :

Wrist :

Hand / fingers :


I certify that the above answers are complete and correct

_____

(Continued)

*Table 5.1* (Continued)

Signed :                                    Dated :

## Physical Examination

| | | | | |
|---|---|---|---|---|
| Height : | Weight : | BMI : | | |
| Pulse : | BP : | PEFR : | | |
| Hearing :  Right : | Left : | Visual Acuity :  Right : | Left : | Colour vison : |
| | | Corrected : | | |
| | | Marfans ?: | | |
| | | Body Fat % : | | |
| | | Beighton score : | | |
| | | Right : | Left : | |

CVS :

Respiratory :

ENT :

Teeth :

Lymph nodes :

Abdomen :

Genitalia :

Skin :

## **Musculoskeletal**

| | | | | |
|---|---|---|---|---|
| **Standing :** | Posture : | Feet : | Pelvic symmetry : | OH squat :  SL Squat : Right : Left : |
| | | | | Duck Walk : Lunge : Right: Left : |
| | | | | KTW:  R  L |
| | | | Calf endurance (25 max)  R  L | |

**Lumbar Spine :**   ROM :   Quadrant :   Neuro :   Power:   Reflexes :   Sensation :   SIJ R / L
**Cervical Spine :**   ROM :   Quadrant :   Spurlings :   Neuro :   Power:   Reflexes :   Sensation :
**Thoracic Spine :**

## Shoulder :

| | | | | | |
|---|---|---|---|---|---|
| ROM : | Abduction | Ext Rotn R / L | Int Rotn R / L | ER/IR Ratio R / L | GIRD : R / L |
| Scapula Rhythm : R / L | Wasting : | | | | |
| Rotator Cuff : | InfSpin : | SupraSp : | Subscap: | Impingement: | ACJ: R / L   SCJ: R / L |
| Stability: | AP stability R / L | Apprehension R / L | Sulcus : R / L | Relocation R / L | X-over R / L |

## Supine

| | | | | |
|---|---|---|---|---|
| Thomas' | Hip Flex R / L | ITB R / L | Flexion R / L | Adductor R / L |
| Slump R / L | SLR R / L | H/S length R / L | Leg Length R / L | |

## Hip

| | | | | |
|---|---|---|---|---|
| ROM IR/ER R / L | Quadrant R / L | Faber R / L | Adductor : Length R / L | Power R / L |
| Squeeze: 0*   60*   90* | Psoas R / L | Pubic Sym: R / L | Inguinal canal R / L | |
| PI / max | add core : | add core : | add core : | |

## Knee

| | | | | |
|---|---|---|---|---|
| ROM : | Effusion R / L | Quads bulk R / L | MCL R / L | LCL R / L |
| Ext / Flex | | | | |
| ACL : Ant Draw R / L | Lachmann: R / L | Pivot: R / L | PCL : R / L | Post Draw : R / L   Lag : R / L |
| Joint Line   tenderness R | McMurray R / L | Apley : R / L | Sup Tib-fib R / L | Dial test R / L |

*(Continued)*

Table 5.1 (Continued)

| Ankle | TCJ ROM PF / DF | R L | STJ ROM | R L | Power | R L | Inv / Ever | R L | Stability : Ant Draw | R L | Talar tilt | R L |
|---|---|---|---|---|---|---|---|---|---|---|---|---|
| Palpation : | Jt Line | R L | Sinus tarsi | R L | Cuboid | R L | 5th MT | R L | Talus | R L | Navicular | R L |
| | | | | | | | | | | | Achilles | R L |
| Syndesmosis | ER stress : | R L | | | Squeeze | R L | Ant Imping | R L | | | | |
| | | | | | | | Post Imping | R L | | | | |

Core stability
(Sahrmann)

Level 1
Level 2
Level 3
level 4
Level 5

**Elbow** R
L

**Wrist** R
L

**Hands** R
L

**Foot** R
L

<u>**Summary of findings**</u>
1
2
3
4
5

<u>**Investigations required :**</u>

<u>**Treatment needs :**</u>

**Prehab needs**

**Rehab needs :**

**Pre-exercise fire-ups :**

**Screening requirements :**

**Recommendations :**

1     Cleared without limitations

2     Cleared after further investigation

3     Cleared but with limitations / precautions

4     Not Cleared

**Signed**         **dated**

## Notes

1  Mayer, F., Bonaventura, K., Cassel, M., Mueller, S., Weber, J., Scharhag-Rosenberger, F., . . . Schar-hag, J. (2012). Medical results of preparticipation examination in adolescent athletes. *British Journal of Sports Medicine 46*, 524–30.

2  Noyes, F. R., & Barber-Weston, S. (2011). Anterior cruciate ligament injury prevention training in female athletes: A systemic review of injury and results of athletic performance tests. *Sports Health: A Multidisciplinary Approach, 4*(1), 36–46. doi: 10.1177/1941738111430203

3  Barber-Westin, S. D., Noyes, F. R., Smith, S. T., & Campbell, T. M.. Reducing the risk of noncontact anterior cruciate ligament injuries in female athletes. *The Physician and Sportsmedicine, 37*(3), 49–61.

4  Ljungqvist, A., Jenoure, P., Engebretsen, L., Alonso, J. M., Bahr, R., Clough, A., . . . Thill, C. (2009). The International Olympic Committee (IOC) Consensus Statement on periodic health evaluation of elite athletes March 2009. *British Journal of Sports Medicine, 43*, 631–43. doi:10.1136/bjsm.2009.064394.

5  Becker, J. M., Rogers, J., Rossini, G., Mirchandani, H., & D'Alonzo, G. E., Jr. (2004). Asthma deaths in sports: A report of a 7-year experience. *Journal of Allergy and Clinical Immunology 113*(2), 264–67.

6  Dickinson, J., McConnell, A., & Whyte, G. (2010). Diagnosis of exercise induced bronchoconstriction. EVH challenges identifies previously undiagnosed elite athletes with exercise induced bronchoconstriction. *British Journal of Sports Medicine, 45*(14), 1126–31.

7  Ansley, L., Kipplelen, P., Dickinson, J., & Hull, J. H. (2011). Misdiagnosis of exercise-induced bronchoconstriction in professional soccer players. *Allergy, 67*(3), 390–95. doi: 10.1111/j.1398-9995.2011.02762.x.

8  Hull, J. H., Ansley, L., Garrod, R., & Dickinson, J. (2007). Exercise-induced bronchoconstriction in Athletes – should we screen? *Medicine and Science in Sports and Exercise, 39*(12), 2117–24.

9  Dickinson, J., McConnell, A., & Whyte, G. (2010). Diagnosis of exercise-induced bronchoconstriction: Eucapnic voluntary hyperpnoea challenges identify previously undiagnosed elite athletes with exercise-induced bronchoconstriction. *British Journal of Sports Medicine, 45*(14), 1126–31.

10  Sharma, S., Whyte, G., & McKenna, W. J. (1997). Sudden death from cardiovascular disease in young athletes: Fact or fiction? *British Journal of Sports Medicine, 31*, 269–76.

11  Maron, B. J., Thompson, P. D., Ackerman, M. J., Balady, G., Berger, S., Cohen, D., . . . Puffer, J. C. (2007). Recommendations and considerations related to preparticipation screening for cardiovascular abnormalities in competitive athletes: 2007 update. *Circulation, 115*, 1643–55.

12  Wilson, M. G., Basavarajaiah, S., & Whyte, G. P. (2008). Efficacy of personal symptoms and family history questionnaires when screening for inherited cardiac pathologies: The role of electrocardiography. *British Journal of Sports Medicine, 42*, 207–11.

13  Papdakis, M., Whyte, G., & Sharma, S. (2008). Preparticipation screening for cardiovascular abnormalities in young competitive athletes. *BMJ, 337*, 806–11.

14  Hodgson, L. (2012). Sudden cardiac death in sport – be prepared part III. *SportEx Medicine, 53*, 20–25.

15  Sheikh, N., & Sharma, S. (2011). Overview of sudden cardiac death in young athletes. *The Physician and Sportsmedicine, 39*(4), 22–36.

16  Maron, B. J., Carney, K. P., Lever, H. M., Lewis, J. F., Barac, I., Casey, S. A., & Sherrid, M. V. (2003). Relationship of race to sudden cardiac death in competitive athletes with hypertrophic cardiomyopathy. *Journal of the American College of Cardiology, 41*(6), 974–80.

17  Corrado, D., Pelliccia, A., Bjørnstad, H. H., Vanhees, L., Biffi, A., Borjesson, M., . . . Thiene, G. (2005). Cardiovascular pre-participation screening of young competitive athletes for prevention of sudden cardiac death: Proposal for a common European protocol. *European Heart Journal, 26*, 516–20.

18  Zipes, D. P., Camm, A. J., Borggrefe, M., Buxton, A. E., Chaitman, B., Fromer, M., . . . Zamorano, J. L. (2006). ACC/AHA/ESC 2006 Guidelines for management of patients with ventricular arrhythmias and the prevention of sudden cardiac death. *Journal of the American College of Cardiology 48*(5), 1–102.

19 Wilson, M. G., & Drezner, J. (Eds.). (2012). Advances in Sports Cardiology. *British Journal of Sports Medicine, 46,* 1–103.

20 Drezner, J. (Ed.). (2013). Seattle Summit on ECG Interpretation: International collaboration to improve cardiac care for athletes. *British Journal of Sports Medicine, 47,* 121–86.

21 Behr, E. R., Papadakis, M., & Sharma, S. (2011). *Cardiac conditions in the young: From ARVC to WPW.* Surrey, UK: Cardiac Risk in the Young.

22 Fuller, C. M. (2000). Cost effectiveness analysis of screening high school athletes for risk of sudden death. *Medicine and Science in Sports and Exercise, 32*(5), 887–90.

# Chapter 6

# The injury risk profiling process

*David Joyce and Dan Lewindon*

## Introduction

For centuries, humans have sought to predict the future in order to ease anxiety about prospective events. Nowadays, this ambition extends to sport and exercise, where performance support teams employ a series of tests in the hope of gaining an insight into future athletic performance or injury risk.

Originally, the purposes of pre-participation evaluations in sport were to assure the coaching staff that their players had commenced the competitive season with a common level of health and fitness and to identify 'treatable' conditions. Whilst these objectives are still present, the scope and ambition of screening has extended to include:

- identification of areas of weakness or pain associated with performance to provide a platform for injury risk management programmes;
- assessment of physical capacities (e.g. aerobic power, acceleration, vertical jump height);
- determination of benchmarks (e.g. what is normal for a certain athletic population based upon age, playing position, etc.);
- assessment of recovery from previous injury (when it is used as a baseline measurement);
- elimination of intrinsic faults prior to coaching technique/training programme changes (such as back squat proficiency or plié technique).

The focus of this chapter is not so much to detail athletic performance testing, as this is covered elsewhere in the text, but rather to demonstrate how a true interdisciplinary approach to athletic profiling can help identify the athlete at risk of injury so that plans can be put in place to mitigate that danger.

The aim of assessing every single aspect of an athlete is unrealistic and not supported by scientific research. The field of tests that *could* be applied is too vast, many of which will be irrelevant to the athlete being tested. It is clear that a strategic approach is required, one that relies on the gathering of intelligence as a method of sifting through all the possible things that 'could go wrong', in order to hone in on those things that are 'most likely to'. In this way, it can be seen that the principal aim of the screening process is for it to yield meaningful *information*, rather than just data.

What is also clear is that screening should not be used as the definitive assessment tool *per se*, but as a method of filtering through all the possible injury scenarios to highlight certain areas of an athlete's profile that require management or further investigation.

This chapter will present a framework for the development of a pragmatic, evidence-based screening tool that is functionally relevant and individually targeted, the fundamentals of which can be applied across all sports and age groups, as well being useful in industrial and military environments.

## Disrupting the injury equation

The occurrence of an injury has wide-ranging effects on the athlete, including:

* reducing time spent training or competing
* imposing a negative effect on sporting performance
* financial costs and psychological implications.

Indirect costs of injury are also evident with impacts sometimes being felt by their team, their family and the wider community. It is clear, therefore, that prevention of injuries in sport and exercise is a worthwhile aim. It is unrealistic to expect all injuries to be preventable. What we can aspire to, however, is a situation where the risk of injury is reduced.

The premise for using screening as a keystone of injury risk reduction relies upon it identifying individuals susceptible to injury. What turns an athlete into a susceptible one is best seen in the following equation:

---

**Injury risk equation 1**

Predisposed individual + extrinsic risk factors
= susceptible individual

---

A predisposed individual is one who is more exposed to injury due to their own intrinsic risk profile. Such intrinsic risks may include past injury, age, reduced joint range of motion (ROM) and muscle weakness. If the predisposed athlete is exposed to extrinsic risk factors, they then become susceptible to injury. Extrinsic risk factors are those that are applied to the athlete, such as training regimen, weather and the nature and laws of the sport itself.

An example of this is a female netballer with hamstring weakness who has poor landing mechanics. In this instance, the athlete is predisposed to knee injuries due to her gender and kinematics, both of which are linked with knee injury risk.[1] Her sport then exposes her further to risk due to the rules promoting sudden decelerations and pivoting. As a result, this athlete is susceptible to an anterior cruciate ligament (ACL) injury.

The second key equation to understand is:

---

**Injury risk equation 2**

Susceptible athlete + injury mechanism
= injury

---

Continuing the above example, should the netballer be exposed to an incident where she has to rapidly decelerate and change direction when catching and passing, all the ingredients are present for an ACL injury.

Each of these three variables (predisposition, extrinsic risk factors and injury mechanism) needs to be identified and either corrected or compensated for if we are to have an impact on reducing overall injury rates. The aim of screening, therefore, is to identify the predisposed individual so that the sum of these injury equations can be minimised.

## Developing a screening tool

### Step 1 – creation of the generic warning index

The first step in developing a pragmatic screening tool, therefore, is to make it as sport-/ activity-specific as possible. In order to do this, it is vital that the injury profile of the sport be examined in detail. The sport's injury profile helps to form the basis of what can be termed a *warning index*. This warning index serves to highlight areas that need special attention paid to them. For example, as a rule, we would look closer at knee injury risk factors in skiers than we would in swimmers. This approach is based on epidemiological findings that tell us that knee injuries result in more competition and training time lost in skiing than in swimming.[2]

Epidemiological studies of injury rates in sport provide the basis for a pragmatic approach to injury risk identification. The governing bodies of many sports commission epidemiological studies into injury incidence and prevalence.

Most sports with a large participation base will have had some epidemiological study published in the scientific literature regarding injury rates over a specified period.

The two key factors to glean from these studies are:

(1) injury incidence, which is usually expressed as number of injuries reported per 1000 hours; and
(2) injury severity, which is usually expressed as games or training days missed.

> A good example is the Australian Football League's injury survey, which is the world's longest running publically released injury survey in sport. Other good examples are the annual injury reports produced by the Rugby Football Union (UK).

It is important to consider both factors because a relatively minor injury may occur frequently, whereas a less common injury may have effects that are more devastating and therefore warrant more investment in preventing it. An example of this is the ACL rupture that, whilst relatively infrequent, accounts for the most number of training days missed in a number of sports.[3] By combining both incidence and severity, a clearer insight into the top priorities for intervention can be gained.

It is vital that the comparison between these statistics and your athletes be valid, however. The sport itself may not be the only variable of interest. Injury patterns often differ depending on factors such as:

• Gender
• Competition level
• Age[4,5,6]

Accordingly, the more these statistics can be broken down the better. In doing this, a true profile of sport-specific injury incidence and severity can be determined, and benchmarks against the population average can be ascertained.

> The downfall of using injury statistics is that often an injury is only recorded if an individual misses training or competing. In many cases, however, an injury may not stop an athlete from participation, although it may reduce their performance when doing so. Using the traditional injury surveillance format, these injuries do not count towards the total statistic and as a result may be under-represented. A more sophisticated method, therefore, is to report on injuries that affect performance, but at present this is not widely presented in the scientific literature.

If possible, it is even more powerful to be not just sport-specific, but also *position-specific*. This helps to account for the varying roles that different players within a team are expected to play, and therefore the varying loads to which they will be exposed. This often translates into a different injury profile. Examples of positional differences in injury profile can be seen in Table 6.1, below.

Once the injuries of greatest significance have been identified, the sport-specific generic warning index has been completed. This forms the basis for screening of the entire group of athletes that is to be tested. The next step is to customise the screen according to the intrinsic risk factors of each individual.

It is important to consider not just the demands of competition, but also the demands of training. In the ice hockey example, whilst ankle sprains do not feature as an injury of high significance, training often involves track running and plyometrics, both of which do have high incidences of ankle injuries.

> By the end of this first step, we aim to identify the 4–5 major injuries that will form the heart of the assessment. The closer your group of athletes is to the groups found in the literature (based on factors such as age, gender, playing position, etc.), the more valid the comparison, which in turn increases the appropriateness of the list of injuries in the *generic warning index*.

*Table 6.1* Examples of the impact of playing position on injury profile

| Sport | Positional differences in injury profile |
| --- | --- |
| Rugby | Higher risk of shoulder instability in five-eight position compared to wing in elite rugby union.[7] A full exploration of injury differences according to playing position in professional rugby union players can be found in Brooks & Kemp (2011). |
| American football | Higher rates of shoulder injury in quarterbacks compared to tight ends.[8] |
| Rowing | Scullers tend to sustain more cervical injuries than sweep rowers.[9] |

## Step 2 – individualising the warning index

Athletes within a group will vary in injury risk profile according to their own intrinsic risk factors. Intrinsic risk factors are those internal to the individual, such as age, gender, race, body mass, muscle strength, physical fitness, biomechanics and history of injury. They can be divided into *modifiable* and *non*-modifiable factors. As the name suggests, non-modifiable factors are those that no manner of interventions can alter, such as age, gender or past injury profile. The presence in an individual of any of these non-modifiable risk factors should filter them into a specific testing pool. Modifiable risk factors will be dealt with in step 3.

The factor that has been shown to be the most powerful predictor of an injury is a past injury to that site. For example it is known the highest risk of a groin injury is a previous groin injury[10] and that individuals with a history of an ankle sprain have a higher chance of re-injuring that ankle.[11] This, therefore, is an area worthy of specific attention, even in a sport such as ice hockey where ankle sprains do not figure as an injury of significance.[12]

Injuries to other areas of the body may also provide a predictive clue to the risk of injuries to other body parts. For example a history of low back pain has been shown to be a powerful predictor of ACL injury in collegiate athletes.[13]

Another example of a targeted approach to screening is in the screening of females for ACL injury risk. Females are between 2–8 times more likely to sustain an ACL injury than males,[14] and it is our view that all females should be assessed for ACL injury risk in any land-based team sport.

By examining the profiles of the athletes or by conducting targeted interviews with them, the presence of many of these risk factors within the group can be ascertained prior to performing any tests. This helps direct the professional to a more targeted and individualised approach to injury screening.

Accordingly, the *interview questionnaire* is the next step in the process. Again, a myriad of factors could be screened for, but it is best to narrow the investigation to the areas of most interest according to the profile of the sport. An example can be seen in appendix 1. Again, it is not designed to be the definitive assessment tool, merely one that acts as a quick method of seeing if a specific injury (past or present) makes its way into the individual-specific warning index. It is a method of filtering information so that the areas of relevance can be distilled and then targeted in a physical examination.

The areas of interest as ascertained by the specific warning index can then be added to those in the generic warning index to give us intelligence-led targets to test during our physical examination. This demonstrates a real advantage of the warning index. Instead of having to examine the literature for risk factors for every single possible injury, our research can now be directed to the examination of those modifiable risk factors that relate specifically to the injuries of greatest significance to the individual.

---

By the end of this second step, we aim to have identified both a generic and an individual-specific warning index. Such an intelligence-led approach enables us to develop a targeted and specific approach to risk factor identification, which increases its diagnostic power.

## Step 3 – determining the risk factors

A myriad of factors have been proposed as being injury risk indicators, but to test for each of them is both unrealistic and unnecessary. The aim should be to make the screening tool as streamlined as possible, which is why we prioritise our modifiable risk factor research to those injuries that we have identified in steps 1 and 2.

In order to conduct the research, scientific databases (such as *Medline, sportdiscuss, Cinahl, Pubmed* and *Web of Knowledge*) need to be accessed with a variety of appropriate keywords entered. These keywords should be used as filters to ensure that the information most relevant to your group of athletes is attained. It is important not to filter too stringently; otherwise, important information may be missed. For example should the area of interest be concussion in lacrosse, it would be prudent to examine the literature regarding concussion in other contact sports as well.

---

### Examples of key search words:

*(name of body part), (name of injury), (sport name), child, youth, senior, amateur, professional, elite, sub-elite, male, female, risk factor, athletic, sport, injury, injuries, modifiable, intrinsic . . .*

---

Table 6.2 below shows some factors that have been identified in previous research as being injury risk factors. These factors were identified using a string of words from the list of examples provided above.

It is vital to know these risk factors, as they direct the next stage of the process of screening tool development, which is to uncover the most valid and reliable assessments of athlete susceptibility to injury.

---

Once this third step has been completed, we should have generated a list of all the risk factors for the injuries that have been identified in the warning index.

---

*Table 6.2* Examples of modifiable risk factors for sporting injuries

| Injury | Modifiable risk factor |
| --- | --- |
| Groin injury | Hip internal rotation[15] |
| Hamstring injury | Hamstring muscle strength[16] |
| Lumbar spine stress fractures in cricket fast bowlers | Asymmetry of quadratus lumborum muscle bulk[17] |
| Concussion in sub-elite rugby league | Aerobic power[18] |

## Step 4 – selection of appropriate assessments of injury susceptibility

It is our belief that the reasons why pre-participation examinations have not been shown to have strong predictive validity[19] is that the screening tests selected are often (a) not specifically targeted at the athlete (therefore failing one of the first two stages) and/or (b) not valid or reliable.

The selection of appropriate tests is critical in the formulation of a screening tool. A number of things must be considered:

- Is the test itself a valid measure of the variable of interest?
- Does the test have sufficient inter- and intra-tester reliability?
- Is the *application* of the test valid?

Table 6.3 below describes these three issues. Ideally, all selected tests would have demonstrated reliability and validity, but it needs to be acknowledged that research often lags behind professional practice, and that clinical experience should not be discarded simply because it is yet to be scientifically proven. Nonetheless, it is reasonable to strive to include only the most appropriate tests. Accordingly, we propose a 3-tiered approach to test selection:

*Tier 1*
*Tests that achieve this status have been shown to be both valid and reliable, may have predictive value as injury predictors and are applicable in a clinical setting.*

*Tier 2*
*These tests have been found to be clinically useful and reliable but may be lacking in scientific proof of their validity or in their ability to be predictive of injury.*

*Tier 3*
*These tests may be clinically useful but may lack convincing scientific validity or reliability.*

*Table 6.3* Essential criteria for test selection

| Issue | When present | When absent |
|---|---|---|
| Test validity | The results of the test are an accurate indication of the variable being investigated. | The results of the test do not provide any true insight into the variable of interest. |
| Test reliability | The results are robust against random error and will be the same when repeated by the same or other people. | Different results may be obtained upon repeated testing by the same person. Equally, the results that one tester achieves may be different from that achieved by another tester. This means that results cannot be compared with confidence and so changes in the variable may not be 'true'. |
| Appropriate test application | This is a form of validity. It means that not only is the type of test selected appropriate, but the performance of the test gives a true indication of the variable of interest. | The test may be appropriate but the way in which it is performed may not give an insight into the variable of interest. For example isokinetic hamstring testing that does not examine its profile at high speeds (300°/sec). |

The core of the screening assessment battery should be comprised of tests in tier 1 and tier 2. Tier 3 tests should be considered only if the high performance professional finds them particularly useful.

Other things that should be considered are the ease and expense of test application. This is particularly the case when there is a group of athletes to be tested on repeated occasions. The aim is to make the entire battery as specific, targeted and user-friendly as possible where the maximum amount of information can be gleaned with a minimum of time or money expenditure.

It is also important to point out that it is our view that all athletes that participate in contact or collision sports should undergo neurocognitive screening at the start of the season. This will serve to act as a baseline measure of higher-order cognitive functioning, one that can be used as a comparison should a concussion be sustained during the course of the season. This view is in keeping with best practice principles as outlined in the Zurich Consensus Statement on Concussion in Sport.[20]

### Step 5 – assessment of movement proficiency

The fifth step requires the selection of tests that examine an individual's ability to perform specific functional tasks, which, in turn, is a display of their proficiency in integrating motion, stability and motor control. This step is essentially an extension of step 3, but we have given it a section of its own to emphasise the functional nature of these tasks.

The analysis of functional movement requires us to examine the system as a whole, which avoids a reductionist approach to examining parts as opposed to patterns. The background and therefore viewpoint of an interdisciplinary performance team is vital here, as is the use of video.

Analysing tasks such as landing control and gait analysis is vital, particularly for dynamic weight-bearing sports. Throwing or bowling technique is also crucial to examine in those

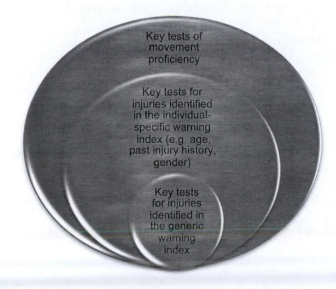

*Figure 6.1* The 'onion skin' of risk factor identification

athletes that rely on such explosive upper limb tasks. Also included should be basic tasks, such as movement dissociation ability and squatting control, especially if loaded squatting will form part of a training regimen.

By this stage, the screening tool of musculoskeletal competencies should be complete. Depending on the level of detail required regarding an athlete, there may be some other pieces of information that can be integrated. Specifically, these may be a psychological profile as well as a medical screening, examining such things as cardiovascular and dental health.

The total screening tool, therefore, is an example of many members of the performance support team providing their expertise.

---

Upon completion of the fifth step, we should have distilled the major intrinsic risk factors for an individual athlete based upon their risk index and movement profile. In essence, we will have developed and individualised an athletic profile and determined all the tests necessary to examine for the susceptible individual.

---

### Step 6 – dealing with the results

The aim of the screening process is to assess risk and to highlight areas that require further investigation. For example a poor performance of an overhead squat, a reduction in shoulder ROM, or asymmetry when running or landing from a drop jump should alert members of the high-performance team to investigate further to ascertain the causes behind these poor results.

To illustrate this further, a poor squat may be due to a number of factors, including insufficient ankle or shoulder ROM, decreased lumbo-pelvic stability or poor technique/motor control. The sports medicine team can assess the relative contributions of ankle ROM to the performance of the squat, whereas the conditioning coach will be able to determine if their inability to squat is due to a technical deficiency. These issues can then be investigated further and managed appropriately.

This demonstrates the real value of the screen; it acts as a filter, whereby risk factors for injuries in the warning index deficits can be deconstructed into their individual parts. It also demonstrates how an interdisciplinary process will provide a thorough insight into the issues at hand. Frequently, a number of factors combine, and it is only through an integrated assessment that these factors can be evaluated and corrected. Again, the value of a multi-faceted screening process is evident.

The results of the screening should provide the high-performance staff with an accurate reflection of an individual athlete's deficiencies that need specific attention. These findings need to be discussed with the entire high-performance team. It is our opinion that this includes both the athlete and coaching staff. This is because all members of the team can provide some insight into the next part of the *injury risk equation,* which deals with the forces they are likely to be subjected to in the future. The marriage of these factors goes some way to providing the high-performance professional with a real insight into injury risk, which is, of course, the necessary first step in injury prevention. These modifiers provide the 'expected future forces' side of the injury risk equation.

Exposure to extrinsic factors known to increase the risk of a specific injury that the athlete is already predisposed to combine to turn the individual into a susceptible one. An example of such an interplay could be a female water polo player with a history of shoulder impingement pain and screening that has revealed anterior instability (predisposed athlete) about to enter a heavy preseason training period involving high-volume-resisted swimming and throwing (extrinsic risk factors). This athlete is now susceptible to further episodes of shoulder pain.

We would not know of her susceptibility to injury had we not understood the two parts of this injury equation. Clearly, all members of the high-performance team need to understand each part of the equation, as all have input into either increasing or decreasing her susceptibility to injury.

The bottom line is, however, that all findings of the screening process must be discussed with the performance and coaching teams and acted upon; otherwise, the entire process is futile. It must be viewed as the crucial first step in a strategic approach to injury risk reduction, but it is useless by itself.

> The completion of this step should provide all members of the interdisciplinary team with a plan of action for addressing any modifiable risk factors.

### Step 7 – review

The screening tool is, by nature, ever-evolving because an individual's risk factors change with time, and the individual will enter or leave various risk groups according to these changes. This may be because during the previous season, they sustained a quadriceps tear, placing them in a risk group for sustaining another one, or they entered a 'high risk' age range (such as being over the age of 23 in the case of hamstring injuries).[21] Also, thanks to appropriate management, their hip ROM may have improved, reducing their risk of groin injuries.

As with any new process, there will be a 'bedding-in' period as the support staff gets used to performing the various assessment items. It is inevitable that some tests will be replaced by others over time due to professional preference or advancements in the scientific rationale for the risk factors of certain injuries. However, the philosophy of an intelligence-led, individually targeted approach to screening, using valid and reliable tests should remain constant.

## How often should screening be performed?

The entire screening process should be completed at the start of each season. This gives the performance professional an indication of the status of a player before training load is applied. This also satisfies one of the other main objectives of screening, and that is to establish baselines, upon which deviations during the season can be measured.

It is considered prudent to repeat the screen in its entirety at the end of the season as well (with any necessary adjustments given any injuries sustained during the season). This can then be used as a means of prescribing off-season programmes. Dependent on time and resources, it could be argued that the process could be performed mid-season as well to ascertain any deviations from the preseason baseline.

It is becoming increasingly common in elite sport for an abridged screening process to be completed on a daily or weekly basis, particularly for those injuries of greatest concern, and using those tests that are most valid and sensitive to change. For example, in sports where groin injuries are of concern, or in an athlete with a recent history of groin injuries, a simple adductor squeeze test can be performed prior to training. It is known that a fall-off in adductor muscle strength precedes a groin injury, and so this test can form part of a quick daily or weekly screen.[22] Other examples may be an assessment of shoulder rotation strength using a handheld dynamometer as an indicator of shoulder function,[23] or a slump test to assess changes in neurodynamics. Fluctuations in these parameters can provide the performance professional with a clear indication of how the athlete is coping with training and competition load. Should there be a dramatic decline in these indices it can provide them with an evidence-based incentive to change programmes prior to an overuse injury occurring.

## Summary

Musculoskeletal injury screening can be a very useful tool in the worthwhile endeavour to reduce injury burden in sport. We have presented a step-by-step framework for the development of an intelligence-led risk assessment tool. It is aimed at examining for the presence of the factors that should be of most concern to the performance professional. It does not, however, seek to be the definitive assessment tool for every injury. It is primarily a method of highlighting the areas of risk that require further attention paid to them. This method of filtering through the vast array of injuries that *could* occur to focus on the injuries that the athlete is most susceptible to will help inform effective management with the ultimate aim of injury risk reduction.

### Case study

Eighteen-year-old female football (soccer) player in an elite development programme. Nil relevant medical history but a past injury history of a left anterior shoulder dislocation four months ago that resulted in three-month absence from competition following a period of conservative management.

### Step 1: Generic warning index (GWI)

We have appraised the literature surrounding women's football. It has revealed the four injuries responsible for most time lost in the sport, which, along with concussion, forms the basis of our generic warning index.

| Area to target | Based upon |
|---|---|
| Knee injury | Knee ligament ruptures are responsible for most training time lost of any injury in female football[24] |
| Lateral ankle sprain | Ankle sprains are the injury of highest incidence in female football[24] |
| Hamstring injury | Hamstring strains being the second-most prevalent injury in elite female football and the most common muscle strain[25] |
| Adductor-related groin pain | Groin muscle strains are the second most common muscular injuries seen in female football[26] |
| Neurocognition deficits | Aiming to set a baseline for neurocognitive competency in the event of a concussive event throughout the season |

## Step 2: Specific warning index (SWI)

Based upon our knowledge of the individual athlete's non-modifiable risk factors, we have been able to generate our specific warning index. For completeness, we have included ACL injury risk, despite the fact that it is found in the GWI.

| Area to target | Based upon |
| --- | --- |
| Shoulder stability | Previous history of a shoulder dislocation. Very high recurrence rates (89%) have been demonstrated in individuals who sustained a traumatic anterior shoulder dislocation aged 30 or less[27] |
| Anterior cruciate ligament (ACL) | Increased risk of ACLI in female football players compared to their male counterparts[1] |

## Step 3: Selection of valid and reliable tests

These tests have been chosen as the most valid and reliable indicators of the risk factors identified for the injuries in the GWI and SWI.

| Area of interest | Test selected | Based upon |
| --- | --- | --- |
| Ankle | Knee-to-wall measurement of ankle dorsiflexion (DF) range of motion | Ankle DF ROM is a strong predictor of ankle sprain[28] |
| | Star excursion balance test | This test has been shown to be sensitive in detecting those with chronic ankle instability[29] |
| Knee | Isokinetic profile of hamstring strength at 300°/sec | Female athletes who have suffered an ACLI demonstrate hamstring weakness on isokinetic testing[30] |
| | Drop vertical jump | A valid and reliable method of assessing lower-limb biomechanics in female football (soccer) players. It has also been shown to be a predictor of ACL injury risk in female athletes[31] |
| Hamstrings | Isokinetic profile of eccentric hamstring strength | Shown to be positively correlated with hamstring muscle strains[32] |
| Adductors | Supine goniometric assessment of hip internal rotation (hip and knee positioned at 90°) | Shown to be a valid indicator of hip ROM, and reductions in internal rotation ROM has been demonstrated to be a powerful predictor of adductor injury risk[22] |
| | Adductor squeeze test | Found to be able to discriminate between athletes with and without groin pain[33] |
| | Active straight leg raise test | Shown to have diagnostic value when assessing adductor-related groin pain[34] |

*(Continued)*

| Area of interest | Test selected | Based upon |
|---|---|---|
| Anterior shoulder stability | Shoulder apprehension and relocation test | Highly specific and sensitive test of anterior shoulder instability[35] |
| Neurocognitive testing | Computerised neurocognitive or digit-symbol substitution test | Shown to be a valid and reliable measure of higher-order cognitive functioning following a concussive event[20] |

## Step 4: Assessment of movement proficiency

These tests have been selected to give an insight into motor control and kinematic competency in football-relevant tasks.

| Test selected | Rationale |
|---|---|
| Landing technique in vertical drop jump | To quantify amount of hip and knee extension and knee valgus, all of which have been shown to be key factors in ACL injuries[31] |
| Analysis of 45° and 90° cutting technique | To quantify the amount of femoral internal rotation and adduction when cutting, factors implicated in ACL injury risk in female soccer players[1] |
| Overhead squat technique | To examine dynamic lumbar spine control and technique in a functional training task |

Once this point is arrived at, we have developed a screening tool that is both sport-relevant and individualised to the specific athlete in question. Depending on the results of these tests, we then have an intelligence-led list of areas requiring in-depth assessment and management.

## Notes

1 Alentorn-Geli, E., Myer, G. D., Silvers, H. J., Samitier, G., Romero, D., Lázaro-Haro, C., & Cugat, R. (2009). Prevention of non-contact anterior cruciate ligament injuries in soccer players. Part 1: Mechanisms of injury and underlying risk factors. *Knee Surgery Sports and Traumatology Arthroscopy Journal*, 17(7), 705–29.
2 Majewski, M., Susanne, H., & Klaus, S. (2009). Epidemiology of athletic knee injuries: A 10-year study. *Knee*, 13(3), 184–88.
3 Hägglund, M., Waldén, M., & Ekstrand, J. (2008). Injuries among male and female elite football players. *Scandinavian Journal of Medicine & Science in Sports*, 19(6), 819–27.
4 Frisch, A., Seil, R., Urhausen, A., Croisier, J. L., Lair, M. L., & Theisen, D. (2009). Analysis of sex-specific injury patterns and risk factors in young high-level athletes. *Scandinavian Journal of Medicine & Science in Sports*, 19(6), 834–41.
5 Gabbett, T. (2003). Incidence of injury in semi-professional rugby league players. *British Journal of Sports Medicine*, 37, 36–44.

6 Foreman, T., Addy, T., Baker, S., Burns, J., Hill, N., & Madden, T. (2006). Prospective studies into the causation of hamstring injuries in sport: A systematic review. *Physical Therapy in Sport*, *7*(2), 101–09.

7 Sundaram, A., Bokor, D. J., & Davidson, A. S. (2011). Rugby Union on-field position and its relationship to shoulder injury leading to anterior reconstruction for instability. *Journal of Science and Medicine in Sport*, *14*, 111–14.

8 Kaplan, L. D., Flanigan, D. C., Norwig, J., Jost, P. & Bradley, J. (2005). Prevalence and variance of shoulder injuries in elite collegiate football players. *British Journal of Sports Medicine*, *33*, 1142–46.

9 Wilson, F., Gissane, C., Gormley, J. & Simms, C. (2010). A 12-month prospective cohort study of injury in international rowers. *British Journal of Sports Medicine*, *44*, 207–14.

10 Ryan, J., DeBurca, N., & McCreesh, K. (2014). Risk factors for groin/hip injuries in field-based sports: a systematic review. *British Journal of Sports Medicine*, *48*, 1089–96.

11 Beynnon, B. D., Murphy, D. F., & Alosa, D. M. (2002). Predictive factors for lateral ankle sprains: A literature review. *Journal of Athletic Training*, *37*, 376–80.

12 Agel, J., Dompier, T., Dick, R., & Marshall, S. (2007). Descriptive epidemiology of collegiate men's ice hockey injuries: National Collegiate Athletic Association injury surveillance system, 1988–1989 through 2003–2004. *Journal of Athletic Training*, *42*(2), 241–48.

13 Zazulak, B. T., Hewett, T. E., Reeves, N. P., Goldberg, B., & Cholewicki, J. (2007). Deficits in neuromuscular control of the trunk predict knee injury risk: A prospective biomechanical-epidemiologic study. *American Journal of Sports Medicine*, *35*(7), 1123–30.

14 Yu, B., & Garrett, W. E. (2007). Mechanisms of non-contact ACL injuries. *British Journal of Sports Medicine*, *41*, 47–51.

15 Verrall, G. M., Slavotinek, J. P., Barnes, P. G., Esterman, A., Oakeshott, R. D. & Spriggins, A. J. (2007). Hip joint range of motion restriction precedes athletic chronic groin injury. *Journal of Science and Medicine in Sport*, *10*, 463–66.

16 Opar, D. A., Williams, M. D., Timmins, R. G., Hickey, J., Duhig, S. J. & Shield, A. J. (2015). Eccentric hamstring strength and hamstring injury risk in Australian footballers. *Medicine and Science in Sport and Exercise*, *67*, 857–65.

17 Ranson, C., Burnett, A., O'Sullivan, P., Batt, M. & Kerslake, R. (2008). The lumbar paraspinal muscle morphometry of fast bowlers in cricket. *Clinical Journal of Sports Medicine*, *18*, 31–7.

18 Gabbett, T. J. & Domrow, N. (2005). Risk factors in subelite rugby league players. *American Journal of Sports Medicine*, *33*, 428–34.

19 Peterson, A., & Bernhardt, D. (2011). The preparticipation sports evaluation. *Paediatric Respiratory Reviews*, *32*(5), 53–7.

20 McCrory, P., Meeuwisse, W. H., Aubrey, M., Cantu, B., Dvo-ák, J., Echemendia, R. J., . . . Turner, M. (2014). Consensus statement on concussion in sport: the 4th International Conference on Concussion in Sport held in Zurich, November 2012. *British Journal of Sports Medicine*, *47*, 250–58.

21 Verrall, G., Slavotinek, G., Barnes, P., Fon, G., & Spriggins, A. (2001). Clinical risk factors for hamstring muscle strain injury: a prospective study with correlation of injury by magnetic resonance imaging. *British Journal of Sports Medicine*, *35*(6), 435–39.

22 Verrall, G. M., Slavotinek, J. P., Barnes, P. G., Esterman, A., Oakeshott, R. D., Spriggins, A. J. (2007). Hip joint range of motion restriction precedes athletic chronic groin injury. *Journal of Science and Medicine in Sport*, *10*, 463–66.

23 Stickley, C. D., Hetzler, R. K., Freenyer, B. G., & Kimura, I. F. (2008). Isokinetic peak torque ratios and shoulder injury history in adolescent female volleyball athletes. *Journal of Athletic Training*, *43*(6), 571–77.

24 Faude, O., Junge, A., Kindermann, W., & Dvorak, J. (2006). Risk factors for injuries in elite female soccer players. *British Journal of Sports Medicine*, *40*, 785–90.

25 Jacobson, I., & Tegner, Y. (2007). Injuries among Swedish female elite football players: a prospective population study. *Scandinavian Journal of Medicine & Science in Sports*, *17*(1), 84–91.

26 Tegnander, A., Olsen, O. E., Moholdt, T., Engebretsen, L., & Bahr, R. (2008). Injuries in Norwegian female elite soccer: a prospective one-season cohort study. *Knee Surgery Sports and Traumatology Arthroscopy Journal, 16*(2), 194–98.

27 Lill, H., Korner, J., Hepp, P., Verheyden, P., & Josten, C. (2001). Age-dependent prognosis following conservative treatment of traumatic shoulder dislocation. *European Journal of Trauma, 27*(1), 29–33.

28 Wright, C. J., Arnold, B. L., Ross, S. E., Ketchum, J., Ericksen, J., & Pidcoe, P. (2013). Clinical examination results in individuals with functional ankle instability and ankle-sprain copers. *Journal of Athletic Training, 48*(5), 581–9.

29 Gribble, P. A., Hertel, J., & Plisky, P. (2012). Using the star excursion balance test to assess dynamic postural-control deficits and outcomes in lower extremity injury: A literature and systematic review. *Journal of Athletic Training, 47*(3), 339–57.

30 Myer, G. D., Ford, K. R., Barber Foss, K. D., Liu, C., Nick, T. G., & Hewett, T. E. (2009). The relationship of hamstrings and quadriceps strength to anterior cruciate ligament injury in female athletes. *Clinical Journal of Sports Medicine, 19*(1), 3–8.

31 Hewett, T., Myer, G. D., Ford, K. R., Heidt, R. S., Jr., Colosimo, A. J., McLean, S. G., . . . Paterno M. V. (2005). Biomechanical measures of neuromuscular control and valgus loading of the knee predict anterior cruciate ligament injury risk in female athletes: A prospective study. *American Journal of Sports Medicine, 33*, 492–501.

32 Fousekis, K., Tsepis, E., Poulmedis, P., Athanasopoulos, S., & Vagenas, G. (2011). Intrinsic risk factors of non-contact quadriceps and hamstring strains in soccer: a prospective study of 100 professional players. *British Journal of Sports Medicine, 45*, 709–14.

33 Malliaras, P., Hogan, A., Nawrocki, A., Crossley, K., & Schache, A. (2009). Hip flexibility and strength measures: reliability and association with athletic groin pain. *British Journal of Sports Medicine, 43*, 739–44.

34 Mens, J. M., Vleeming, A., Snijders, C. J., Koes, B. W., & Stam, J. (2002). Validity of the active straight leg raise test for measuring disease severity in patients with posterior pelvic pain after pregnancy. *Spine 27*(2), 196.

35 Lo, I. K., Nonweiler, B., Woolfrey, M., Litchfield, R., & Kirkley, A. (2004). An evaluation of the apprehension, relocation, and surprise tests for anterior shoulder instability. *American Journal of Sports Medicine, 32*(2), 301–307.

# Chapter 7

# Assessing and developing the kinetic chain

*Ian Prangley*

## Introduction

The human body continues to achieve amazing athletic feats of precision, power and speed. How does a baseball pitcher accurately throw a baseball at over 100 mph, a sprinter run 100 m in under 10 seconds or a high jumper leap well over 2 m? At the highest level, what separates the good from the great? Many of these answers can be found by exploring the concept of the human kinetic chain.

The concept of the kinetic chain originated from a German engineering scientist named Franz Reuleaux to describe how components of a system that are interlinked by pin joints can be affected by movement of just one component. In sport, the kinetic chain concept is often used when describing athletic movements, such as throwing, running and jumping. In theory, throwing darts involves a kinetic chain, although it would be rare to hear this term used in this context. The kinetic chain becomes of more interest in sports that involve powerful and/or repetitive propulsion, either of the distal segment (a fist in boxing), an external object (throwing a baseball) or of one's own body (sprinting or jumping).

In this chapter we will uncover how the kinetic chain contributes to performance and relates to injury. With regards to performance, the summation of forces and movement efficiency will be presented as two primary outcomes of an effective kinetic chain. Furthermore, distribution of load over multiple joints has implications for injury prevention and will be discussed extensively. Ultimately, those working directly with athletes need to be able to appropriately assess and develop the kinetic chain, and therefore a significant section of this chapter is devoted to this. Before delving into this, a brief introduction of the types of kinetic chain movements are presented and discussed below.

## Types and variations of the athletic kinetic chain

There are two types of kinetic chain movement patterns: push-like movement patterns and throw-like movement patterns. Push-like patterns are more often used when shifting heavy objects, such as a rugby union scrum, or where the distal segment is pushing against a heavy resistance, such as when cycling. Throw-like patterns are used for developing high movement speed, which is often transferred to an external object, such as pitching a baseball or kicking a football. In throw-like patterns, proximal segments of the body accelerate the distal segments, and finally contribute to the velocity of the object being thrown. This has also been referred to as the 'whip-like effect' and the 'proximal-to-distal sequence'.[1] Gross athletic movements of running and swimming involve a series of kinetic chains in order to propel the body. In

*Table 7.1* Kinetic chain variations

| Load on distal segment | Mobility of distal segment | Kinetic chain type | Example |
|---|---|---|---|
| No load | Moveable | Open | Kicking a football |
| External load | Fixed | Closed | Stance phase to push off in sprinting |
| External load | Moveable | Combination | Wrestling |

all cases, the primary outcome is that there is a transfer of energy from one body segment to another, resulting in the *summation* of forces.

An alternate classification of the different kinetic chain movements, specifically closed and open chains, is also very commonly employed. The term 'open kinetic chain' refers to when the distal segment is free to move, while the 'closed kinetic chain' refers to when the distal segment is fixed, and force is produced against the fixed object in order to move the proximal segments and therefore the body. However, these terminologies become confusing, particularly when complex movements involve a combination of closed and open kinetic chains.

By considering variables of load and mobility of the distal segment, a more complete classification of kinetic chains is available. A summary of this classification with comparison to open and closed kinetic chains is presented in Table 7.1.

Under this classification system, human movement is a product of open, closed or combination kinetic chains working either in isolation or simultaneously. A seemingly simple activity such as running involves both open and closed kinetic chains. The stance leg is a closed kinetic chain resulting in propulsion, while the swing leg is an open kinetic chain movement.[2] Similarly, passing a rugby ball while running involves an additional open kinetic chain in order to propel the ball.

## The effective and ineffective kinetic chain and performance

Top-level athletes provide the best examples of the human kinetic chain working effectively. The ability to produce repetitive, powerful and energy-efficient movement is almost a prerequisite for success at the highest level in sport. Efficiency is the ratio of energy output to input, and is therefore improved when the energy output increases relative to the input.[3] The concept of kinetic chain power and efficiency applies to sports requiring power and speed, as well as endurance-based activities.

Power-based sports demand an effective kinetic chain in order to transfer muscle energy into a powerful movement. Think of the stock whip, which, when used correctly, results in immense speed of the tip due to transfer of energy from the arm and down the length of the whip. This is why world-class coaches and athletes spend considerable time refining technique in order to improve intermuscular coordination and optimise elastic energy storage and release through the kinetic chain.

While movement technique is key to kinetic chain performance, equally important is the need for well-developed basic physical attributes, such as balance, stability and strength. For example a stable trunk is required for elite sprinting performance, and strong periscapular muscles are important to provide a base for energy to be transferred effectively during a boxer's punch. When a significant 'energy leak' is present, the movement speed is compromised, and for the athlete to increase their power and speed, other muscles must be recruited to a greater extent in order to make up for the energy leak in the system.

In endurance sports, conservation of energy through efficient movement is critical to success. Leaks in the kinetic chain can be highly detrimental, as the musculature must work harder to make up for the lost energy, accelerating fatigue and compromising performance. An example of this is a long-distance runner with weak lateral stabilisers of the hip. During the stance phase, energy is lost through this weak link in the chain, resulting in reduced running efficiency. Therefore this runner needs to expend greater energy in order to maintain the same running speed of a highly efficient runner.

Psychology and tactics aside, when performing a desired movement, individuals who are able to effectively transfer energy through the kinetic chain, with minimal leaks or wasted energy, are the most likely to succeed. Coaches, trainers and physiotherapists who are experts in a particular sport are able to visually assess this to a high level, and it is generally discussed in terms of technical proficiency. Methods to assess the kinetic chain will be discussed in greater detail later in this section.

---

An efficient kinetic chain is key to performance.

Roger Federer's ability to produce almost 'effortless' movement and stroke power is well regarded amongst tennis professionals. This is a reflection of his ability to use his kinetic chain effectively to produce power with minimal wasted energy in both stroke production and movement around the court. By producing power without unnecessary energy loss, he has a significant advantage when playing less technically proficient opponents during matches, where fatigue could be the determining factor in the result. Furthermore, considering that in Grand Slam tournaments players are required to win seven matches in two weeks in order to win the tournament, conservation of energy becomes all the more important, to maximise recovery prior to the next match.

---

## The effective and ineffective kinetic chain and injury

The kinetic chain has an extremely important association with injury susceptibility, and the study of biomechanics has been used extensively to identify movement faults that result in injury. Inefficient movement mechanics lead to injury in the following ways:

### Accelerated muscle fatigue

As previously discussed, energy leaks in the kinetic chain can lead to accelerated muscle fatigue. Amongst other effects, fatigue has been shown to reduce proprioceptive sense in shoulders,[4,5,6] alter scapulothoracic and glenohumeral motion,[7] increase tibial translation in healthy knees,[8] reduce postural control[9] and change impact loading characteristics when running.[10] Fatigue, therefore, features as a significant injury risk factor in endurance-based, repeat-effort sports, which is why optimising the kinetic chain is so important.

## Excess stress on links (joints) in the chain

Dysfunctional movement mechanics can increase stress on joints and soft tissues of the kinetic chain. In particular, poor utilisation of proximal segments to generate or transfer energy can place greater stress on distal segments. For example, elbow pathologies in tennis are often the result of technical problems on the serve, particularly a lack of an effective leg drive and a 'falling away' from the ball, resulting in the elbow joint taking on greater valgus forces. In the same manner, baseball research has shown correct pitching biomechanics reduces elbow valgus load and improves pitching efficiency.[11] It is therefore of no surprise that optimising the throwing kinetic chain is vital in the rehabilitation of shoulder and elbow injuries. In the lower body, excessive rear foot eversion and hip adduction has been shown to be a risk factor in people with patellofemoral joint pain,[12] demonstrating how movement aberrations at proximal and distal linkages can produce abnormal forces and stresses on a joint.

Whilst the kinetic chain is often discussed in relation to producing movement, the concept can also be extended to explain how the body can absorb forces during movement deceleration, such as landing from a jump. Deceleration of the body and the eccentric muscle action can place excessive forces on tendons, making the athlete susceptible to the development of tendinopathies. Optimising the use of the kinetic chain to absorb forces across multiple linkages will reduce the potential for overload. Stiff landing strategies and altered hip sequencing upon landing have been shown to be more present in athletes with patella tendinopathy.[13,14] In this situation the kinetic chain is not used effectively to decelerate the body in such a manner that forces are spread across anatomical structures. Instead, the patterning results in overload of the quadriceps/patella tendon and increases injury susceptibility. This is discussed in greater detail in chapter 16.

Clearly, then, optimising the human kinetic chain is an important component in injury prevention and rehabilitation. The following sections outline the means by which the kinetic chain can be assessed and developed.

---

An efficient kinetic chain is key to preventing injury: Continuing from the previous example regarding Roger Federer and his extremely efficient movement mechanics, it is unsurprising that he has completed a career almost entirely injury-free. So far in his career, he has not missed any of the four grand slam events in any year since he began competing in them in 1999.[15]

---

## Assessing the kinetic chain

We have established the relationship between biomechanics, performance and injury. It is therefore intuitive that the ability to assess the kinetic chain becomes very important for the coach, trainer or physiotherapist in order to improve performance or reduce the risk of injury/re-injury. Assessing the kinetic chain should include a three-pronged approach involving field-based performance testing, movement analysis and musculoskeletal screening.

## Performance measures

As a starting point, we can use simple performance tests as a means of assessing the output of the kinetic chain. It is important that the tests replicate the key movements of the sport. While these tests will be influenced by factors such as gross muscle power, a significant reduction in performance relative to previous performance measures and current power profile may indicate a dysfunction within the kinetic chain. Table 7.2 describes some common tests of kinetic chain performance.

While undertaking these tests is most commonly done when the athlete is fresh, it is also worth considering conducting them when the athlete is fatigued. In sports that require repetition of the same movements over a prolonged period, neuromuscular

*Table 7.2* Tests of the kinetic chain

| Field test | Aspects of kinetic chain analysed | Example of kinetic chain breakdown | Related sports |
|---|---|---|---|
| Medicine ball sidearm throw distance | Transfer of energy from ground – leg drive – trunk rotation – throw | Insufficient leg and hip drive, reducing power of the throw | Sports requiring rotational throwing power, such as tennis (groundstrokes), judo, rugby |
| Overarm throw distance | Transfer of energy from ground – leg drive – trunk extension/flexion – throw | Poor spine extension resulting in reduced distance over which the ball can be accelerated during the throw | Overhead throwing sports, such as cricket, baseball, softball, javelin, badminton |
| 20 m sprint time | Transfer of energy from ground – foot/ankle – knee extension – hip extension – trunk – forward propulsion | Poor core and pelvic stability – insufficient transfer of energy to forward propulsion | Sports requiring maximal acceleration (soccer, hockey, bob skeleton, baseball) |
| 50 m kickboard time | Transfer of energy from trunk – hips – feet/ankles – forward propulsion and lift | Reduced ankle plantarflexion range to maximise propulsion and lift | Swimming |
| Kicking distance | Transfer of energy from trunk – hip flexion – knee extension – ball | Poor stance leg stability, reduced hip extension, reduction in the summation forces that contribute to foot contact speed | Soccer, rugby, American football |
| Single leg hop for distance | Transfer of energy from ground – foot/ankle plantarflexion – knee extension – hip extension – forward & upward propulsion | Poor hip stability and hip extension reducing transfer of energy. Reduced distance achieved compared to other side may be indicative of this | Power-based sports, such as sprinting and long jump |

fatigue can have detrimental effects on the kinetic chain. By comparing performance in these tests while under fatigue as well as fresh, the decay in kinetic chain competency can be assessed.

## Biomechanical analysis

Whilst the undertaking of regular biomechanical analysis would be wonderful, we know that in practice this is often not feasible. In the immediate coaching environment, video motion analysis tools can be utilised frequently and contain features to analyse movements and trajectories, calculate speeds and demonstrate key techniques and positions. This type of technology is invaluable to the coach when assessing athletic kinetic chain performance. Furthermore, continued technological advancement is making this process less time-consuming to perform, particularly with the trend towards the use of mobile devices and smartphones to perform the video analysis with several free apps now available to download. As the field of biomechanics is very broad, we will not discuss it any further, and we will assume that the benefits of biomechanical analysis in the context of the kinetic chain is well appreciated.

## Musculoskeletal screening

Elements such as muscle strength, control, flexibility and joint range of motion may positively or negatively impact on the kinetic chain and therefore need to be assessed. Musculoskeletal screening is a means for doing this and is a valued component of athletic preparation in almost every sport. This is discussed in greater detail in chapter 6.

Movement-based screening tools that examine movement quality provide a good starting point for assessing the kinetic chain, as it is reasonable to assume that, if the athlete is unable to maintain appropriate alignment and joint positioning in a controlled and slow manner, then this will be accentuated during high-velocity movements, resulting in poor biomechanics, reduced power production and energy leaks through the kinetic chain.

Beyond these movement screens, more focused assessment of joint ranges and individual muscle strengths should follow, to more accurately identify specific deficiencies that have potentially detrimental consequences for athletic movement mechanics. For example, in baseball, a difference in passive hip range has been associated with various pitching biomechanical parameters of the hips and pelvis.[16] Table 3 outlines some examples of common musculoskeletal findings and their impact on biomechanics and injury.

The musculoskeletal screening process forms an integral part of assessing the function of the kinetic chain and highlights specific deficiencies that need to be addressed in order to improve kinetic chain performance and reduce injury risk.

While undertaking performance measures and biomechanical analysis are accepted assessments that can help determine performance success, often less well appreciated is the value of musculoskeletal screenings. Screenings can identify issues that may place an athlete at risk of injury, but equally, they may also help determine athletic performance. Therefore, it is very important that the practitioner has an excellent understanding of the demands of the sport the athlete participates in, and can relay the information back to the coaches from both an injury-prevention and performance perspective.

*Table 7.3* Common screening findings and relationship to injury

| Screening finding | Impact on the kinetic chain and injury implications |
| --- | --- |
| Reduced ankle dorsiflexion | • Increased risk of patellar tendon injury due to reduced absorption of load[17]<br>• Reduced knee flexion displacement due to reduced dorsiflexion displacement at the ankle, resulting in greater ground reaction forces. Implied increased risk of ACL injury[18]<br>• Reduced dorsiflexion displacement causing decreased quadriceps activation, increased medial knee deviation and knee valgus. Implied increased risk of developing patellofemoral joint pain[19] |
| Proximal hip weakness (especially hip abductors) | • Increased knee valgus on single squatting and landing. This has implications for development of patellofemoral joint pathology, ACL tears and ITB syndrome[20] |
| Scapular dyskinesis | • Altered glenoid positioning and mechanics possibly increasing risk of developing rotator cuff impingement and labral pathology[21] |

## Developing the kinetic chain

Once deficiencies in the kinetic chain are identified, the next step is to design interventions to correct the faulty mechanics. The interventions selected will depend on the sport, the individual athlete needs and the situation (i.e. competition, training or rehabilitation phase). The coach, strength and conditioning coach and physiotherapist should all contribute during this stage.

Quite often, the intervention is left to the coach, as deficiencies in the kinetic chain are likened to specific technical issues, which is considered the coach's expertise. However, strength and conditioning coaches can have a significant impact on the development of the kinetic chain by utilising full body, multi-segment exercises in athlete preparation programs. In a similar manner, physiotherapists can contribute significantly, particularly where musculoskeletal deficiencies are impacting on movement mechanics. Furthermore, during late stage rehabilitation, programs integrating whole body exercises that utilise the kinetic chain are important as steps towards returning to full training and competition. It should go without saying that a strength base is critical to the success of any programme looking at integrated kinetic chain enhancement, and so we will not discuss this rationale any further. Instead, the following sections will look at different means by which the kinetic chain can be developed.

## Training movements, not muscles, and sport-specific training

There has been a recent shift in philosophy amongst many strength and conditioning coaches to 'train movements, not muscles', as part of the functional training approach. Established coaches are less likely to prescribe strength and power exercises that target only one muscle group, such as the quadriceps on the knee extension machine. This is not to say that these exercises are ineffective, as they may be critical during such times as early stage knee rehabilitation. However, they are far less effective for developing the kinetic chain.

Whilst specificity of training is desirable, it is important to recognise that some sport-specific interventions may actually be detrimental, and therefore care needs to be taken by the coach when prescribing these types of exercises. Intuitively, we would not ask a golfer to train with a particularly heavy club in order to improve club head speed, nor a sprinter to train in mud. The reasoning behind this is that the exercise with its subtle biomechanical variations may negatively impact on the athlete's technique and therefore be counterproductive. Excessively loaded sled pulls are a good example. Many sprint coaches employ this drill due to its highly specific nature. However, the concern with this exercise is that too much resistance may disrupt sprint mechanics, with suggestions that a low load of 12.6 per cent of body weight is best used to minimise change in sprint kinematics.[22]

Whilst this may be true particularly for maximal velocity training, very recent research has demonstrated that acceleration over 5 m is better trained with higher loads of 30 per cent of body weight.[23] This finding is not unexpected, as the large power output required during initial acceleration phases may be better developed with high load training.

The key point is that when choosing sport-specific drills, it is important that the coach is confident that the drill will improve and not impair performance of the kinetic chain movement. If this is doubtful, then it may be better to prescribe exercises of a less specific nature that still target kinetic chain function. Weightlifting is one such training modality and is discussed in the following section.

## Weightlifting to improve the kinetic chain

One highly effective method to develop power in the kinetic chain is through the use of weightlifting, which is commonly, but incorrectly, referred to as Olympic lifting. Weightlifting includes the snatch and clean and jerk, as well as their training derivatives.

The defining difference between weightlifting and other methods of strength training is that they are performed in an explosive, high-speed manner and deceleration at the end of the lift does not occur. During the traditional back squat, deceleration must occur at the top of the squat. In comparison, the clean involves deceleration only during the catch phase, and the acceleration phase engages the calf muscles such that the feet may leave the ground, even under high load. Triple extension of the hips, knees and ankles, a critical requirement for lower-body power and propulsion, is a key feature of weightlifting and is therefore an excellent means of training the lower-body kinetic chain. To support the theory, practical research has demonstrated that a ballistic lifting program that includes weightlifting is superior to a traditional resistance training program for inducing gains in vertical jump height.[24,25]

One of the downfalls of weightlifting is that the lifts are difficult to learn and require considerable practice and feedback. Additionally, it is considered by many that weightlifting places the athlete at risk of injury, particularly if undertaken with poor technique.[26] However, with correct technique and supervision, weightlifting is considered a safe training modality.[27,28]

## Plyometric training to improve the kinetic chain

In the elite athlete with a well-developed strength base, plyometric training is an excellent means to improve kinetic chain functioning. As well as stimulating favourable muscle adaptations, these exercises aim to optimise the use of elastic properties of tendons for the storage and recoil of energy. This can help to improve the transfer of energy through the kinetic chain, leading to higher power output and efficiency. Even in well-trained endurance runners, a period of plyometric training can improve efficiency and reduce the energy cost of running.[29]

## Training the core to improve the kinetic chain

The musculature around the trunk and pelvis, commonly referred to as the core, plays a vital role in the generation and transfer of energy in the kinetic chain. Poor active stability in this region impairs the ability of the pelvic girdle to transfer loads between the trunk and legs. When sprinting, 'stiffening' of the core is essential to transfer energy from the hips for propulsion and to avoid 'energy leaks'.[30] Furthermore, its combined stabilising/moving functions are key to transferring energy from the legs to the upper limb during throwing actions. Deficiencies in strength or timing of core musculature can result in unwanted movement through the trunk and a reduction in performance.

The ability for the core to effectively transfer load can be assessed through a variety of tests. For example the active straight leg raise (ASLR) is a reliable test to check the quality of load transfer from the trunk to leg.[31] Whilst we feel that this is a very helpful test in the athletic population and is particularly useful in individuals with a history of low back, pelvic and sacroiliac joint (SIJ) dysfunction, most research into its use has been on post-partum women and therefore care must be taken when applying these same results to elite athletes.

The hip and pelvis is another very common area where energy may be lost through the kinetic chain. The lateral stabilisers of the hip – in particular gluteus medius – are a common area of weakness in athletic populations. Most athletic movements involve propulsion or stabilisation through one leg, such as the stance phase during sprinting, the stance leg during a kick in taekwondo or a high jumper's leap, and therefore large forces must be transferred effectively. To assess the integrity and function of the lateral stabilisers, observation of posture and muscle size, as well as functional movement and strength testing, is recommended.[32] In athletes, assessment of the single leg squat and hop is effective at assessing any strength deficiencies of the gluteal muscles that may be a source of energy leaks. Medial deviation of the knee, hip adduction and dropping or hitching of the pelvis on one side are indicative of weaknesses.

## Flexibility training to improve the kinetic chain

Both joint range of motion and muscle length will have an impact on athletic movement and must be considered in the development and optimisation of the kinetic chain. The degree of flexibility needed will largely depend upon the movement demands of a sport. Some sports demand greater flexibility in particular body regions and muscles, and less in others. For example a swimmer will require large range of motion through the shoulders and thoracic spine, whilst an ankle dorsiflexion limitation may be of less concern. Therefore, once the demands of a sport are well understood, it is then a process of screening the athlete to identify where deficiencies are, and implementing a programme to improve these areas. Of course, not all inflexibilities are easily rectified, particularly structural limitations, such as a fixed block in the hip that limits its ability to internally rotate. In these cases, it is important that this information is conveyed to coaches so they understand that the impact of these inflexibilities on the kinetic chain cannot be rectified. The topic of flexibility is covered in more depth in chapter 13.

## Technical correction to improve the kinetic chain

Through technical correction, coaches often attempt to 'fine-tune' an athlete's kinetic chain segments and thus propulsion of an object, limbs or the body. To demonstrate, consider the tennis athlete who is failing to achieve the cocking position early enough on the serve. This is commonly referred to as the 'trophy' position, and when obtained at or prior to leg drive, results in the arm being driven back into external rotation, as the leg drives the body upwards to the ball (see Figure 7.1). The leg drive therefore contributes significantly to the elastic recoil of the throwing arm (see Figure 7.2). However, if the athlete fails to get the arm in the trophy position, regardless of how powerful the leg drive is, it will not contribute as significantly

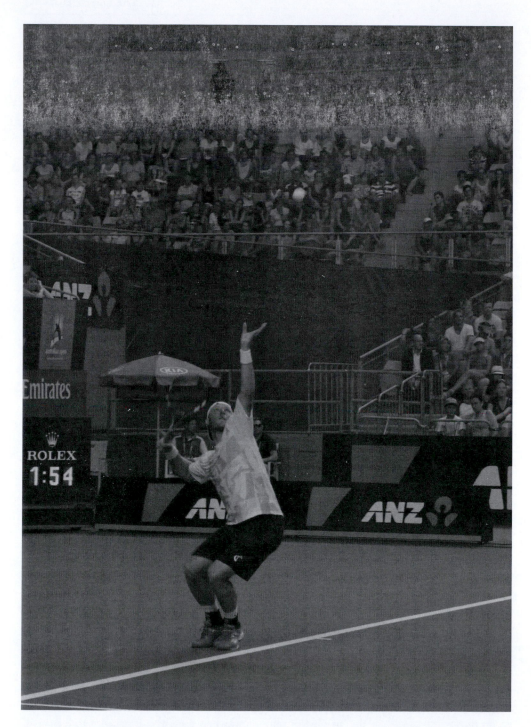

*Figure 7.1* Samuel Groth, who recorded the fastest ever tennis serve in May 2012, in the cocking or 'trophy' position of the service action

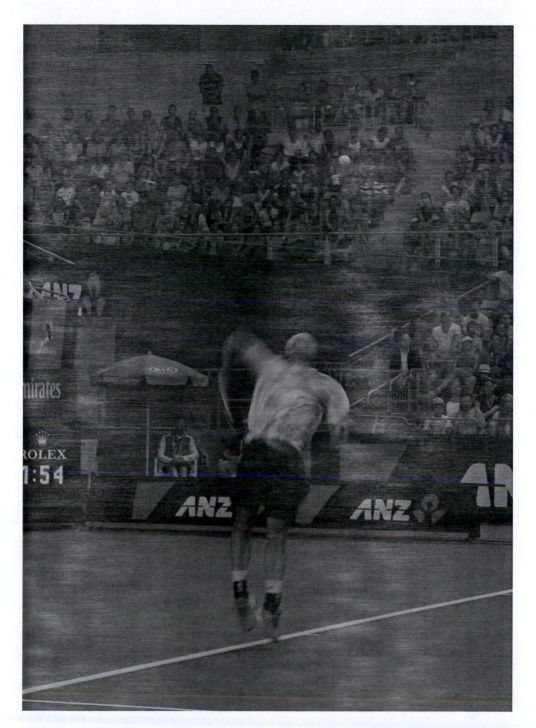

*Figure 7.2* The leg drive has helped to drive the throwing arm into external rotation therefore assisting the elastic recoil during the serve

Courtesy of Tennis Australia

to the throwing action. Energy is not transferred optimally through the kinetic chain and therefore requires technical intervention. The coach may address this by having the athlete alter the take-back speed or path in order to find the appropriate position just prior to the initiation of leg drive.

Technical correction should typically be undertaken with the assistance of video analysis tools that are widely available on the Web or as mobile device applications. They allow the coach to accurately determine the technical issue that is affecting the kinetic chain. Furthermore, ongoing assessment and feedback is possible to assist the coach and athlete during the process of change.

> There are many coaching interventions that can lead to an improvement in kinetic chain function. The assessment of each athlete, combined with an understanding of the demands of their sport, position or style of play is critical to ascertaining which intervention/s will prove to be most effective. This can only be achieved through a co-ordinated approach of the coach, strength and conditioning coach, physiotherapist and the athlete.

## Asymmetries and imbalances

It is the natural response of the human body to adapt to athletic demands by increasing mass, developing strength or altering flexibility of soft tissues placed under stress. Due to this, athletes may develop asymmetries or imbalances of corresponding soft tissues, such as bone, muscle or tendon. For the purposes of clarity, 'asymmetries' refers to side-to-side differences in strength, size, flexibility, range of motion or positioning of the same anatomical structure. 'Imbalance' indicates abnormalities in predetermined acceptable ratios of muscle strength or flexibility for agonist and antagonist muscles.

## Asymmetries

In the majority of cases, asymmetries are a natural and essential by-product of an athlete's training and competition demands. As an example, there are significant differences in single leg jump performance and thigh circumference in snow boarders due to the asymmetrical nature (rear versus front foot) of the activity.[33] Furthermore, with ongoing participation in asymmetrical sports, it may prove difficult to reverse or correct musculoskeletal asymmetries.

From a performance perspective, a study on Australian footballers demonstrated a reduction in kicking accuracy in those with a side-to-side asymmetry in lower limb mass.[34] It was implied that a lower lean muscle mass of the supporting leg might affect kicking accuracy due to a reduction in stability of the supporting leg when executing the kick. In this case, interventions to rectify the asymmetry are warranted. Furthermore, there are asymmetries that are a proven risk factor for injury, such as hip rotation range of motion asymmetries and low back pain in rotational sports.[35] These asymmetries may have developed due to postural or mechanical dysfunction or poor training methods, or have genetic origins, and interventions to correct these asymmetries should be implemented, or, at least, accommodated for.

However, the relationship of asymmetries to injury is not always clear. If an asymmetry is not of close proximity to the spine, or is not considered to have a bearing on the spine, then it would be unlikely to be predictive of injury. However, even asymmetries of the soft tissues of the spine have produced conflicting results as it relates to injury predictability. An example of this is the increase in mass of *quadratus lumborum* in the dominant side of cricket fast bowlers. Initially, presence of an asymmetry was shown to be associated with lumbar injury.[36] However, more recent research has been conflicting, demonstrating that those fast bowlers who remained uninjured over the course of a cricket season actually had larger asymmetries.[37] The reasons for the conflicting results may be attributed to differences in the methods and timing of data collection. Significant asymmetries of the *quadratus lumborum*, lateral abdominal wall, *iliopsoas* and gluteals are also present in the elite tennis player but not proven to be an injury risk factor.[38,39] Similarly, asymmetries in psoas major and quadratus lumborum muscle size are noted in Australian Football League (AFL) players, and do not appear to be related to the number of injuries.[40] In summary, there is potential for asymmetries of muscles attaching to the spine to cause injury, but if the asymmetry occurs naturally due to appropriate sport-specific training, then it should not be of a major concern.

### Asymmetries of the upper limb in the throwing athlete

Unilateral sports, such as racket and throwing sports, are prime examples of how the demands of the sport can lead to asymmetries. In tennis players, the dominant arm has been demonstrated to be of significantly greater volume when compared to the non-dominant arm due to muscle hypertrophy.[41] This is a natural development and the asymmetry should have no impact on injury. In fact, the increase in muscle mass of the forearm is an adaptation to the sporting demands and therefore will be more likely to be protective of injury.

One of the more heavily researched asymmetries in unilateral overhead throwing athletes is the presence of glenohumeral internal rotation deficiency (GIRD) of the throwing arm. Previously, it was accepted that the internal rotation deficit was largely due to tightening of the posterior capsule that occurs naturally due to microtrauma during the follow-through phase of the throw.[42] However, more recent research has revealed that the internal rotation deficit can be attributed to torsion of the humerus that occurs gradually over a long period of time via the repetitive forces generated during the acceleration phase of the throw.[43,44] There is still a substantial amount of research required to provide definitive answers regarding the implications of this asymmetry. However, for throwing athletes, the increase in shoulder external rotation could be deemed favourable from a performance perspective. A more in-depth discussion on this is provided in chapter 12.

Scapular positioning and function is regarded as an important component in preventing injury and rehabilitating the injured shoulder. In a clinical setting, the dominant scapula is typically assessed with reference to the non-dominant side or the clinician's opinion on the 'ideal' position and function. In volleyballers, tennis players and baseball pitchers, the dominant scapula has been shown to rest in greater anterior tilt and internal rotation and may be considered as a normal 'adaptation'.[45] Although research has demonstrated differences in scapula function between injured and non-injured shoulders, there has yet to be convincing evidence of scapula dysfunction as a cause of injury.[46] This adds some weight to the argument that subtle differences in positioning and function are a normal adaptation to the demands of the sport.

In summary, side-to-side asymmetries are a natural and potentially favourable adaptation to athletic demands and, for the most part, have little impact on injury risk. It is up to the clinician to determine whether an asymmetry is of concern and warrants addressing, or if indeed it can be addressed while the athlete continues to participate in the sport. Factors such as the nature of the sport, injury history and extent of the asymmetry, as well as research or anecdotal supporting evidence, should all be considered when making this decision.

## Imbalances

Asymmetries of the same anatomical structure are easy to define. Imbalances, on the other hand, are more difficult to identify, as they require an 'acceptable' agonist/antagonist ratio to be determined. Additionally, there is still much argument regarding the predictive nature of imbalances, and whether they are, in fact, just normal adaptations to sporting demands.

A reduction in strength of the hip adductors relative to abductors is suggested to be a predictor of adductor muscle strains in ice hockey players.[47] In soccer players, this same reduction is also present in those with groin pain, and rehabilitation should be directed at restoring an ideal adduction to abduction ratio of 1.05.[48] Interestingly, this 'ideal' ratio differs from the 0.95 ratio calculated in the ice hockey players, and is most likely due to the differing demands of the sport. Therefore, care should be taken when applying the results of studies to other sports, as the demands of each sport may result in small differences to strength ratios.

Reduced strength of the hamstrings relative to the quadriceps has also been proposed as a risk factor for hamstring tears. While some studies have proven that this is the case,[49,50] there is also evidence to refute this claim.[51] This ratio is also of interest as a risk factor for ACL injury. A reduction in hamstring to quadriceps strength ratio has been shown to be predictive of ACL injury in female athletes.[52]

In the throwing athlete, it is well established that the shoulder internal rotators are significantly stronger relative to the external rotators of the shoulder when compared with individuals from the general population, or the non-dominant arm.[53,54,55] It is suggested that this ratio imbalance places the throwing shoulder at risk of injury and therefore should be targeted in rehabilitation and preventative programmes. However, substantial evidence of its predictive capacity is lacking with only one study providing some proof of this in baseball players.[56] Anecdotal case studies of professional tennis players with long-standing weakness of the *infraspinatus* due to *suprascapular* nerve damage paint an interesting picture. Despite the large shift in the strength ratio favouring internal rotation strength, there does not appear to be a difference in both performance and shoulder injury susceptibility when compared with other players without *infraspinatus* strength deficits.

The implication of soft tissue imbalances and asymmetries on athletic performance and injury remains unclear. The repetitive and often highly asymmetrical movements of many sports often lends to the natural development of asymmetries and imbalances. In many cases, this is purely an adaptation to the physical demands and therefore protective of injury. However, certain imbalances and asymmetries, particularly those that have not arisen from sporting demands, may result in abnormal biomechanics or kinetic chain disruptions. In these cases, the athlete is placed at a high risk of injury. Table 7.4 demonstrates a number of known asymmetries and imbalances and their potential relationship to injury.

*Table 7.4* Asymmetries/imbalances and relationships to injury

| Asymmetry/Imbalance | Relationship to injury |
| --- | --- |
| Concentric hamstring: quadriceps strength ratio at 180 deg/sec | Reduced ratio increases risk of hamstring injury in sprinters[49] |
| Concentric hamstring: quadriceps strength ratio at 300 deg/sec | Reduced hamstring strength but not quadriceps strength relative to matched male controls increases risk of ACL injury in female soccer and basketball athletes[52] |
| Trunk flexor & extensor strength | Teenagers with LBP have stronger flexors and weaker extensors compared with controls[57] |
| Hip rotation ROM | Side-to-side asymmetry is prevalent in those with lower back pain in rotation sports[35] Reduced lead hip medial rotation compared with non-lead hip in golfers with LBP[58] |
| Shoulder internal and external rotation strength | Reduced ER:IR ratio is predictive of in-season shoulder injury in baseball pitchers[56] |

To assess whether an imbalance or asymmetry is detrimental to performance or places the athlete at risk of injury, it is important to consider the demands of the sport. Never assume that an asymmetry will necessarily lead to injury. In fact, the opposite may actually be the case. However, if the asymmetry results in altered or suboptimal functioning of the kinetic chain, and is changeable, then interventions to correct them are certainly warranted.

## Summary

The kinetic chain concept is an excellent framework for describing complex athletic movements. Using this framework allows those working in athletic development to assess the relationships of the components of muscle power, flexibility, stability, balance, intermuscular co-ordination and elastic energy to producing energy-efficient, powerful and accurate movements. Once the interactions of these components are understood and assessments have taken place, the coaching team can put together a development plan for the athlete. Refining technique, correcting detrimental imbalances, improving flexibilities of key areas and strengthening 'links' within the chain become the starting point. As these building blocks are put in place, and the athlete becomes robust, training for power through weightlifting, plyometrics and sport-specific exercises will develop the kinetic chain to the highest level.

## Notes

1  Hirashima, M., Kadota, H., Sakurai, S., Kudo, K., & Ohtsuki, T. 2002. Sequential muscle activity and its functional role in the upper extremity and trunk during overarm throwing. *Journal of Sports Sciences*, 20, 301–310.

2   Maclester, J., & Pierre, P. S. 2008. *Applied biomechanics: concepts and connections*. Retrieved from Cengage-Brain.com

3   Blazevich, A. J. 2010. *Sports biomechanics: the basics: optimising human performance*. London, UK: A & C Black.

4   Carpenter, J. E., Blasier, R. B., & Pellizzon, G. G. 1998. The effects of muscle fatigue on shoulder joint position sense. *The American Journal of Sports Medicine*, 26, 262–265.

5   Myers, J. B., Guskiewicz, K. M., Schneider, R. A., & Prentice, W. E. 1999. Proprioception and neuromuscular control of the shoulder after muscle fatigue. *Journal of Athletic Training*, 34, 362.

6   Lee, H. M., Liau, J. J., Cheng, C. K., Tan, C. M., & Shih, J. T. 2003. Evaluation of shoulder proprioception following muscle fatigue. *Clinical Biomechanics*, 18, 843–847.

7   Ebaugh, D. D., McClure, P. W., & Karduna, A. R. 2006. Effects of shoulder muscle fatigue caused by repetitive overhead activities on scapulothoracic and glenohumeral kinematics. *Journal of Electromyography and Kinesiology*, 16, 224–235.

8   Wojtys, E. M., Wylie, B. B., & Huston, L. J. 1996. The effects of muscle fatigue on neuromuscular function and anterior tibial translation in healthy knees. *The American Journal of Sports Medicine*, 24, 615–621.

9   Gribble, P. A., & Hertel, J. 2004. Effect of lower-extremity muscle fatigue on postural control. *Archives of Physical Medicine and Rehabilitation*, 85, 589–592.

10  Christina, K. A., White, S. C., & Gilchrist, L. A. 2001. Effect of localized muscle fatigue on vertical ground reaction forces and ankle joint motion during running. *Human Movement Science*, 20, 257–276.

11  Davis, J., Limpisvasti, O., Fluhme, D., Mohr, K. J., Yocum, L. A., Elattrache, N. S., & Jobe, F. W. 2009. The effect of pitching biomechanics on the upper extremity in youth and adolescent baseball pitchers. *The American Journal of Sports Medicine*, 37, 1484–1491.

12  Barton, C. J., Levinger, P., Crossley, K. M., Webster, K. E., & Menz, H. B. 2012. The relationship between rearfoot, tibial and hip kinematics in individuals with patellofemoral pain syndrome. *Clinical Biomechanics*, 27, 702–705.

13  Bisseling, R. W., Hof, A. L., Bredeweg, S. W., Zwerver, J., & Mulder, T. 2007. Relationship between landing strategy and patellar tendinopathy in volleyball. *British Journal of Sports Medicine*, 41, e8.

14  Edwards, S., Steele, J. R., McGhee, D. E., Beattie, S., Purdam, C., & Cook, J. L. 2010. Landing strategies of athletes with an asymptomatic patellar tendon abnormality. *Medicine & Science in Sports & Exercise*, 42, 2072–80.

15  ATP. 2014. *Roger Federer: playing activity* [Online]. Available from http://www.atpworldtour.com/Tennis/Players/Top-Players/Roger-Federer.aspx?t=pa&y=0&m=s&e=gs#.

16  Robb, A. J., Fleisig, G., Wilk, K., Macrina, L., Bolt, B., & Pajaczkowski, J. 2010. Passive ranges of motion of the hips and their relationship with pitching biomechanics and ball velocity in professional baseball pitchers. *The American Journal of Sports Medicine*, 38, 2487–2493.

17  Malliaras, P., Cook, J. L., & Kent, P. 2006. Reduced ankle dorsiflexion range may increase the risk of patellar tendon injury among volleyball players. *Journal of Science and Medicine in Sport*, 9, 304–309.

18  Fong, C. M., Blackburn, J. T., Norcross, M. F., McGrath, M., & Padua, D. A. 2011. Ankle-dorsiflexion range of motion and landing biomechanics. *Journal of Athletic Training*, 46, 5.

19  Macrum, E., Bell, D. R., Boling, M., Lewek, M., & Padua, D. 2012. Effect of limiting ankle-dorsiflexion range of motion on lower extremity kinematics and muscle-activation patterns during a squat. *Journal of Sport Rehabilitation*, 21, 144.

20  Powers, C. M. 2010. The influence of abnormal hip mechanics on knee injury: A biomechanical perspective. *Journal of Orthopaedic & Sports Physical Therapy*, 40, 42–51.

21  Burkhart, S. S., Morgan, C. D., & Kibler, W. B. 2003. The disabled throwing shoulder: spectrum of pathology Part III: The SICK scapula, scapular dyskinesis, the kinetic chain, and rehabilitation. *Arthroscopy: The Journal of Arthroscopic & Related Surgery*, 19, 641–661.

22  Lockie, R. G., Murphy, A. J., & Spinks, C. D. 2003. Effects of resisted sled towing on sprint kinematics in field-sport athletes. *The Journal of Strength & Conditioning Research*, 17, 760–767.

23 Kawamori, N., Newton, R.U., Hori, N., & Nosaka, K. 2014. Effects of weighted sled towing with heavy versus light load on sprint acceleration ability. *Journal of Strength and Conditioning Research*, manuscript ahead of print.

24 Channell, B. T., & Barfield, J. 2008. Effect of Olympic and traditional resistance training on vertical jump improvement in high school boys. *The Journal of Strength & Conditioning Research*, 22, 1522–1527.

25 Hoffman, J. R., Cooper, J., Wendell, M., & Kang, J. 2004. Comparison of Olympic vs. traditional power lifting training programs in football players. *The Journal of Strength & Conditioning Research*, 18, 129–135.

26 Lavallee, M. E., & Balam, T. 2010. An overview of strength training injuries: Acute and chronic. *Current Sports Medicine Reports*, 9, 307–313.

27 Hamill, B. P. 1994. Relative safety of weightlifting and weight training. *The Journal of Strength & Conditioning Research*, 8, 53–57.

28 Hedrick, A., & Wada, H. 2008. Weightlifting movements: Do the benefits outweigh the risks? *Strength & Conditioning Journal*, 30, 26–35.

29 Berryman, N., Maurel, D., & Bosquet, L. 2010. Effect of plyometric vs. dynamic weight training on the energy cost of running. *The Journal of Strength & Conditioning Research*, 24, 1818–1825.

30 McGill, S. 2010. Core training: Evidence translating to better performance and injury prevention. *Strength & Conditioning Journal*, 32, 33–46.

31 Mens, J. M., Pool-Goudzwaard, A., Beekmans, R. E., & Tijhuis, M. T. 2010. Relation between subjective and objective scores on the active straight leg raising test. *Spine*, 35, 336–339.

32 Grimaldi, A. 2011. Assessing lateral stability of the hip and pelvis. *Manual Therapy*, 16, 26–32.

33 Danielsson, T. 2010. *Asymmetry in Elite Snowboarders: A study comparing range of motion in the hip and spine, power in lower extremities and circumference of thigh* (Unpublished student thesis). School of Business and Engineering, Halmstad University, Sweden.

34 Hart, N. H., Nimphius, S., Cochrane, J. L., & Newton, R. U. 2013. Leg mass characteristics of accurate and inaccurate kickers – an Australian football perspective. *Journal of Sports Sciences*, 31(15), 1647–1655.

35 van Dillen, L. R., Bloom, N. J., Gombatto, S. P., & Susco, T. M. 2008. Hip rotation range of motion in people with and without low back pain who participate in rotation-related sports. *Physical Therapy in Sport*, 9, 72–81.

36 Engstrom, C. M., Walker, D. G., Kippers, V., & Mehnert, A. J. 2007. Quadratus lumborum asymmetry and L4 pars injury in fast bowlers: A prospective MR study. *Medicine & Science in Sports & Exercise*, 39, 910–917.

37 Kountouris, A., Portus, M., & Cook, J. 2013. Cricket fast bowlers without low-back pain have larger quadratus lumborum asymmetry than injured bowlers. *Clinical Journal of Sport Medicine: Official Journal of the Canadian Academy of Sport Medicine*, 23(4), 300–304.

38 Sanchis-Moysi, J., Idoate, F., Izquierdo, M., Calbet, J. A., & Dorado, C. 2013. The hypertrophy of the lateral abdominal wall and quadratus lumborum is sport-specific: An MRI segmental study in professional tennis and soccer players. *Sports Biomechanics*, 12, 54–67.

39 Sanchis-Moysi, J., Idoate, F., Izquierdo, M., Calbet, J. A., & Dorado, C. 2011. Iliopsoas and gluteal muscles are asymmetric in tennis players but not in soccer players. *PloS ONE*, 6, e22858.

40 Hides, J., Fan, T., Stanton, W., Stanton, P., McMahon, K., & Wilson, S. 2010. Psoas and quadratus lumborum muscle asymmetry among elite Australian Football League players. *British Journal of Sports Medicine*, 44, 563–567.

41 Lucki, N. 2006. Physiological adaptations of the upper limb to the biomechanical environment of playing tennis. Proceedings of the National Conferences on Undergraduate Research, 2006, University of North Carolina at Asheville, Asheville NC, 3466–3472.

42 Myers, J. B., Laudner, K. G., Pasquale, M. R., Bradley, J. P., & Lephart, S. M. 2006. Glenohumeral range of motion deficits and posterior shoulder tightness in throwers with pathologic internal impingement. *The American Journal of Sports Medicine*, 34, 385–391.

43 Whiteley, R. J., Ginn, K. A., Nicholson, L. L., & Adams, R. D. 2009. Sports participation and humeral torsion. *The Journal of Orthopaedic and Sports Physical Therapy*, 39, 256–263.

44 Taylor, R., Zheng, C., Jackson, R., Doll, J., Chen, J., Holzbaur, K., Besier, T., & Kuhl, E. 2009. The phenomenon of twisted growth: Humeral torsion in dominant arms of high performance tennis players. *Computer Methods in Biomechanics and Biomedical Engineering*, 12, 83–93.

45 Oyama, S., Myers, J. B., Wassinger, C. A., Ricci, R. D., & Lephart, S. M. 2008. Asymmetric resting scapular posture in healthy overhead athletes. *Journal of Athletic Training*, 43, 565.

46 Kibler, W. B., Sciascia, A., & Wilkes, T. 2012. Scapular dyskinesis and its relation to shoulder injury. *Journal of the American Academy of Orthopaedic Surgeons*, 20, 364–372.

47 Tyler, T. F., Nicholas, S. J., Campbell, R. J., & McHugh, M. P. 2001. The association of hip strength and flexibility with the incidence of adductor muscle strains in professional ice hockey players. *The American Journal of Sports Medicine*, 29, 124–128.

48 Thorborg, K., Serne, R, A., Petersen, J., Madsen, T. M., Magnusson, P., & Hölmich, P. 2011. Hip adduction and abduction strength profiles in elite soccer players – implications for clinical evaluation of hip adductor muscle recovery after injury. *The American Journal of Sports Medicine*, 39, 121–126.

49 Yeung, S. S., Suen, A. M., & Yeung, E. W. 2009. A prospective cohort study of hamstring injuries in competitive sprinters: Preseason muscle imbalance as a possible risk factor. *British Journal of Sports Medicine*, 43, 589–594.

50 Orchard, J., Marsden, J., Lord, S., & Garlick, D. 1997. Preseason hamstring muscle weakness associated with hamstring muscle injury in Australian footballers. *The American Journal of Sports Medicine*, 25, 81–85.

51 Bennell, K., Wajswelner, H., Lew, P., Schall-Riaucour, A., Leslie, S., Plant, D., & Cirone, J. 1998. Isokinetic strength testing does not predict hamstring injury in Australian Rules footballers. *British Journal of Sports Medicine*, 32, 309–314.

52 Myer, G. D., Ford, K. R., Foss, K. D. B., Liu, C., Nick, T. G., & Hewett, T. E. 2009. The relationship of hamstrings and quadriceps strength to anterior cruciate ligament injury in female athletes. *Clinical Journal of Sport Medicine*, 19, 3–8.

53 Yildiz, Y., Aydin, T., Sekir, U., Kiralp, M., Hazneci, B., & Kalyon, T. 2006. Shoulder terminal range eccentric antagonist/concentric agonist strength ratios in overhead athletes. *Scandinavian Journal of Medicine & Science in Sports*, 16, 174–180.

54 Saccol, M. F., Gracitelli, G. C., da Silva, R. T., Laurino, C. F. D. S., Fleury, A. M., Andrade, M. D. S., & da Silva, A. C. 2010. Shoulder functional ratio in elite junior tennis players. *Physical Therapy in Sport*, 11, 8–11.

55 Ellenbecker, T., & Roetert, E. 2003. Age specific isokinetic glenohumeral internal and external rotation strength in elite junior tennis players. *Journal of Science and Medicine in Sport*, 6, 63–70.

56 Byram, I. R., Bushnell, B. D., Dugger, K., Charron, K., Harrell, F. E., & Noonan, T. J. 2010. Preseason shoulder strength measurements in professional baseball pitchers identifying players at risk for injury. *The American Journal of Sports Medicine*, 38, 1375–1382.

57 Bernard, J. C., Boudokhane, S., Pujol, A., Chaléat-valayer, E., Le Blay, G., & Deceuninck, J. 2013. Isokinetic trunk muscle performance in pre-teens and teens with and without back pain. *Annals of Physical and Rehabilitation Medicine*, 57(1), 38–54.

58 Murray, E., Birley, E., Twycross-Lewis, R., & Morrissey, D. 2009. The relationship between hip rotation range of movement and low back pain prevalence in amateur golfers: An observational study. *Physical Therapy in Sport*, 10, 131–135.

# Chapter 8

# Assessing athletic qualities

*Nick Winkelman*

## Introduction

The assessment of athletic qualities is one of the most important aspects of a comprehensive athletic development model. Objective assessments provide an integrated understanding of an athlete's current physical capabilities and the underpinning relationship of each unique quality being tested. This in turn allows for the development of a physical profile for each athlete.

Each *athletic profile* is based on a series of assessments that measure distinct movement qualities with common strength and power needs. This allows us to:

- identify performance deficits
- prioritize the training process
- identify talent
- discriminate between playing ability based on physical competencies
- monitor player readiness
- provide return-to-performance (RTP) objectives following injury.

Each profile represents a unique athletic signature that is anchored against normative information. Norms can be based on an individual's current capabilities, where the profile represents changes from one testing session to the next. This is valuable when population norms are not available and we want to identify if training is making effective changes to the athlete. Norms can also be based off specific populations (e.g. sport, age and position) where performance capabilities are represented in relation to a group of individuals that exemplify a standard.

In both cases, the results are used to drive the prioritization within the training process. It should be noted that this is a very linear approach that assumes all variables being measured are of equal importance to performance. More complex models can be generated to account for weighted importance of certain variables over others. This discussion is beyond the scope of this chapter but is important for the overall understanding of athletic profiling.

Every athletic profile should be relevant to sport and position. When determining which qualities are most important for sporting performance, we should consider primary contributing factors and their relationship to both each other and the performance. If the assessments selected do not capture the full scope of the sport and position needs, then gaps may exist when trying to identify performance capabilities and RTP readiness.

The inadequacies of our RTP criteria have challenged us to re-evaluate the way we assess athletic qualities. A shift from the reductionist point of view to an integrated systems approach to assessment is warranted. An integrated systems approach looks at phenomenon from a multifaceted standpoint and examines the interrelationship of variables across various conditions. Integrated models need to consider all underpinning strength and power qualities, movement qualities, relevant environmental factors and associated cardiovascular needs of the sport and position.

Based on the scope of this chapter, the following sections will discuss relevant strength, power, sprinting, agility, aerobic fitness and anaerobic fitness assessments as part of an integrated performance and RTP testing model. Considerations for performance and therapy will be discussed. While anthropometric, movement screening, and cognitive testing are not discussed, the inclusion of such assessments play an equally important role in generating a comprehensive athletic profile.

## Maximal strength

Strength is critical for sporting performance and injury resilience. The ability to generate large forces in the correct direction is an essential aspect of athletic performance. Specifically, the expression of force relative to body weight is a primary determinant of movement speed.

There are many ways to assess the force generating capabilities of an athlete, but in all cases, the measure of interest is maximal strength. *Maximal strength* can be defined as the maximal voluntary contractile force the neuromuscular system is capable of producing in a single effort, irrespective of time.[1]

---

The importance of maximal strength can be seen in the strong correlations to sprinting speed,[2] agility[3] and jumping[4] and the role it plays in RTP following injury.[5,6]

---

Maximal strength is classically assessed by having an athlete perform a one-repetition maximum (1RM) on a movement of interest (e.g. bench press). *Relative strength* can then be calculated from the 1RM by dividing by the individual's body mass (BM) in kilograms (i.e. 1RM/BM). Protocols to directly test 1RM will use incremental loads that go from low to high with adequate rest between sets until a final repetition maximum is achieved.[7] An alternative to the direct testing of a 1RM to assess maximal strength is the prediction of a 1RM based on a higher repetition structure. Research has shown that the best prediction equations are based on performing 4–6 repetition maximums.[8,9] This is commonly used in an effort to avoid the perceived injuries that may be caused by 1RM testing and can be less time consuming when dealing with a larger group of athletes.

## Rate of force development

While maximal strength and the ability to generate large forces are important, of equal importance is the rate at which force can be generated. From a testing standpoint maximal force is exhibited at $\geq 300$ms,[10] whereas sporting type movements including sprinting,[11] jumping[12] and cutting occur in $\leq 250$ms.

> By definition, *rate of force development* (RFD) is the slope of the force-time curve, where the change in force is divided by change in time ($\Delta$Force/$\Delta$Time).[13]

The RFD at the onset of a movement has been termed *starting strength*[14] and is measured during the first 0–50ms of a movement action, whereas, the point where peak RFD occurs has been termed *explosive strength* and is measured at 50–200ms of a movement action.[13,15] RFD is measured using a force platform (FP) or isokinetic dynamometer (IKD) across a variety of movements. The isometric mid-thigh pull is a common exercise used to assess lower body RFD and maximal force using a force platform, while isometric leg extensions are commonly used to assess lower body RFD using an IKD.[16]

From an RTP standpoint, RFD is an important measure to examine. Research has shown that following anterior cruciate ligament (ACL) reconstruction surgery, elite soccer players demonstrated a recovery in peak force six months post-op, but RFD at 30 per cent, 50 per cent and 90 per cent of maximum voluntary isometric contraction (MVIC) only achieved 80 per cent, 77 per cent and 63 per cent of pre-injury levels.[17] By 12 months both MVIC and all RFD values achieved or exceeded 90 per cent of pre-injury levels. This provides us with the understanding not only that an athlete needs to regain maximal strength, but also of the specific strength qualities represented by improved RFD capabilities.

## Maximal power

The expression of maximal power is one of the most important determinants of athletic performance. Power is a function of an athlete's ability to generate force and velocity against a given load (i.e. power (watts) = force × velocity). By definition, *maximal power* can be considered the highest wattage an individual can generate at a given load during a specific movement (e.g. power clean).

Similar to maximal strength, there are direct and indirect measurements of maximal power. The primary tools used to directly measure maximal power include linear position transducers (LPT) and FP. The LPT can accurately measure displacement and is a valid measure of velocity, while the FP can accurately measure ground reaction force (GRF). Further, power can be measured across a range of movement and exercise types, including: (a) plyometrics (e.g. jump squat), (b) ballistic exercises (e.g. bench throws), and (c) Olympic lifts (e.g. power snatch). All of these exercise types can be used in concert with an LPT, FP or a combination of both measurement tools.

When assessing maximal power, it is very common to identify the load that optimizes maximal power production. Specifically, the load that optimizes maximal power is likely dependent on training level, training modality and specific movement.

> Maximal power is commonly achieved between 40 and 60 per cent of 1RM,[18,19] but it should be noted that loads as low as 10 per cent of 1RM have been shown to elicit maximal power in untrained individuals.[20]

To identify the load that optimizes maximal power, the assessment of a power profile is often recommended. The literature supports the use of weightlifting,[21] ballistic exercises[18,19] and plyometrics[22] as appropriate exercise modes for this type of assessment. Specifically, athletes will perform the identified exercise under a range of low load and high load conditions. This data provides critical insights around the training loads that an athlete should focus on to improve their overall power production capabilities relative to sport and position.

While the direct assessment of power qualities is ideal, this is not always practical based on equipment, time and space limitations. Therefore, jump and hop assessments are common field tests that provide an indirect measurement of power characteristics. Moreover, jump- and hop-based assessments allow for a more specific assessment of movement within the context of the sporting environment (i.e. field or court).

## Jump and hop assessment

Jump and hop assessments are commonly used for sports performance testing and as RTP markers of readiness. Jump and hop protocols will use the following initiation types which each represent a distinct strength quality demand: (a) non-countermovement (NCM), (b) countermovement (CM), or (c) depth (or drop) jump (DJ). An NCM requires the athlete to descend to a desired position (e.g. squat position) and hold for 1–2 seconds before rapidly moving in the desired direction (i.e. vertically or horizontally). A CM requires the athlete to rapidly lower to a desired position with no pause before rapidly moving towards the desired direction. Finally, the DJ involves the same mechanism as a CM with the only difference being the athlete is dropped from a designated box height before initiating movement.

The NCM-jump/hop, CM-jump/hop, and DJ are all measures of explosive strength qualities. Specifically, the NCM is a strong indirect measure of starting and explosive strength, the CM is a strong indirect measure of explosive strength and the DJ can be considered a strong indirect measure of explosive and reactive strength. *Reactive strength* can be considered a measure of explosive strength under the conditions of a fast stretch-shortening cycle (i.e. <250ms ground contact time).[14] The DJ is commonly used to assess an athlete's reactive strength due to the higher stretch-shortening loads and lowered ground contact times (i.e. <200ms).[23]

The vertical jump is one of the most common assessments used to test NCM and CM power capabilities. The vertical jump can be assessed using a traditional jump-and-reach device or a permanent measuring device on a wall. A second testing option is the use of a jump (switch) mat. When using a jump mat, the coach can have the athlete jump with or without arms (i.e. hands on hips or holding dowel on shoulders), noting that the testing protocol should be consistent to ensure that results can be compared between individuals and over time. In addition to assessing jump height, alternative assessment methods have been suggested for measuring reactive strength during a DJ. A common measure of reactive strength during the DJ is the reactive strength index (RSI). The RSI is calculated by dividing jump height by ground contact time (i.e. RSI = [JH/GCT]).[24] Note that the RSI can only be measured when using a force plate or jump mat that can calculate ground contact time.

When assessing the DJ, it is best to test over a range of drop heights from 30–60 cm. It has been suggested that the selected drop heights be based on athlete experience, with a practical recommendation that drop heights should not exceed an athlete's CM jump height.

Within DJ testing, the instruction during a DJ is critical to the strength quality being measured (i.e. 'jump as high as you can' vs. 'jump as high as you can while spending the least amount of time on the ground').[25] When assessing a DJ where the instruction is to 'jump as high as you can', the athlete will move in a manner that is biomechanically similar to that of a CMJ. Therefore, this form of instruction instigates a type of jump that is an indirect measure of explosive strength. Conversely, when assessing a DJ where the instruction is to 'jump as high as you can while spending the least amount of time on the ground', the athlete will move through a smaller range of motion while producing significantly less ground contact times. This form of DJ instruction allows for a more accurate measurement of reactive strength.

The broad jump is another classic assessment of lower body explosive strength. While it can be argued that vertical and horizontal jumps are underpinned by the same strength qualities, they differ in the directional specificity of the movements. For example the broad jump is a better predictor of sprinting and agility than the vertical jump.[26]

Vertical hopping assessment provides similar insights about underlying explosive strength capabilities and allows us to evaluate left versus right symmetry. Vertical hopping can be assessed using the same jump and reach techniques or jump mat. Absolute hop heights can be calculated and compared for left versus right symmetry. A side-to-side asymmetry of ≤10–15 per cent should be pursued both for RTP and as a general recommendation for injury prevention.[27,28] Additionally, combined left and right vertical hop heights show a strong correlation to sprinting and may have more functional relevance to predicting RTP than bilateral vertical jumping.[29]

Horizontal hopping assessments provide the same benefits as vertical with the benefit of directional specificity to many sporting movements. The most common test is the single hop test, where subjects hop out and land on the same leg for maximal distance. Similar to the vertical hop, left versus right is compared, with ≤10–15 per cent difference being the cut-off point for injury prevention and RTP. A different version of this test involves the athlete stepping off a 20 cm box before hopping out as far as they can and landing on two legs. Further, strong support has shown that the single leg horizontal drop hop (SLHDH) predicts sprinting performance with significant correlations over 0–10m.[26]

In summary, jumping and hopping provide indirect measurement of maximal power and associated specific strength qualities (i.e. starting, explosive and reactive strength). Further, jumping and hopping correlate to specific field tests due to similar ground contact times, ground reaction forces and direction of force. Therefore, the assessment of jumping and hopping can be considered essential tests for a comprehensive athletic profile model and as RTP criteria before releasing an athlete to sprinting and agility testing.

## Sprinting speed

Sprinting is a fundamental task in almost every land-based sport and has high functional relevance within an athletic profiling model and as RTP criteria. Depending on the distance run, there are different strength- and movement-specific requirements. From a testing standpoint, we should consider the following variables:

(a)  testing equipment
(b)  testing distance
(c)  start type.

There are two primary ways of testing sprinting performance that include the use of timing gates or stopwatches. When at all possible, it is better to use timing gates, as the reliability and validity is higher than stopwatches.[30] If using stopwatches is unavoidable, an average time of two or more people timing is preferable.

When selecting a test distance, the athlete's position and general sport requirements should be considered. In most field and court sports, the two distinct speed qualities of interest include acceleration and maximal velocity sprinting.[31]

> Acceleration is characterized by a large increase in velocity with associated forward-body lean and piston-like leg action. This quality is best measured over 0–10m. Maximal velocity sprinting, on the other hand, is characterized by an upright posture and a cyclical type leg action and is best measured from 20–30m or 20–40m.

Therefore, a distance of 30m or 40m can be recommended for most assessment protocols, as splits at 0–10m and 20–40m will provide distinct information about acceleration and max velocity sprinting capabilities.

The final consideration when testing sprinting is the type of start that is used. The two categories include a flying start and the static start. The flying start requires the athlete to start one metre behind the first timing gate (i.e. start line), which will be activated once the athlete crosses the beam. For dynamic sports that do not require a large amount of starting strength (e.g. soccer), this is the preferred start method. The second start type is a static start from a two or three point stance. This start type is preferred for sports that present with sudden bursts of sprinting from static or semi-static positions (i.e. American football and rugby). Two or three point starts can be selected based on the most relevant positions adopted within the specific sport of interest.

> The assessment of sprinting provides distinct information about acceleration and max velocity capabilities. The information gained from these tests can direct the prioritization of the performance training process and provides critical insights concerning RTP readiness and overall athlete confidence.

# Agility

The ability to change direction is fundamental to many sports and is an underpinning determinant of sporting success. Measures of agility can be considered distinct motor abilities that must be assessed as a part of a comprehensive athletic profiling model. Further, a high incidence of lower body injuries occur during cutting and pivoting sports, and for this reason it has been recommended that agility assessment be integrated into performance testing as an important criteria for RTP following injury.[32,33]

The term agility has carried a diversity of definitions over the years, and therefore it is important that we define the various categories of agility. *Agility* is a 'rapid whole body movement with change of velocity or direction' of movement under non-reactive or reactive conditions in response to a stimulus.[34,35] Under non-reactive conditions, the major emphasis is pre-planned change of direction. Under reactive conditions, there is an increased cognitive demand, as we need to perceive and respond to a specific stimulus (i.e. sight, sound or touch) prior to changing direction. Therefore, the terms non-reactive agility and reactive agility should be used to define the specific performance test being used.

Many tests have been proposed for the assessment of non-reactive agility, including:

- T-test
- 5–10–5 (Pro Agility)
- L-drill (3-cone drill)
- 505 agility test
- Illinois agility test
- Zigzag run test.

All tests can be completed using timing gates or stopwatches with a relevant playing surface, space and set of cones. All of these tests are highly correlated, which allows us to pick 1–2 tests that capture the movement distances and directions that are relevant to sport and position.[36] The two major limiting factors across these tests include the inability to assess reactive decision making and to accurately distinguish left and right change of direction (COD) symmetry.

The reactive agility test (RAT) has been proposed as a solution for the assessment of reactive decision making and can provide critical insights about left versus right symmetry.[34,37,38] The RAT test assesses non-reactive and reactive agility within the context of the same drill (i.e. set-up and distances travelled). While different protocols exist, the RAT generally includes a 4m linear sprint followed by a 45° cut to the left or right, which results in an additional 4m run. The test is first performed under non-reactive conditions, where the athlete knows the direction they are running following the linear sprint. The second iteration involves the athlete reacting to an opponent, video or light system that directs them to the left or right following the linear sprint. The difference in left versus right can be calculated for the non-reactive and reactive conditions.

The difference between the non-reactive and reactive times can be compared to provide an understanding of reactive-based decision making. Additionally, this information allows the bucketing of athletes into the following categories:[38]

(a)   slow mover/slow thinker
(b)   slow mover/fast thinker
(c)   fast mover/slow thinker
(d)   fast mover/fast thinker.

Each bucket provides us with the insight to know whether an athlete struggles with decision making or has specific speed and strength deficits related to change of direction.[39]

> The assessment of non-reactive and reactive agility provides a more robust under-standing of an athlete's on-field capabilities. The ability to compare left versus right symmetry under reactive and non-reactive conditions provides complete visibility into the scenarios where injury is most likely to occur.

## Aerobic and anaerobic energy system assessment

The final components needed for a comprehensive athletic profile is the assessment of aerobic and anaerobic fitness capabilities. While the strength, power and movement qualities discussed underpin an athlete's potential, the ability to endure and express repeated performance within and across a sport match is critical.

> We know that the majority of injuries occur toward the second half of a sport match,[40] with endurance likely being a contributing factor. These and other results highlight the importance of aerobic capabilities matched with movement quality.

The importance of aerobic and anaerobic capacity as measured by multistage fitness testing has been recently recommended as an important RTP criteria following ACL reconstruction.[41]

Many aerobic tests are available, including step tests, walking tests and various running tests.[42] More recently, multistage fitness testing has been recommended as a valid and reliable way to predict maximal aerobic capabilities, with peak heart rates attained matching those achieved during $VO_2$ analysis testing.[43,44,45] The Yo-Yo Intermittent Recovery 1 (Yo-Yo IR1) test uses $2 \times 20m$ runs of increasing speed progressed with an auditory signal and interspersed with 10 s rest between stages.[43,44] Each test takes 10–20min, with the peak heart rate and stage achieved being recorded. Based on the results, equations have been created to predict $VO_2$ max.[44]

The aerobic system and anaerobic systems contribute during all fitness testing, but there are certain tests that provide greater insights concerning the anaerobic capacities of the athlete. Some of the most common tests include the Yo-Yo IR2 test and the running-based anaerobic sprint test (RAST).[46] The RAST test involves the athlete performing $6 \times 35m$ sprints at maximal speed with 10 s rest between repetitions. Based on the weight of the individual and the time of each repetition, calculations can provide average power per repetition, maximal power, minimum power, average power and a fatigue index score (watts/sec).[47]

Both aerobic and anaerobic tests should be used within an athletic profiling model, with the results providing RTP criteria following injury. Developing specific aerobic and anaerobic qualities supports an athlete's ability to repeatedly express strength and power within movement.

## Summary

It is vital that all members of a human performance team have a thorough understanding of physical testing. The assessments discussed allow the coach and medical team to develop comprehensive athletic profiles that can be used to improve performance and as RTP criteria. Similar to cognitive baseline testing for concussions, each athletic profile can be used as a standard that must be met before complete RTP is achieved. Further, it may be recommended that, rather than an athlete achieving ≥90 per cent of performance compared to the pre-injury athletic profile, the athlete must achieve 100+ per cent of the pre-injury athletic profile, as original deficits may have been an underpinning determinant of the injury in the first place. This systems-based approach to the assessment of athletic qualities allows the coach and medical team to evaluate each quality within the context of the whole system, permitting an integrated perspective on athletic performance and RTP.

## Notes

1 Poliquin, C. (1989). Classification of strength qualities. *Journal of Strength & Conditioning Reasearch*, *11*(6):48–50.

2 Young, W., McLean, B., & Ardagna, J. (1995). Relationship between strength qualities and sprinting performance. *Journal of Sports Medicine and Physical Fitness*, *35*(1):13–19.

3 Nimphius, S., McGuigan, M. R., & Newton, R. U. (2010). Relationship between strength, power, speed, and change of direction performance of female softball players. *Journal of Strength & Conditioning Research*, *24*(4):885–895.

4 Young, W., Wilson, G., & Byrne, C. (1999). Relationship between strength qualities and performance in standing and run-up vertical jumps. *Journal of Sports Medicine and Physical Fitness*, , *39*(4):285–293.

5 Barber-Westin, S. D., & Noyes, F. R. (2011). Objective criteria for return to athletics after anterior cruciate ligament reconstruction and subsequent reinjury rates: A systematic review. *The Physician and Sportsmedicine*, *39*(3):100–110.

6 Thomee, R., Kaplan, Y., Kvist, J., et al. (2011). Muscle strength and hop performance criteria prior to return to sports after ACL reconstruction. *Knee Surgery, Sports Traumatology, Arthroscopy*, *19*(11):1798–1805.

7 McBride, J. M., Triplett-McBride, T., Davie, A., & Newton, R. U. (2002). The effect of heavy- vs. light-load jump squats on the development of strength, power, and speed. *Journal of Strength & Conditioning Research*, *16*(1):75–82.

8 Reynolds, J. M., Gordon, T. J., & Robergs, R. A. (2006). Prediction of one repetition maximum strength from multiple repetition maximum testing and anthropometry. *Journal of Strength & Conditioning research*, 20(3):584–592.

9 Dohoney, P., Chromiak, J. A., Lemire, D., Abadie, B. R., & Kovacs, C. (2002). Prediction of one repetition maximum (1-RM) strength from a 4–6 RM and a 7–10 RM submaximal strength test in healthy young adult males. *Journal of Exercise Physiologyonline*, 5(3):54–59.

10 Thorstensson, A., Karlsson, J., Viitasalo, J. H., Luhtanen, P., Komi, P. V. (1976). Effect of strength training on EMG of human skeletal muscle. *Acta Physiologica Scandinavica*, 98(2):232–236.

11 Kuitunen, S., Komi, P. V., & Kyrolainen, H. (2002). Knee and ankle joint stiffness in sprint running. *Medicine and Science in Sports and Exercise*, 34(1):166–173.

12 Luhtanen, P., & Komi, P. V. (1979). Mechanical power and segmental contribution to force impulses in long jump take-off. *European Journal of Applied Physiology and Occupational Physiology*, 41(4):267–274.

13 Aagaard, P., Simonsen, E. B., Andersen, J. L., Magnusson, P., & Dyhre-Poulsen, P. (2002). Increased rate of force development and neural drive of human skeletal muscle following resistance training. *Journal of Applied Physiology*, 93(4):1318–1326.

14 Schmidtbleicher, D. (1992). Training for power events (pp381–395). In P. V. Komi (Ed.), *Strength and power in sport*. London: Blackwell Scientific.

15 Stone, M. H., Stone, M., & Sands, W. A. (2007). *Principles and practice of resistance training.* Champaign, IL: Human Kinetics.

16 Zebis, M. K., Andersen, L. L., Ellingsgaard, H., & Aagaard, P. (2011). Rapid hamstring/quadriceps force capacity in male vs. female elite soccer players. *Journal of Strength & Conditioning Research, 25*(7):1989–1993.

17 Angelozzi, M., Madama, M., Corsica, C., et al. (2012). Rate of force development as an adjunctive outcome measure for return-to-sport decisions after anterior cruciate ligament reconstruction. *The Journal of Orthopaedic and Sports Physical Therapy, 42*(9):772–780.

18 Baker, D., Nance, S., & Moore, M. (2001). The load that maximizes the average mechanical power output during explosive bench press throws in highly trained athletes. *Journal of Strength & Conditioning Research, 15*(1):20–24.

19 Baker, D., Nance, S., & Moore, M. (2001). The load that maximizes the average mechanical power output during jump squats in power-trained athletes. *Journal of Strength & Conditioning Research, 15*(1):92–97.

20 Stone, M. H., O'Bryant, H. S., McCoy, L., Coglianese, R., Lehmkuhl, M., & Schilling, B. (2003). Power and maximum strength relationships during performance of dynamic and static weighted jumps. *Journal of Strength & Conditioning Research, 17*(1):140–147.

21 Comfort, P., Udall, R., & Jones, P. A. (2012). The affect of loading on kinematic and kinetic variables during the mid-thigh clean pull. *Journal of Strength & Conditioning Research, 26*(5), 1208-14.

22 Sheppard, J. M., Cormack, S., Taylor, K. L., McGuigan, M. R., & Newton, R. U. (2008). Assessing the force-velocity characteristics of the leg extensors in well-trained athletes: The incremental load power profile. *Journal of Strength & Conditioning Research, 22*(4):1320–1326.

23 Young, W. B., Pryor, J. F., & Wilson, G. J. (1995). Effect of instructions on characteristics of counter-movement and drop jump performance. *The Journal of Strength & Conditioning Research, 9*(4):232–236.

24 Flanagan, E. P., Ebben, W. P., & Jensen, R. L. (2008). Reliability of the reactive strength index and time to stabilization during depth jumps. *Journal of Strength & Conditioning Research, 22*(5):1677–1682.

25 Young, W., Cormack, S., & Crichton, M. (2011). Which jump variables should be used to assess explosive leg muscle function? *International Journal of Sports Physiology and Performance, 6*(1):51–57.

26 Fairchild, B. P., Amonette, W. E., & Spiering, B. A. (2011). Prediction models of speed and agility in NFL combine attendees. *The Journal of Strength & Conditioning Research, 25*:S96. 10.1097/1001.JSC.0000395730.0000368106.a0000395739.

27 Impellizzeri, F. M., Rampinini, E., Maffiuletti, N., & Marcora, S. M. (2007). A vertical jump force test for assessing bilateral strength asymmetry in athletes. *Medicine and Science in Sports and Exercise, 39*(11):2044–2050.

28 Wilk, K.E., Romaniello, W. T., Soscia, S. M., Arrigo, C. A., & Andrews, J. R. (1994). The relationship between subjective knee scores, isokinetic testing, and functional testing in the ACL-reconstructed knee. *The Journal of Orthopaedic and Sports Physical Therapy, 20*(2):60–73.

29 McCurdy, K. W., Walker, J. L., Langford, G. A., Kutz, M. R., Guerrero, J. M., & McMillan, J. (2010). The relationship between kinematic determinants of jump and sprint performance in division I women soccer players. *Journal of Strength & Conditioning Research, 24*(12):3200–3208.

30 Hetzler, R. K., Stickley, C. D., Lundquist, K. M., & Kimura, I. F. (2008). Reliability and accuracy of handheld stopwatches compared with electronic timing in measuring sprint performance. *Journal of Strength & Conditioning Research, 22*(6):1969–1976.

31 Little, T., & Williams, A. G. (2005). Specificity of acceleration, maximum speed, and agility in professional soccer players. *Journal of Strength & Conditioning Research, 19*(1):76–78.

32 Myer, G. D., Paterno, M. V., Ford, K. R., & Hewett, T. E. (2008). Neuromuscular training techniques to target deficits before return to sport after anterior cruciate ligament reconstruction. *Journal of Strength & Conditioning Research, 22*(3):987–1014.

33 Myer, G. D., Schmitt, L. C., Brent, J. L., et al. (2011). Utilization of modified NFL combine testing to identify functional deficits in athletes following ACL reconstruction. *The Journal of Orthopaedic and Sports Physical Therapy, 41*(6):377–387.

34   Sheppard, J. M., Young, W. B., Doyle, T. L., Sheppard, T. A., & Newton, R. U. (2006). An evaluation of a new test of reactive agility and its relationship to sprint speed and change of direction speed. *Journal of Science and Medicine in Sport, 9*(4):342–349.

35   Sheppard, J. M., & Young, W. B. (2006). Agility literature review: Classifications, training and testing. *Journal of Sports Sciences, 24*(9):919–932.

36   Stewart, P. F., Turner, A. N., & Miller, S. C. (2012). Reliability, factorial validity, and interrelationships of five commonly used change of direction speed tests. *Scandinavian Journal of Medicine & Science in Sports, 24*(3):500–506

37   Farrow, D., Young, W., & Bruce, L. (2005). The development of a test of reactive agility for netball: A new methodology. *Journal of Science and Medicine in Sport, 8*(1):52–60.

38   Gabbett, T., & Benton, D. (2009). Reactive agility of rugby league players. *Journal of Science and Medicine in Sport, 12*(1):212–214.

39   Gabbett, T. J., Kelly, J. N., & Sheppard, J. M. (2008). Speed, change of direction speed, and reactive agility of rugby league players. *Journal of Strength & Conditioning Research, 22*(1):174–181.

40   Gabbett, T. J. (2004). Incidence of injury in junior and senior rugby league players. *Sports Medicine (Auckland, N.Z.), 34*(12):849–859.

41   Barber-Westin, S. D., & Noyes, F. R. (2011). Factors used to determine return to unrestricted sports activities after anterior cruciate ligament reconstruction. *Arthroscopy, 27*(12):1697–1705.

42   Reiman, M. P., & Manske, R. C. (2009). *Functional testing in human performance.* Champaign, IL: Human Kinetics.

43   Krustrup, P., Mohr, M., Amstrup, T., et al. (2003). The Yo-Yo intermittent recovery test: Physiological response, reliability, and validity. *Medicine and Science in Sports and Exercise, 35*(4):697–705.

44   Bangsbo, J., Iaia, F. M., & Krustrup, P. (2008). The Yo-Yo intermittent recovery test: A useful tool for evaluation of physical performance in intermittent sports. *Sports Medicine (Auckland, N.Z.), 38*(1):37–51.

45   Buchheit, M. (2008). The 30–15 intermittent fitness test: Accuracy for individualizing interval training of young intermittent sport players. *Journal of Strength & Conditioning Research, 22*(2):365–374.

46   Keir, D. A., Theriault, F., & Serresse, O. (2012). Evaluation of the running-based anaerobic sprint test as a measure of repeated sprint ability in collegiate level soccer players. *Journal of Strength & Conditioning Research, 27*(6):1671-8.

47   Mckenzie, B. (1998). RAST. Retrieved from http://www.brianmac.co.uk/rast.htm.

## Chapter 9

# Running mechanics in injury prevention and performance

*Frans Bosch and John IJzerman*

## Introduction

Running is the activity that is most commonly associated with sports injury. It is likely that a variety of intrinsic and extrinsic running-related risk factors combine to produce running-related injuries. However, this process remains poorly understood. Although the long list of potential contributing factors makes prevention and management of running injury extremely challenging, optimising running technique is likely to be critical to both maximising performance and minimising injury risk. With that in mind, achieving safe and efficient running technique is the primary focus of this chapter.

The running motion is complex, and firm links between aspects of running technique and specific injury types are yet to be established. Although kinetic and kinematic measurements are commonly used to identify important rules for correct technique, they fail to account for other influences and constraints that help to determine ideal technique, such as anatomical factors, musculotendinous mechanical properties and motor control mechanisms. As such, isolated mechanical models are inadequate. An example of this can be seen with the movement of the lead leg prior to foot contact, in which the leg first swings forwards and then backwards before meeting the ground (Figures 9.1 and 9.2). In mechanical models the only function of this so-called 'swing-leg' retraction is to produce stance phase horizontal and vertical ground reaction forces required to propel the body. Rather than explaining the efficiency of swing-leg retraction in purely mechanical terms, the importance of swing-leg retraction in factors such as the ability to resist perturbations (e.g. due to mis-timing or mis-placement of foot contact and the need for co-variation) and musculotendinous self-regulation of spring mass behaviour during the running action[1] need to be integrated with mechanical models in order to better understand sound running technique.

To take account of such constraints in technique models, this chapter will describe running at constant high speed, integrating influences such as the architecture of the musculoskeletal system and relevant neurophysiological factors. The concepts of muscular co-contractions and muscle synergies within a robust running action will be described in order to explain the determinants of top-speed running performance and how deviation from anatomically efficient technique may lead to injury.

## The running cycle

The breakdown of the 'anatomical' running cycle identifies the main points at which technique is shaped by muscle control and action. This breakdown differs from traditional models in a number of respects. Traditional descriptions of the cycle seldom distinguish between

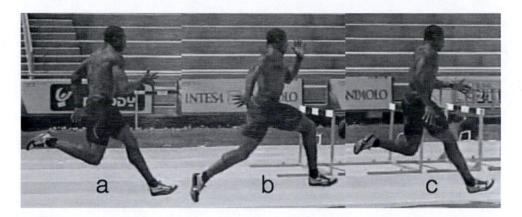

*Figure 9.1* Right lower limb swing phase: a) forward swing, b) reversal, c) backward swing (swing-leg retraction)

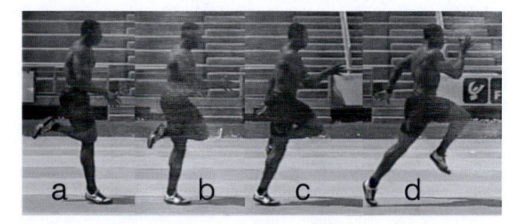

*Figure 9.2* Right lower limb stance phase: a) full contact, b) mid-stance, c) heel-off, d) toe-off

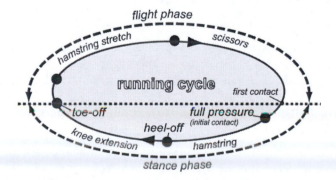

*Figure 9.3* The running cycle

*Table 9.1* Key events in the running cycle

| Action | |
| --- | --- |
| First contact | The point at which the foot makes contact with the ground |
| Full pressure (initial contact) | The point at which full weight is resting on the stance leg |
| Hamstring dominant stance | Hamstring directing ground reaction force (more horizontal) |
| Heel-off | The point at which the heel leaves the ground |
| Knee extension | Energy transport (from knee to ankle) |
| Toe-off | The point at which the foot leaves the ground |
| Hamstring stretch | Elastic loading of the hamstring when the lower leg rotates forward |
| Scissors | Repositioning of the front leg (swing-leg retraction) |

'initial contact' and 'full contact'. However, the point at which the foot first touches the ground (initial contact) is a relatively unimportant point in the cycle, for it cannot be linked to a crucial change in the organisation of muscle action. In contrast, the point at which the full weight of the body is transferred to the foot (full contact) *is* important, for it is the point at which the muscles of the stance leg are loaded with elastic energy by external forces.

Other key events in the anatomical cycle include:

- *Heel off* (particularly, the transport of energy by the bi-articular muscles of stance leg)
- *Toe-off* (involves a sudden major change in muscle activity)
- *Forward rotation* of the lower leg during 'flight phase' (when large amounts of elastic energy are transported from the trailing leg to the hamstring of the leading leg).

Of course, there are other important 'events' (such as pelvic movements and their associated muscle actions) that are linked to the critical points in the cycle described above.

The model used in this chapter explicitly refers to the correct *structure* of the technique, rather than the ideal *technique*, for there is no 'ideal' technique in the sense of a precisely described outward form of the motion, in which ideal joint angles can be prescribed.[2] Here, reference is to the *structure* of the running technique, meaning the underlying organising *principles* that govern muscle function and control. It should be noted, however, that the outward appearance of the technique may differ among individuals even if the underlying generic principles are respected.

Individuality is more evident in low-speed running than high-speed running, hence the greater similarity in the technique of elite sprinters.

## Determining running technique quality – the positive running model

Running is a cyclical motion. This makes it difficult to start just anywhere in the cycle when explaining causes and effects, for the start is itself the effect of a previous cause. The most practical starting point is toe-off (the point at which the foot leaves the ground at the end of

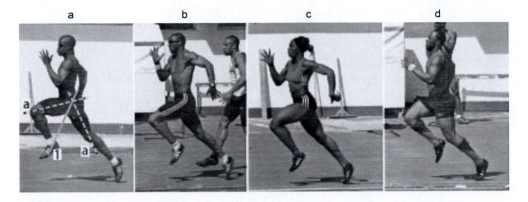

*Figure 9.4* Positive running technique

the stance phase). This is the point at which the greatest and most sudden change in muscle activity during the cycle takes place (Figure 9.2d). Toe-off is also the point at which the quality of the motion can be measured within a model that is based on posture – the 'positive running' posture. Positive running can be measured by drawing a line through each of the athlete's thighs in a side-on video still at toe-off. The angle between the two lines is then bisected. The further forward the bisecting line points, the better the running technique (Figure 9.4a). This concept will be explored in greater detail later in this chapter.

## The running cycle and injury

### The toe-off posture

When running, it is essential to stabilise the hip and pelvis. Moreover, because of the high forces generated during running (especially at toe-off), the muscles involved need to be facilitated to work at length and contraction speeds that provide optimum resistance to opposing forces. The hip movements also require stability of the sacroiliac joint, which is achieved by the *gluteus medius* and the contralateral *latissimus dorsi*, together with the *transversus abdominis* and the *obliquus internus*. These all have an important part to play in stabilising the pelvic girdle by generating force closure.[3]

The hip adductor muscles are critical to the stability of the hip and pelvis but it is important to note that not all the adductor muscles function in the same way during hip motion. *Gracilis* and *adductor longus* are lengthened during hip extension, whilst *adductor magnus* and *semitendinosus* are lengthened when the hip flexes. The differences in location of these muscles mean that, in conjunction with *gluteus medius*, the adductor muscle group act to stabilise the hip and pelvis in three dimensions.[4]

All these stabilising qualities of muscles depend on a good 'positive running' posture at toe-off, optimising muscle length and hence hip and pelvic stability.

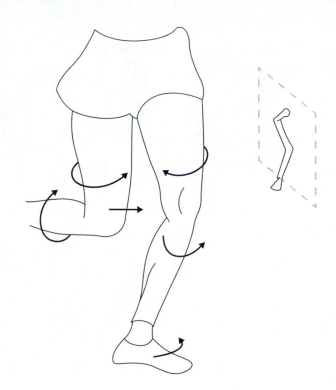

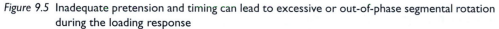

*Figure 9.5* Inadequate pretension and timing can lead to excessive or out-of-phase segmental rotation during the loading response

The hip provides the main driving force in running through the activity of strong muscles, such as the *iliopsoas*, the hip adductors, the gluteals and the hamstrings. The movements of the distal leg joints are initiated from here. This means that if hip motion forces are inadequate, it can lead, for example, to rotational discrepancies around the knee joint, abnormal shear forces around the patellofemoral joint and insufficient stiffness of the foot joint at subsequent points in the running cycle.

## The importance of the pelvis to injury-free running

The pelvis works like a large central lever, exerting a considerable moment of force on the attached muscles. It is for this reason that motion in this area plays a major role in running effectiveness. During the stance phase, the pelvis moves in all three anatomical planes: forward movement of the free (swing) side of the pelvis in the transverse plane (manifesting as internal rotation of the stance leg), upward movement of the free side of the pelvis in the frontal plane and anterior tilt of the pelvis in the sagittal plane.

The degree and speed of anterior tilt of the pelvis at the end of the stance phase is of critical importance to the quality of technique at toe-off. Excessive and uncontrollable tilt must be avoided. It occurs when, in the stance phase, the thigh extends further than functional extension in the hip would normally allow (Figure 9.6). Positive running seeks to limit this

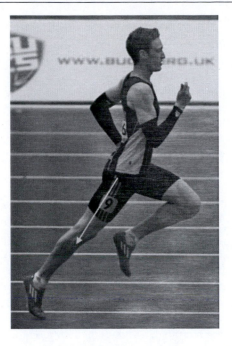

*Figure 9.6* Excessive thigh extension at toe-off (combination of hip extension and anterior pelvic tilt)

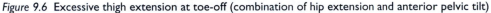

excessive stance leg thigh extension such that the thigh is relatively vertical at toe-off. Two factors are critical in achieving this:

1   Transport of energy, early in the stance phase, from the hip to the ankle via the knee by the biarticular *rectus femoris* and *gastrocnemius*. Owing to the early activity of the *gastrocnemius*, transport of energy occurs with the knee relatively flexed, and the stance phase can be ended early, i.e. before the knee extends. Top-level sprinters therefore have shorter contact times than less accomplished sprinters, resulting in a higher stride frequency.[5,6,7]

2   Early and sufficiently strong activity of the *abdominal/iliopsoas* complex. These muscles have to 'absorb' significant pelvic rotational (tilting) forces in the running motion. Given the force-length relationship of the abdominal muscles, whose force production is rapidly reduced when their length is not within the optimum range, this is only possible if the muscle group is working close to its optimum length. If contraction does not occur well before toe-off, or insufficient force is produced, excessive anterior pelvic tilt will occur.

Earlier and sufficient contraction of the abdominal muscles to prevent excessive anterior pelvic tilt, and early hip-to-knee energy transfer via the rectus femoris and gastrocnemius will allow 'toe-off' to occur with the thigh in a more vertical position.

In addition to reducing ground contact times, this facilitates more efficient, safer and faster recovery of the leg during swing as

1   There is less distance (shorter arc)
2   The 'swing-leg' lever is shorter
3   The muscles flexing the hip are in a more favourable length-tension range.

## Injury and the toe-off posture

It is vital to prevent uncontrolled, excessive anterior tilt of the pelvis at toe-off. When stabilisation of this forward tilt is inadequate, running efficiency is reduced and local structures are vulnerable to both acute and overload injury.

Injuries related to this uncontrolled tilt include:

- Traction-related injuries to the lower abdominal tissue, including inguinal disruption *rectus abdominus* insertion injury (enthesopathy)[8]
- Simple strains to the biarticular adductor muscles[9] and lower abdomen
- Hip joint overload, including femoroacetabular impingement[10]
- Pubic symphysis joint/capsular overload[11]
- Traction- and compression-related injuries to the ilioinguinal or genitofemoral nerves[2]

### The hamstring loading phase

During the initial part of the forward swing phase, there is little tension in the hamstrings and they effectively hang underneath the thigh (Figure 9.1 a–b). This is termed 'muscle-slack' and must be overcome before the elastic elements of the hamstring can be loaded effectively later in the swing phase. After toe-off, the distal end of the swing-leg shank rotates forward. At this time, the hamstrings are recruited, lengthening the musculotendinous unit and subjecting it to elastic stretch. This distal stretching moment should be accompanied by a proximal stretching moment from forward tilt of the pelvis. Both stretching moments should be distributed through the proximal and distal hamstring attachments in a coordinated manner.

---

**Muscle slack**

At rest, muscles are not taut. In fact, they dangle somewhat between origin and insertion. Given this 'dangling', the contractile elements of a muscle must shorten substantially at the first stage of contraction (or its attachment points must move further apart because of external forces) before significant forces can be produced in order to move or stabilise a joint.[12] In other words, the slack must first be taken up before the muscle can contribute meaningfully to force production.

---

Swing phase stretch and loading of the proximal end of the lead leg hamstring (Figure 9.5) occurs in response to anterior tilt of the pelvis. This anterior tilt is due to forceful contraction of the contralateral iliopsoas to initiate flexion of the trail leg hip. Stretch and loading of the distal hamstring occur as the knee extends (Figure 9.1b – reversal).

It is often assumed that the hamstring acts 'eccentrically' during the forward swing and reversal phases (Figures 9.1 and 9.2); however whilst the musculotendinous unit is lengthening, the hamstring muscles will be acting isometrically or even contracting slightly in the production of very high muscular forces.

Besides these requirements for isometric contractions, it is important to bear in mind that the negative muscle-tendon work of the hamstrings increases substantially with sprinting speed.[13]

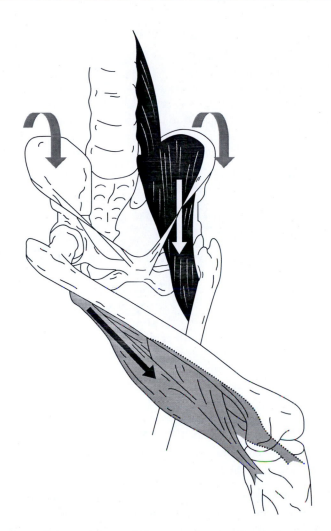

*Figure 9.7* Contraction of the m. iliopsoas (white arrow) causes forward rotation of the pelvis (grey arrows), which in turn leads to loading of elastic parts of the muscle during contraction of the contralateral hamstring (black arrow)

## Injury and the hamstring loading phase

If anterior tilt of the pelvis is not well-controlled at toe-off, the pelvis will subsequently tilt posteriorly after toe-off and during hamstring loading, which interferes with control of the hamstring loading phase described above. Practical experience shows that constant uncontrolled forward rotation of the pelvis in runners often leads to reduced force production in the hamstrings. Together with insufficient or badly timed trail leg hip flexion immediately after toe-off, this can lead to intramuscular disturbance and strain of the hamstrings or the co-contracting adductor muscles. Under these circumstances, fatigue may also play an important part,[14] and therefore, it is recommended that running whilst fatigued be postponed until the final stages of rehabilitation, after sound technique has been firmly re-established.

---

**Why leg curls are bad for running technique**

When considering training and rehabilitation, it is sensible to apply the principles of *specificity*. In running, the muscle fibres of the hamstrings act isometrically, at the optimum length and at the optimum pennation angle. Strength exercises including leg curls utilise the hamstrings in a non-functional manner as they emphasise concentric and eccentric muscle actions as opposed to the isometric conditions they are required to operate in during locomotion. These types of exercises may therefore impair the optimal muscle action control systems, having a negative effect on the contribution of the hamstrings during running.[15]

---

## The scissors motion

In the scissors motion, the trail leg moves forward, mainly owing to forceful activity of *iliopsoas*. At the same time, the extended lead leg swings backwards (swing leg retraction). This backward swing of the leg makes a major contribution to stability during the following stance phase. By extending the leg before initial contact, the athlete develops tension in the limb. This 'pre-tension' action that occurs just prior to initial foot contact serves to optimise proximal to distal energy transport and neuromuscular firing via a sequence of stretching down the kinetic chain from the hip to the ankle. During this immediate pre-contact phase, precise timing of ankle plantar flexion can be observed in the best sprinters. This 'scissoring' sequence is closely linked, in a reflex pattern, to the movement (hip and knee flexion) of the trailing leg.[16]

This 'swing-leg retraction' with a tensioning effect can only really be achieved if the leading leg is in the right position at toe-off and there is sufficient vertical movement to execute the scissors motion. This can be seen in Figures 9.6 and 9.8.

### Injury and the scissors motion

In the scissors motion, elastic loading in the hamstring is continued and is followed by unloading of elastic energy after the knee has extended. This loading and unloading takes place while the stance leg is stabilised by the muscle-tendon complex.[1] This is the point at which

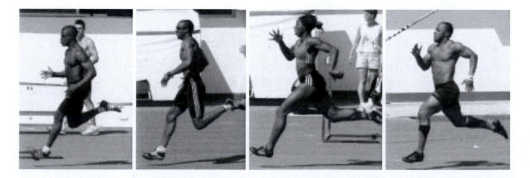

*Figure 9.8* The scissors motion, from left to right: a positive running posture (far left) gets progressively more negative

hamstring strain may occur if the preceding actions fail to achieve sufficient stability in the leading leg. The biceps femoris is especially at risk, with the greatest peak excusion of the hamstrings during sprinting.[17]

---

### The danger of over-striding

Over-striding as a result of insufficient scissors motion may put the hamstrings at greater risk of injury, and perhaps also the *adductor magnus* as a co-contractor in hip extension. During rehabilitation, running with a tail wind should be postponed until the final phase, when it will help to emphasise active landing and to de-emphasise over-striding.

---

## *Full contact*

Landing with active plantar flexion of the foot results in optimum tension in the leg at the point of full contact. This largely reduces muscle slack in the muscles that are about to be loaded with elastic stretching, and the complex energy transport pattern can be initiated almost immediately. During this initial stance phase, it is crucial that the ground reaction force must also have a horizontal component, brought about by transport of energy from the knee to the hip by the hamstrings. The hamstrings will thereby be active from the point at which the lower-leg rotates forward in the flight phase (Figure 9.1 a–b) until well into the stance phase (Figure 9.2a–c).[18]

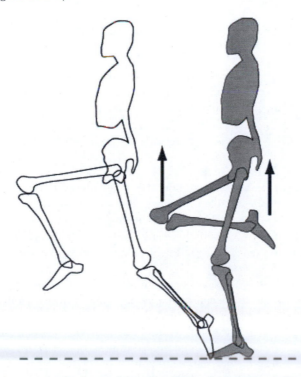

*Figure 9.9* In positive running the knee of the swing leg at mid-stance must have clearly moved past the knee of the stance leg

Muscular co-contractions in the stance leg, which are built up just before ground contact, provide the necessary stiffness in the knee and ankle. In positive running, this is supported by the position of the swing leg; at the point when the foot is directly below the hip, the knee of the swing leg is already well in front of the knee of the stance leg (see Figure 9.7). In this position, the movement of the swing leg (flexed at the hip with the knee upwards and the heel moving towards the hamstring/buttock) will reinforce the tension in the stance leg through a spinal reflex arc. The stance leg can thus exert more force and hence is optimally protected against the influence of unpredictable external forces.

## The importance of foot placement in preventing running injuries

Foot placement is critical to assess in the running athlete, and improvements should be coached if deemed sub-optimal. Forces associated with mis-timing and/or mis-placement of the foot that are either excessive or poorly absorbed can lead to injuries and dysfunctions, such as patellofemoral pain, patellar and Achilles tendinopathy, leg and foot bone stress injury and iliotibial band syndrome. Although these injuries are more commonly seen in middle-distance runners, athletes with malalignment are also at risk during high-speed running. As a consequence, an obvious place to start within rehabilitation is to improve pelvic muscle function.

Moreover, it is important to consider running form. In particular, the anterior knee is especially vulnerable to injury at full contact because of the braking forces that develop if the trailing leg does not catch up fast enough with the leading leg during the scissor motion, or because of inadequate activity of the vastus muscles.[19] Unstable ankle joints or forefoot pronation due to forefoot varus alignment may also interfere with normal variability in leg segment movements during the full contact phase if the scissor motion is inadequate.

A correlation has been found between reduced segment variability and patellofemoral pain in runners,[20] while reducing hip adduction during hip flexion through real-time feedback leads to substantially reduced patellofemoral pain.[21]

### Heel-off

In good technique, the foot plantar flexes early in the stance phase, so that there is no, or very little, dorsiflexion of the ankle throughout the stance phase. This means that the elastic parts are loaded and unloaded, while the contractile elements of the muscles contract isometrically at their optimum length. This is especially important in the calf muscles, owing to the large counteracting forces (3–4 x body weight) and the critical force-length relationship of, for example, soleus, so that even slight dorsiflexion is enough to place the muscle outside its effective range.

The quadriceps are unlikely to play a significant part in generating positive work during running, as they act primarily as a facilitator for energy transfer from the hip to the ground.[22] Transport of energy from the knee to the ankle is optimal when plantar flexion of the foot takes place as early as possible in the stance phase when the knee is still relatively flexed and the 'rope function' (due to high musculotendinous stiffness) of the *gastrocnemius* may be very effective. At the same time as the heel elevates (Figure 9.2.c–d), the free side of the pelvis must also be raised. This increases the vertical component of the heel-off.

A rule for proper timing of the movement of the free side of the pelvis is that the free (swing leg) side must be higher than the stance leg side when the heel has clearly left the ground.

## Injury and heel-off

At toe-off, the ankle joint is plantar flexed in order to facilitate forward thrust of the body. This places great strain on the forefoot, the arch of the foot and the tarsal bones, and may even lead to stress fractures of the navicular or metatarsals. As the arch of the foot acts like a spring, which unloads in the second half of the stance phase, incorrect foot placement during high-speed running may result in high forces in the longitudinal aponeurosis, where partial ruptures may occur.

As activity of *quadratus plantae* plays a part in tensioning *flexor digitorum*, incorrect foot placement may also interfere with this function and may eventually predispose the athlete to medial biomechanical overload syndrome (discussed in greater detail in chapter 25).

High tension in the ankle and foot joints is specifically important during the contact phase (Figure 9.2 b–d) for maximal elastic loading of the Achilles tendon. This loading may be determined by the timing of the contractile element (the calf muscles) in generating force, rather than the force itself.[23] During high-speed running, the limited time from mid-stance to toe-off may thus restrict performance, because the time window for unloading the tendons becomes too short.[7]

If sufficient time is not available to load the elastic element and/or overcome muscle slack, the tendon is at great risk of injury, and Achilles tendon injuries are therefore frequently seen in high-speed running. Calf muscle strains also occur, for the actions of these muscles load the Achilles tendon. With insufficient stability of the forefoot and hindfoot, and excessive dorsiflexion of the ankle joint, the calf muscle strain is mostly on the medial side, making the medial musculotendinous junction a common injury site. Therefore, exercises that condition the feet to be stable and strong are clearly essential for mastering high-speed running.

## Movements in the transverse plane

Rotations in the transverse plane appear more or less isolated from movements in the other planes. However, there is a close link between transverse plane rotations and swing-leg retraction. Rotation of the trunk causes the free (swing) side of the pelvis to move forward. The resulting internal rotation in the extending (stance) lower limb has an eccentric influence on the *gluteus maximus*. This muscle has to extend the hip with great speed and force during the flight and stance phases, which is a problem given the force-speed characteristics of muscles. This eccentric impact of torsion in the trunk to some extent facilitates the *gluteus maximus*, for it reduces the contraction speed of the muscle and hence increases its contraction force.

In conjunction with internal or external rotation of the lower leg, internal rotation of the stance-leg hip performs a second function during the stance phase. These rotations in the transverse plane make running stable and resistant to disruption,[24] and hence are essential to execution of the technique.

A third function of trunk rotation in high-speed running may be to store elastic energy in the vertebral column by increasing and decreasing curvature, compressing and decompressing intervertebral discs and stretching and shortening intervertebral ligaments during trunk rotation and counter-rotation.[25]

## Injury and movement in the transverse plane

If the running technique involves insufficient or excessive trunk, pelvic, thigh or lower-leg transverse plane rotation, it causes imbalance in the optimum length of agonistic and antagonistic muscles, reducing the efficiency and safety of key propulsive movements such as hip flexion.

In the trunk, rotational dysfunction of the vertebral column, or reduced elasticity of the intervertebral discs may lead to abdominal muscle strain and cumulative injury to the intervertebral and facet joints of the lower back.

Because rotation occurs relatively high in the lumbar spine, thoracolumbar dysfunction may play a part in symptoms that may even be manifested as abductor strain, or lumbosacral or sacroiliac pain. Although not frequently mentioned, this dysfunction, which is due to repeated excessive rotation of the trunk, may well cause referred pain in the area of the corresponding spinal nerves (T12 and L1).

Excessive hip adduction may cause the foot to cross the mid-line on landing and lead to compensating contralateral trunk side-flexion with eccentric activation of the hip abductors occurring to control this movement.

Excessive pelvic drop (the 'Trendelenburg' sign) may be seen as compensation for weakness of the contralateral hip abductors, possibly due to previous injury. However, there is poor correlation between pelvic drop and hip abductor strength,[26] so weakness of other components in the closed kinetic chain may play a part, as may deficits in neuromuscular timing. In rehabilitation, assessing and addressing key deficits along the kinetic will be important.

## Heel-off to toe-off

At the end of the stance phase, many of the main muscles (gluteus maximus, hamstrings and calf) display greatly decreasing or even totally absent EMG activity. This occurs at the same time as increasing activity in other muscles, such as the abdominals and the *iliopsoas*. The relatively low activity in one muscle group and increasing activity in the other must be well timed, and may well be the component of the running cycle during which the system comes under greatest pressure.

## Injury and heel-off to toe-off

### Lack of hip stability

Injury problems around the hip area may originate in the hip joint itself, i.e. a range-of-motion (ROM) deficit due to femoroacetabular impingement or intra-articular pathologies. Combined lesions with adductor strain also occur, because these muscles can no longer perform their stabilising function around the hip, partly because of reduced stiffness and perhaps also due to proprioceptive deficits. As leg muscle activity is low during heel-off to toe-off, passive stability is of the utmost importance.

The pelvis therefore needs to be in the correct position, and so the athlete must have sufficient strength and neurodynamic timing in the abdominal muscles to generate force closure of the sacroiliac joint and prevent excessive anterior tilt of the pelvis. In poor running technique, the abdominal muscles are often activated after toe-off and hence fail to protect the hip/pelvic area.

## Lack of hip mobility

The athlete must obviously have sufficient hip flexion to initiate powerful movement in high-speed running. However, the range of hip extension is often overlooked. Reduced hip extension may result in insufficient action of the stance leg and disrupt forward motion of the hip due to insufficient pretension of the psoas muscle. Athletes will try to maintain an upright trunk position, and compensation for reduced hip extension may manifest in anterior tilt of the pelvis. This may lead to compression lesions of the low lumbar intervertebral disc and facet joints, and in some cases compression of the fifth lumbar nerve root in the lumbosacral tunnel.[27] Besides lower back pain, this may also make the athlete vulnerable to hamstring strain.

Another consequence of limited hip mobility might be excessive stance-leg rotational strain. Maltracking of the patella producing anterior knee pain is a potential consequence. Hyperlaxity of the knee joint may increase this risk, especially since in top-level sprinters, the knee never reaches full extension. As a result, plantar flexion of the ankle is less pronounced in top-level sprinters, and the joint is rapidly dorsi-flexed into a neutral position after toe-off.[18]

## Summary

As an answer to the lack of effective ways to treat many of the running injuries, we focussed on improving running form and skills by the model of positive running, a model which explicitly refers to the correct structure of the technique. Toe-off is the point at which the quality of the motion in this model is measured.

The differences between good, protective technique and poor, injury-prone technique are discussed and also the possible injuries that can occur. Pointing these injuries to a certain moment in the running cycle, however, always remains arbitrary.

The stabilising qualities of muscles are emphasized because the 'positive running' posture optimises muscle length and hence hip and pelvic stability.

It is from here that energy is transported early in the stance phase via the knee by the biarticular rectus femoris and gastrocnemius.

Also, the importance is shown of the link between movements in the transverse plane and swing-leg retraction. The latter also facilitates the optimal use of the elastic properties of the tendons as important speed facilitators.

As a result, the positive running model has a positive influence on the first part of the stance phase, which appears to be the most important period in generating speed and preventing injury.

## Notes

1 Seyfarth A., Geyer, H., & Herr, H. (2003), Swing-leg retraction: A simple control model for stable running. *Journal of Experimental Biology*, *206*: 2547–55.
2 Davids, K., Glazier, P., Araújo, D., & Bartlett, R. (2003). Movement systems as dynamical systems: The functional role of variability and its implications for sports medicine. *Sports Medicine*. *33*: 245–60.
3 Vleeming, A., Snijders, C. J., Stoeckart, R., & Mens, J.M.A. (1997). The role of the sacroiliac joints in coupling between spine, pelvis, legs and arms. In A.M.V. Vleeming, T. Dorman, C. Snijders, & R. Stoeckart (Eds.). *Movement, Stability & Low Back Pain*. New York: Churchill Livingstone.
4 Morrenhof, J. W. (1989). *Stabilisation of the human hip joint, a kinematical study*. Leiden, The Netherlands: Leiden University Press.

5  Dorn, T. W., Schache, A. G., & Pandy, M. G. (2012). Muscular strategy shift in human running: dependence of running speed on hip and ankle muscle performance. *Journal of Experimental Biology, 215*: 1944–56.

6  Miller, L. H., Umberger, B. R., & Caldwel, G. E. (2012). Sensitivity of maximum sprinting speed to characteristic parameters of the muscle force–velocity relationship. *Journal of Biomechanics, 45*: 1406–13.

7  Weyand, P. G., Sternlight, D. B., Bellizzi, M. J., & Wright, S. (2000). Faster top running speeds are achieved with greater ground forces not more rapid leg movements. *Journal of Applied Physiology, 89*: 1991–9.

8  Kluin, J., den Hoed, P. T., van Linschoten, R., IJzerman, J. C., & van Steensel, C. J. (2004). Endoscopic Evaluation and Treatment of Groin Pain in the Athlete. *American Journal of Sports Medicine, 32*: 944–9.

9  Weir, A., Veger, S.A.S., van de Sande, H.B.A., Bakker, E.W.P., de Jonge, S., & Tol, J. L. (2009). A manual therapy technique for chronic adductor-related groin pain in athletes: a case series. *Scandinavian Journal of Medicine & Science in Sports, 19*: 616–20.

10  Fricker, P. A. (2007). How do you treat chronic groin pain? In D. MacAuley, & T. M. Best (Eds.), *Evidence-based sports medicine* (p. 389–404). London: BMJ Publishing Group.

11  Choi, H., McCartney, M., & Best, T. M. (2011). Treatment of osteitis pubis and osteomyelitis of the pubic symphysis in athletes: A systematic review. *British Journal of Sports Medicine, 45*: 57–64.

12  Higashihara, A., Ono, T., Kubota, J., Okuwaki, T., & Fukubayashi T. (2010). Functional differences in the activity of the hamstring muscles with increasing running speed. *Journal of Sports Sciences. 28*: 1085–92.

13  Thelen, D. G., Chumanov, E. S., Sherry, M. A., & Heiderscheit, B. C. (2006). Neuromusculoskeletal models provide insights into the mechanisms and rehabilitation of hamstring strains. *Medicine & Science in Sports & Exercise, 38*: 135–41.

14  Pinniger, G. J, Steele, J. R., & Groeller, H. (2000). Does fatigue induced by repeated dynamic efforts affect hamstring muscle function? *Medicine & Science in Sports & Exercise, 32*: 647–53.

15  Proske, U., & Allen, T. J. (2005). Damage to skeletal muscle from eccentric exercise. *Exercise and Sport Sciences Reviews, 33*: 98–104.

16  Kyröläinen, H., Avela, J., & Komi, P. V. (2005). Changes in muscle activity with increasing running speed. *Journal of Sport Sciences, 23*: 1101–9.

17  Thelen, D. G., Chumanov, E. S., Hoeerth, D. M., Heiderscheit, B. C., Best, T.M., & Swanson, S. C. (2004). Hamstring muscle kinematics during sprinting. *Medicine & Science in Sports & Exercise, 36*: S2.

18  Novacheck, T. F. (1998). The biomechanics of running. *Gait and Posture. 7*: 77–95.

19  Montgomery III, W. H., Pink, M., & Perry, J. (1994). Electromyographic analysis of hip and knee musculature during running. *American Journal of Sports Medicine, 22*: 272–8.

20  Hamill, J., van Emmerik, R.E.A., Heiderscheit, B. C., & Li, L. (1999). A dynamical systems approach to lower extremity running injuries. *Clinical Biomechanics, 14*: 297–308.

21  Noehren, B., Scholz, J., & Davis, I. (2011). The effect of real-time gait retraining on hip kinematics, pain and function in subjects with patellofemoral pain syndrome. *British Journal of Sports Medicine, 45*: 691–6.

22  Bezodis, I. N., Kerwin, D. G., & Salo, A. T. (2008). Lower-Limb Mechanics during the Support Phase of Maximum-Velocity Sprint Running. *Medicine & Science in Sports & Exercise, 40*: 707–15.

23  Kubo, K., Kanehisa, H., Kawakami, Y., & Fukunaga, T. (2001). Influences of repetitive muscle contractions with different modes on tendon elasticity in vivo. *Journal of Applied Physiology, 91*: 277–82.

24  Glazier, P. S., Wheat, J. S., Pease, D. L., & Bartlett, R. M. (2006). Movement system variability. In K. Davids, S. Bennett, & K. Newell (Eds.), *The interface of biomechanics and motor control: Dynamics systems theory and the functional role of movement variability* (p. 49–69). Champaign: Human Kinetics.

25  Abitol, M. (1995). The integrated function of the lumbar spine and sacroiliac joint. In A. Vleeming, V. Mooney, C. Snijders, & T. Dorman (Eds.). *Second interdisciplinary world congress on low back pain* (pp. 61–73). San Diego, CA: University of California, San Diego, School of Medicine.

26  Burnet, E., & Pidcoe, P. (2009). Isometric gluteus medius muscle torque and frontal plane pelvic motion during running. *Journal of Sports Science and Medicine, 8*: 284–8.

27  Orchard, J. W., Farhart, P., & Leopold, C. (2004). Lumbar spine region pathology and hamstring and calf injuries in athletes: is there a connection? *British Journal of Sports Medicine, 38*: 502–4.

## Chapter 10

# Landing mechanics in injury prevention and performance rehabilitation

*Julie Steele and Jeremy Sheppard*

## Introduction

Landings are an extremely common athletic manoeuvre, whether they be a single-limb landing during a running stride or after leaping to catch a ball, a two-footed landing following a vertical jump, or landing on an unstable surface, such as a surfboard, after performing an aerial manoeuvre. Irrespective of the task, the landing phase starts the moment an athlete contacts the supporting surface[1] and continues until their centre of mass stops moving downward and their momentum is zero. From a biomechanical perspective, landings require optimal technical performance while ensuring efficient absorption of the impact forces generated at foot-ground contact to minimise the potential for injury. Landing tasks, particularly those involving high impact forces, have been associated with a variety of injuries, especially ankle ligament sprains, patellar tendon injuries and anterior cruciate ligament (ACL) ruptures.

Despite being a fundamental component of so many movement skills, it is only in recent years that coaching manuals and the sports science literature has included precise instructional information on the biomechanics of landings. However, we need to understand biomechanical principles underlying landings if we are to effectively instruct athletes on how to maximise their performance while minimising their injury risk.

By the end of this chapter, the reader should understand:

- The biomechanics of landings
- What happens when landings go wrong
- The role of landing training in athletic performance and injury prevention
- How to design a well-considered landing training program for elite athletes.

## Biomechanics of landings

### Types of landings in sport

The type of landings performed in sport are influenced by numerous factors, including:

- constraints imposed by the rules of a sport (e.g. not being able to take another step after receiving a pass, such as in netball)
- the need to simultaneously perform another skill (e.g. catch a ball)
- positioning of teammates or opponents
- the environment in which you perform the landing (e.g. landing on a narrow beam in gymnastics requires a different strategy from landing on a wide soft mat).

It is imperative to appreciate the multifaceted nature of landing tasks. Landing biomechanics studies typically focus on tasks that can easily be standardised in the laboratory, such as drop landings, where study participants simply step off a platform before landing. The landing strategy employed in these tasks, however, is very different from what we see in sport. Therefore, implications arising from research investigating drop-landing tasks should be treated with caution when considering what happens in whole jump-landing tasks.

Other aspects of landings should also be considered when appraising research studies. For example:

- Was the landing a single- or double-limb landing, because these landings differ with respect to important biomechanical considerations? The greater ground reaction forces generated when landing on one limb and an inability to effectively attenuate this force can increase the risks for injuries, such as cartilage lesions, ligament ruptures, bone bruises and menisci tears in single-limb landings.[2]
- What must an athlete do following the landing? If a gymnast or volleyball player has to jump upward immediately following foot-ground contact, the duration of the landing is likely to be brief and the amount of knee flexion less. This is due to the need to maximise the stretch-shortening cycle characteristic of rebound type activities. However, if the landing is the terminal phase of the task, the athlete can focus on shock absorption and regaining stability at foot-ground contact.

> Ideally, a whole jump-landing task that replicates the movement of interest should be used to investigate the biomechanics of a specific landing task, and laboratory-based investigations should replicate game-like movements.

### Biomechanical considerations governing landings

In jump-landing tasks we propel ourselves upward until we momentarily reach the peak of our flight above the ground. It is at this point that we possess maximum potential energy. The amount of potential energy will depend upon our body mass ($m$), our acceleration due to gravity ($g$) and the height ($h$) our centre of mass is above the ground ($mgh$). The higher above the ground and the greater our body mass, the greater our potential energy (see Figure 10.1).

After reaching the flight peak we begin to 'fall' back towards the ground, converting our potential energy into kinetic energy. Immediately prior to ground contact, our kinetic energy is equivalent to half our body mass multiplied by our velocity ($v$) squared ($\frac{1}{2}mv^2$). Because mass and gravity is constant for a given landing, it is the height that we raise our centre of mass above the ground that ultimately governs our potential, and in turn, our kinetic energy at foot-ground contact. An upward force from the ground, which we generate at foot-ground impact, must then dissipate this kinetic energy when our foot contacts the ground.

The first 50 milliseconds of a landing are often referred to as the passive or impact phase because you are unlikely to be able to activate your muscles in response to the sudden, high-frequency impact forces that are applied when your foot collides with the ground.[3] During the subsequent active phase of landing, however, additional eccentric muscle activity can be generated to resist the lower-extremity 'collapsing' into flexion and, in turn, assist in bringing your body's momentum to zero. Interestingly, humans can predict impact forces and then use complex multijoint solutions to try and attenuate the loads experienced at foot-ground contact. The

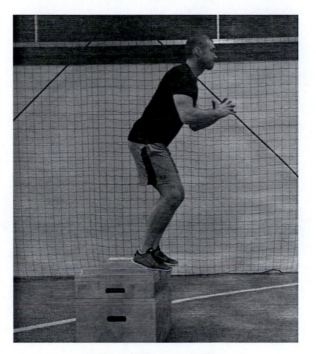

$$PE = Mb \times g \times H$$

*Figure 10.1* Variables that contribute to potential and kinetic energy

ankle, knee and hip joints are the primary contributors to shock absorption, with muscles crossing the joints assisting to dissipate energy. The spine, intervertebral discs, and trunk muscles also contribute to shock absorption, albeit to a lesser extent than the lower limb joints. Because the human body is a kinetic chain, if one of the major joints is compromised during a landing, the energy is likely to be transferred proximally to the next joint within the chain (see chapter 7).

The vertical ground reaction forces generated during the impact phase of landings range from about two times body weight (BW) in activities such as jogging (Figure 10.2) to approximately 4–11 BW in abrupt activities such as landing after catching a ball in netball or double-limb gymnastic landings from various heights. Simulated parachute landings with vertical descent velocities between 4.6 and 6.7m/s can cause vertical ground reaction forces exceeding 11 BW.[4]

Irrespective of the task, the vertical ground reaction forces generated at foot-ground contact increase in direct response to increases in drop height and descent velocity. The rate at which the vertical ground reaction force is applied to the lower limb is also important, because the tissues responsible for absorbing force, such as muscle, bone and the heel pad, are viscoelastic (i.e. they are sensitive to the rate of loading). As the loading rate increases, the stiffness of these tissues increases so they are able to absorb more force per unit of deformation.

Each time your foot contacts the ground at landing it also generates a horizontal frictional or 'braking' force component. In fact, to stop going forward rapidly upon landing can only be achieved by applying an appropriate opposing horizontal frictional force; the greater the desired deceleration, the larger must be the frictional force.[5] This is why it is more difficult

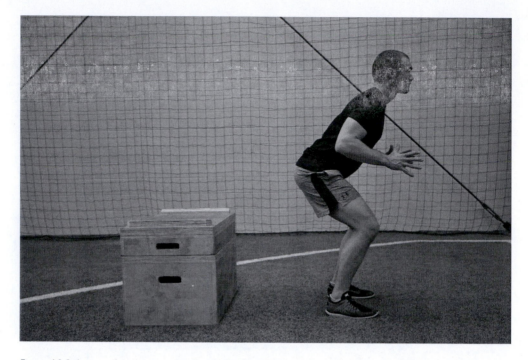

*Figure 10.2* Impact forces generated upon landing may be up to 11 times body weight

to land and stop sliding forward on ice than on grass. The horizontal ground reaction force component during tasks such as running is, on average, 0.45 BW.

In tasks where athletes must stop abruptly, such as after leaping forward to catch a netball, peak braking forces as high as 6.5 BW have been recorded and are thought to contribute to injuries such as anterior cruciate ligament (ACL) ruptures.[5] These forces, however, are influenced by factors such as the pathway of your centre of mass at initial foot-ground impact and the frictional characteristics between the landing surface and your footwear. To reduce excessive braking forces at landing, you should encourage athletes to jump upwards more than horizontally, therefore converting some of their horizontal momentum to vertical momentum at landing. Also, ensure their footwear is appropriate to the surfaces they train and compete upon.

Excessive and repeated ground reaction forces combined with a high loading rate can increase the risk for ligament damage, articular degeneration and chronic musculoskeletal disorders. Although most athletes can withstand the ground reaction forces generated in their sport, individuals with a musculoskeletal misalignment or unusual landing technique are at risk of injury.[5] Understanding key factors that affect the ground reaction forces generated in jump-landing sports and teaching good landing technique is imperative to ensure these forces are minimised to reduce loading of the body and to optimise performance.

## Key considerations for good landing technique

Although it is beyond the scope of this chapter to highlight every biomechanical factor likely to influence landing technique, some of the key considerations that will influence loading are outlined below.

### Actively bend your ankles, knees and hips

During landings, the lower limb is commonly depicted as a spring, which is used to absorb external loading via a complex multijoint solution. The lower limb spring must have both compliance and strength to be able to absorb the impact forces generated at landing, but in a controlled manner so that the lower limb does not collapse. If an athlete displays a low range of motion, particularly in the ankle, knee and hip joints during impact absorption, it is generally described as a 'stiff landing'.

Landings with too much leg stiffness, combined with high ground reaction forces and rapid loading rates, have been associated with catastrophic bone injuries, whereas too little leg stiffness where there is excessive joint range of motion can lead to soft tissue injuries.[6] It is therefore important that athletes actively bend their ankles, knees and hips during the impact absorption phase of foot-ground contact to cushion the ground reaction forces. Numerous studies have confirmed that *active* lower limb flexion is the key factor in impact force attenuation and energy absorption, rather than just having a bent but rigid knee (see Figure 10.3).[7,8]

Athletes who contact the ground with an extended knee and then actively flex the joint increase the time over which the forces are absorbed and, in turn, reduce peak loading. Increasing knee flexion during landing will also affect the musculature surrounding the knee. For example the antigravity muscles, such as the quadriceps muscles, are in a more advantageous position to absorb kinetic energy at impact when knee flexion is increased, thereby reducing reaction forces that propagate up the lower limb kinetic chain.[7]

Actively bending the lower limb joints when landing also increases your stability by lowering your centre of mass, assuming that your line of gravity remains well within your base

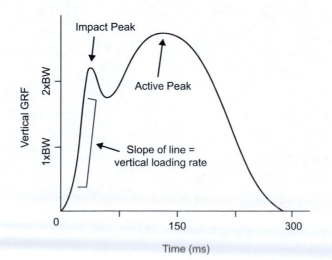

*Figure 10.3* Force-time graph

of support. Research has shown that female soccer players who display low flexion motion in the sagittal plane during a drop landing task also exhibit greater frontal plane loading at the knee.[8] Females who have limited flexion motion in the sagittal plane are thought to rely on passive restraints in the frontal plane to control deceleration of their total body centre of mass, possibly predisposing them to risk of ACL injury.[8]

While encouraging increased knee flexion, athletes should avoid postures that have excessive external foot rotation, internal or external tibial rotation, knee valgus or an abducted and internally rotated hip, because these postures have also been associated with higher valgus and internal rotation loads at the knee and, in turn, an increased risk of injury.[9]

Although it fosters impact absorption, increased knee flexion during landing has been identified as a strong predictor of patellar tendinopathy, whereby athletes with that condition land with more knee flexion, which increases patellar tendon loading.[10] Coaches involved in sports that have high rates of patellar tendinopathy, such as volleyball, should closely monitor the jump-landing load (frequency) of their athletes to reduce patellar tendon loading and, in turn, the likelihood of developing patellar tendinopathy (see chapter 15).

### Avoiding exaggerated 'striding out'

During single-limb landings in which you have high horizontal momentum prior to contacting the ground, it is imperative that you avoid adopting an exaggerated 'striding out' posture (see Figure 10.4) because this posture has been associated with excessively high horizontal braking forces and, in turn, ACL injury. Encouraging athletes to jump upward rather then merely forward can reduce these high braking forces. Jumping upward on the move enables some of your horizontal momentum to be converted to vertical momentum, thereby decreasing the horizontal distance you travel and, in turn, decreasing the braking forces generated at landing.[5]

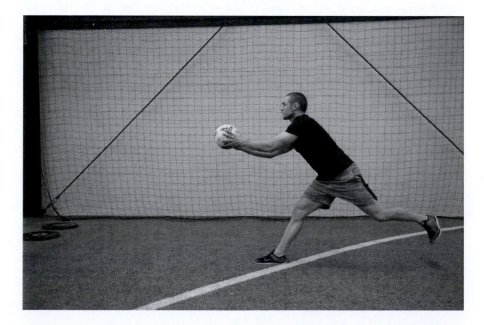

*Figure 10.4* Catching with an incorrect striding out posture

Jumping upward also allows you to eliminate the exaggerated 'striding out' position by reducing the foot-hip distance at ground contact, and allowing greater knee flexion. This is particularly important in single-limb landing tasks, as single-limb landing manoeuvres are typically much stiffer than double-limb landings, due to a relative lack of knee flexion.[2]

## Maintain a neutral foot posture

The ground reaction forces generated at landing are also influenced by whether you initially contact the ground on your heel, forefoot or some other part of your foot. In recent years there has been extensive debate in the scientific literature, stimulated by the barefoot running trend, about the influence of foot biomechanics on the impact forces generated at landing. Although most would agree that athletes should land with the foot neutrally aligned to eliminate excessive ankle add-abduction, internal rotation or dorsiflexion, their footfall pattern is affected by numerous factors, including the peak height attained above the ground, their approach momentum and the nature of the landing surface and footwear.

When the predominant direction of movement during descent is vertical, and when landing from a higher height, athletes tend to plantar-flex their feet and contact the ground with the forefoot, followed by rapid dorsiflexion after ground contact. In a study of trained paratroopers, 69 per cent landed on their forefoot, despite all having been trained to use a flatfoot landing technique. Landing on the forefoot enables an extra segment, the foot, to be included at foot-ground contact and, in turn, the ability to dissipate the landing forces over increased time.[4] When landing on the forefoot, however, the high-impact forces are borne by the small bones of the foot and can lead to bone injuries. In single-limb leaps to land, athletes typically hold their foot in dorsiflexion and land on the heels first, creating a stiffer landing, as discussed previously. It is important to acknowledge that motion of the foot at the ankle will also influence the range of motion over which the ankle joint plantar flexor muscles can act, in turn causing the knee and hip extensor muscles to contribute more to force dissipation.

## Ensure coordinated neuromuscular control

Efficient neuromuscular control during landing tasks is an important factor to ensure knee joint stability and protection at foot-ground contact. During high impact landings involving a predominantly vertical descent, the ground reaction force will cause the lower limb joints to flex. The antigravity extensor muscles, such as the quadriceps and calf muscles, eccentrically resist this flexion to prevent the lower limb 'collapsing' and to dissipate energy during landing. Because this muscular force development takes time, our motor control system behaves in a predictive manner, recruiting the relevant muscles before initial foot-ground contact in order to set the initial lower limb compliance to a level deemed appropriate to withstand the ensuing impact force.[4]

During single-limb horizontal leaping movements, the hamstring muscles are typically activated before initial foot-ground contact and before the quadriceps.[11] This helps provide a counterbalancing force to resist the quadriceps-induced anterior tibial translation and, in turn, play an important role as synergists to reduce ACL stress and decrease injury susceptibility. Flexing the knee during landing also helps to increase the hamstring's ability to generate posterior tibial drawer and to provide secondary restraint to anterior tibial translation (see Figure 10.5).[12]

Coordinated quadriceps-hamstring muscle recruitment is essential to dynamically stabilise the knee. A study of athletes who had ruptured their ACL but could still perform abrupt

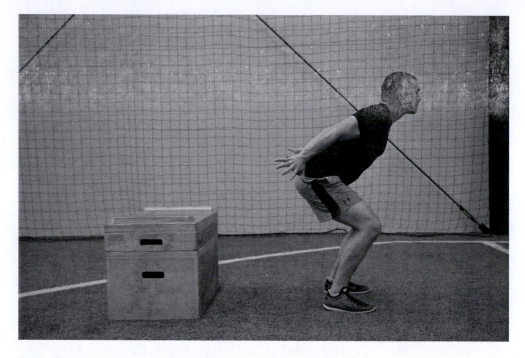

*Figure 10.5* Landing from a jump with hamstrings contracted reduces translational stress on the ACL

single-limb landings showed that these athletes were able to synchronise their peak hamstring muscle activity to better coincide with the high anterior shear forces generated at the knee joint just after initial foot-ground contact.[11] This better synchrony enables the hamstring muscles to stabilise the limb against giving-way episodes via increased joint compression and posterior tibial drawer, at a time when the ACL would be most vulnerable to injury.

Interestingly, males have been shown to display muscle synchrony patterns that are thought to be more protective of the ACL than females, possibly accounting for the higher susceptibility of females to non-contact ACL injuries compared to males.[13] Athletes need training activities to enable them to develop optimal muscle recruitment strategies, combined with adequate muscle strength, to ensure joint integrity during landings associated with their sport.

### Don't neglect trunk motion

Traditionally, athletes were encouraged to land with an erect trunk to enhance their stability by ensuring the line of gravity remained well within the limits of their base of support. In team sports, however, trunk posture at landing is often dictated by the need to avoid making contact with an opponent or equipment (such as the net in volleyball), or the need to catch a ball. For this reason we recommend that you should land with your torso upright and facing

Landing mechanics 129

forwards (i.e. not laterally flexed) and with your knees and feet pointing in the direction of travel.[9] However, active trunk flexion during landing can produce concomitant increases in knee and hip flexion and, in turn, less injury risk compared to landing with an erect trunk.[12]

Increased knee and hip flexion can also favourably alter the insertion angle and increase passive tension in the hamstring muscles, potentially providing the hamstring muscles with a mechanical advantage for resisting anterior tibial translation.[12] However, whether active trunk flexion should be encouraged will depend upon the skill level and physical conditioning of your athletes, and the constraints of their sport described above.

## When landings go wrong

Landing-related injuries frequently occur in sports that involve repetitive landings, such as volley-ball, basketball and gymnastics or following high-velocity descents, such as landings after para-chuting from a plane. Many of these injuries are associated with inadequate shock attenuation during the landing action, which leads to injuries, such as articular cartilage damage, ligament ruptures, bone bruises and menisci tears.[2] Apart from the short-term disruption to an athlete's training and competing schedule as a result of injury, injuries can have devastating long-term consequences and terminate involvement in sport for life. For example, after an ACL rupture, many athletes are predisposed to the lifelong negative health consequences associated with osteo-arthritis. Interestingly, approximately 70 per cent of ACL injuries do not involve direct physical contact between athletes at the time of injury but are more related to poor landing biomechan-ics. For this reason, we believe that good landing biomechanics and proper physical preparation can prevent many of the lower-limb injuries that are common in jump-landing sports.

## The role of landing training in athletic performance and injury prevention

Research has shown that athletes can accurately respond to verbal instructions to alter their landing biomechanics. In fact, simply asking an athlete to 'land softly' can significantly increase their hip and knee flexion and decrease the peak ACL load.[14] Although video and audio feedback (especially when combined with verbal instructions) are helpful in modifying landing strategies, we are usually unable to respond appropriately to complex instructions, such as consciously contracting specific muscles when landing.

Altering the activity of specific muscle groups during dynamic landings requires more specialised muscle activation training. In fact, comprehensive lower-limb injury prevention programs should combine landing-technique instruction with neuromuscular and proprio-ceptive training, together with physical conditioning activities designed to produce long-term neuromuscular and biomechanical adaptations. In a meta-analysis of programs designed to reduce the incidence of ACL injuries in female athletes, it was concluded:

- training effects of neuromuscular preventive programs were more pronounced in par-ticipants under 18 years of age;
- pre- and in-season training was more effective than either pre-season or in-season train-ing alone; and
- plyometric and strengthening components of exercise protocols were found to be more essential than balancing activities, although the optimal combination of neuromuscular-biomechanical components remains to be verified.[15]

## How to design a landing training program for elite athletes

### Physical factors underpinning landing

Although physical factors and technical execution of landings can be addressed independently, these factors are interdependent. That is, physical limitations can retard the acquisition or execution of proper technique, yet high physical aptitude does not inherently manifest into technique improvements. Clearly, technical aptitude and physical capacities are directly related, and we need to ensure our athletes develop appropriate physical abilities to underpin and promote technical skill in landing.

### Interplay of mobility and strength qualities

To effectively absorb force and stabilise the body during landings, adequate joint range of motion, whole-body mobility and strength are critically important. However, the *available* range at a joint does not necessarily provide controlled mobility through that available range. General and specific strength qualities are required for an athlete to be able to effectively decelerate force in a controlled manner when landing. Athletes must therefore have an *effective* range of motion accompanied by the appropriate strength and neuromuscular control strategy to land correctly and safely. The practise and mastery of this technique must be supported by adequate physical capabilities.

### Strength qualities development

To develop capacity to land safely, strength training is essential, particularly training that develops lower-body strength, as well as strength of the torso and upper body. As a primary aim in landing is to effectively absorb the high forces generated at initial contact, high force capabilities must be a primary consideration. General and maximal strength training methods provide foundation components upon which technique can be built, as high force production/force absorption is influenced by the maximal capability to produce force.

To maximise the transfer of strength training to landing performance, we encourage free-weight exercises as the primary training method. This is because exercises such as squats using free-weights require whole-body balance and control through an eccentric and concentric action, allowing the athlete to gain strength and stability during actions and postures that are relevant to landing. It is useful to include both bilateral and unilateral exercises. Bilateral exercises (e.g. squats) are highly effective in developing strength, whilst supplementary unilateral exercises (e.g. single-leg squats and calf raises) develop an athlete's ability to balance and control force on one leg, an important consideration for sports where single-limb landings are common.

Further supplementary exercises such as decline (heel lift) single-leg squats with an emphasised eccentric action (e.g. additional load or 3–4-second eccentric) are also an effective means to promote positive tendon adaptation, as well as muscular strength and control.[16] When used properly, Olympic lifts (i.e. snatch, clean and jerk) are particularly good for improving power, but also a safe and effective means for training athletes to dynamically absorb force. Essentially, Olympic lifting is not a jump *per se*, but the lifts require compression and absorption in the catch phase, which is relevant to a bilateral landing sequence (see Figure 10.6).

Along with strength training and Olympic lifting, concurrent or subsequent development of high stretch-load tolerance (i.e. plyometric capability involving the stretch shorten cycle) is important to augment the application of strength to the relative velocity of jumping and

(a)

(b)

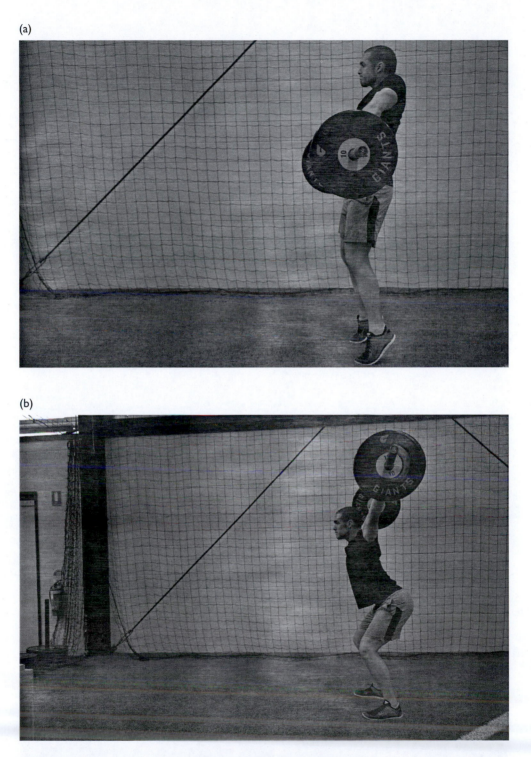

*Figure 10.6* (a) The end of the propulsive phase of the snatch; (b) The initial arresting of the load in the snatch; (c) The full squat position of the snatch; (d) The completed snatch

(c)

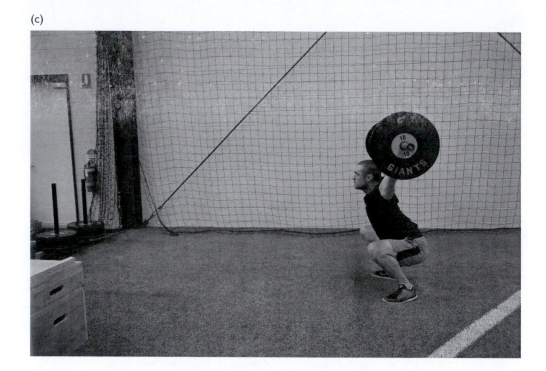

(d)

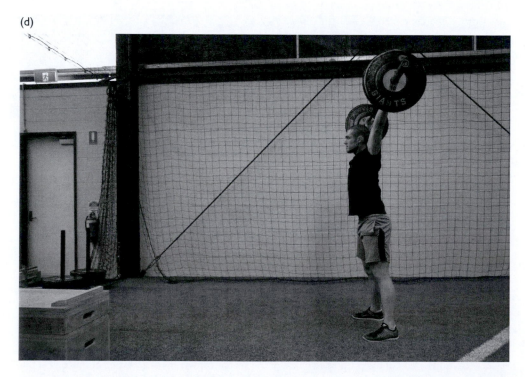

*Figure 10.6* (Continued)

landing. Impactful exercises, such as single- and double-leg hops over distance, alternating bounds, tuck jumps and depth jumps, are excellent exercises to develop plyometric ability whilst allowing for coaching of good landing technique. Therefore, including plyometric exercises with athletes who have a background in strength training is a highly effective way to develop tolerance and control of high eccentric loads, a critical aspect of landing.

> Strength is a foundational physical quality and must be developed to underpin effective landing. To develop specific strength qualities relevant to landing requires:
>     Strength Qualities for Landing = Maximal Strength + Olympic Lifting + Plyometric Training + Supplementary Exercise

### Mobility development

Effective mobility is required to achieve the positions that support good landing technique, with particular importance placed on the range of motion at the ankle, knee and hip. For example limited knee flexion can result in a stiffer landing (and increased force) and/or increased hip flexion in order to compensate. Similarly, poor dorsiflexion range of motion will reduce the available amount of force that can be absorbed through the ankle joint upon landing and, in turn, increase the force that must be absorbed through the rest of the body (i.e. in the knee, hip and back). Although ankle dorsiflexion range in a 'knee to wall' test is commonly between 6 and 8cm, athletes in jump and land sports should aim for higher values. For example elite surfers generally achieve values >12cm, with national team male volleyball players achieving >15cm.

> Although mobility of the ankle, knee and hip are particularly important, your body is an integrated apparatus. Whole body mobility requires stretching exercises combined with dynamic mobility activities and soft-tissue care, such as myofasical release, mobilisation, manipulation therapies, and foam rolling.

### Developing landing ability

As with any skill, training to land must be coached and practiced. However, landing in many sporting contexts cannot be perfectly controlled, and the ideal landing and what actually happens in sport may differ. For example in team sports every landing would ideally involve both feet contacting the ground simultaneously in order to distribute the force across both lower limbs. However, this rarely happens due to inherent aspects of the game (e.g. a volleyball player changing their body-position during a spike to avoid a block). Furthermore, the 'safest' landing in sport is not necessarily the most effective, and so we train to achieve the safest landing that is effective for the circumstance. Nonetheless, specific landing practise and reviewing landing technique is important, as the foundation skill helps underpin safe and effective landings whether they are 'ideal' or not.

The simplest and most effective way to isolate a landing is to perform separate landing-oriented drills. For athletes with lower strength or less skill, simple jump landings from a stationary position, forward hops or multiple hops with a 'hold' are effective, with the intention of landing effectively (see Figure 10.7). As increases in skill and physical conditioning permit, more challenging landing tasks should be introduced.

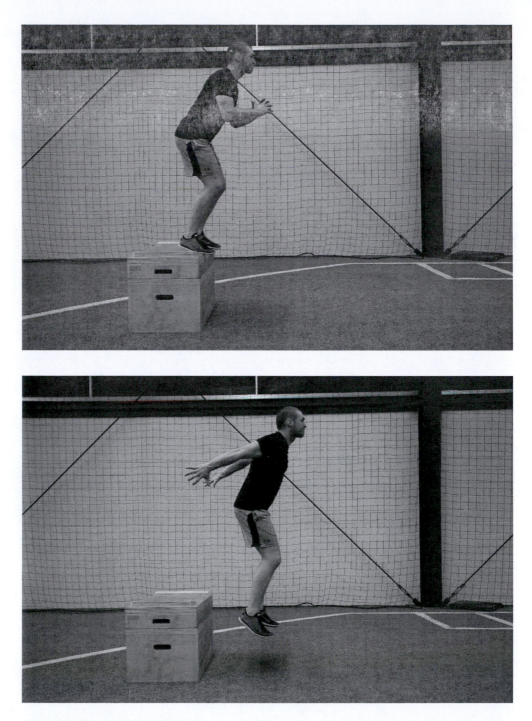

*Figure 10.7* Effective altitude landings

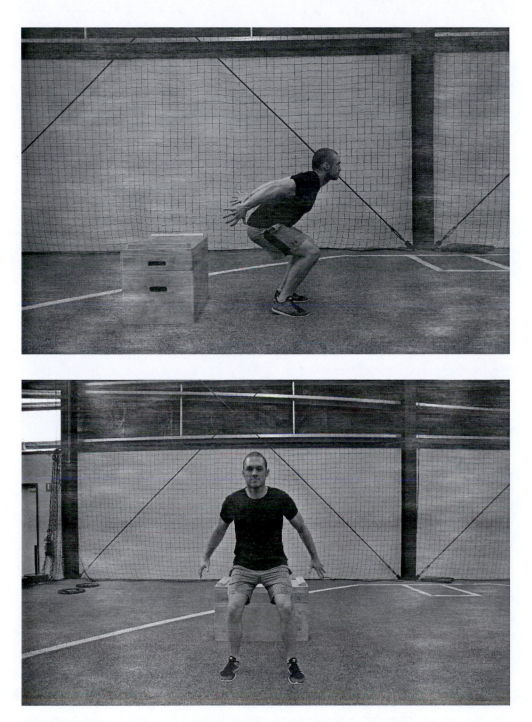

*Figure 10.7* (Continued)

A combination of implicit and explicit coaching can be employed, depending on the context, with, however, a bias towards implicit learning techniques and external coaching cues (e.g. 'land softly', 'land quietly' or 'land like a spring to absorb' rather than 'bend your hips and knees more'). Video is easily combined in the training setting for intermediate feedback to foster skill development. For example, during skill practise such as volleyball spike attempts, after each attempt, the spike and landing can be replayed and displayed on a video screen, and the athlete can self-evaluate the safety and effectiveness of their landing. The athlete can then articulate this information to the coach, or by answering specific questions about their landing such as: 'Did I absorb the force like a spring?' or 'Was I active in the landing?' The athlete can then use their knowledge of the skill to solve other movement problems they experience, with long-lasting impact, compared to explicit coaching that is dominated by internal cues.

## Monitoring landing load

In high-volume jump-land sports (e.g. volleyball, basketball and netball), monitoring and manipulating the training load, and therefore the landing load of the athletes, is a critical factor in reducing chronic injury risk, as well as promoting continued adaptation. This is not to say that we should reduce training load as a rule. In fact, in some cases, a high training load is required to develop skills that are necessary to achieve success at the elite level. Whilst better jumpers may be more at risk of injury, this should be seen as the *consequence* of the required high training load and high-jump heights that elite athletes undertake, and astute management rather than avoidance is recommended.

The way in which we manipulate the load within each training unit (day, week or block), as well as increase volume progressively with training age and physical preparedness, are important considerations in avoiding unnecessary chronic injuries common to high-volume jump-land sports.

**Monitoring Training Load:** The monotony of *training* load can be calculated as the average daily load (e.g. for 1 week) divided by the standard deviation of the daily load of that time period.[17] We can also calculate the monotony of the jump and land load in a similar fashion, with lower monotony (i.e. <1.5) desirable. The example below is for a senior national team volleyball player, whose weekly training load included 3,800 jump-and-landing activities, and varied from 0–1,200 jumps per day:

Jump-Land Monotony = Average Jumps per Day/Standard Deviation of Jumps in the week

Monotony = 543/450, or 1.2

It is also important to consider undulations of this load over the training weeks. From our experience, large and continuous increases (i.e. >10%/week) in jump-and-landing load, as well as infrequent 'unloading' weeks where total load is sharply reduced, tend to be associated with injury onset. Therefore, periodisation of training load is fundamental to sports preparation. This medium-term planning process must also reflect the athlete's long-term development, and their preparedness for the loads based on maturation, physical competency and training history.

# Summary

As a fundamental component of many sporting tasks, landings require optimal technical performance while ensuring efficient absorption of the impact forces generated at foot-ground contact to minimise the potential for injury. It is imperative that we understand the biomechanical principles underlying different types of landing techniques to effectively instruct athletes on how to safely absorb the impact forces generated on landing. Technique tips for a safe landing include actively bending your ankles, knees and hips; avoiding an exaggerated striding-out action or excessively flexed trunk posture; maintaining a neutral foot; and ensuring coordinated neuromuscular control. Training programs aimed at improving the effectiveness and safety of landings must also consider an athlete's physical development, as landing performance requires both highly developed physical qualities combined with technical mastery. Adequate and effective joint range of motion, whole-body mobility and strength are all critically important physical qualities that must be developed to underpin effective landing technique so athletes can safely achieve their performance goals.

# Notes

1   Although athletes land on a variety of surfaces, including fixed apparatus and equipment that is free to move (e.g. a skate board), for ease of explanation we will refer to landings in which the athlete's foot contacts the ground.
2   Yeow, C. H., Lee, P.V.S., & Goh, J.C.H. (2011). An investigation of lower extremity energy dissipation strategies during single-leg and double-leg landing based on sagittal and frontal plane biomechanics. *Human Movement Science*, *30*(3): 624–635.
3   Nigg, B. M., Cole, G. K., & Bruggemann, G. P. (1995). Impact forces during heel toe running. *Journal of Applied Biomechanics*, *11*(4): 407–432.
4   Whitting, J. W., Steele, J. R., Jaffrey, M., & Munro, B. J. (2009). Does foot pitch at ground contact affect parachute landing technique? *Military Medicine*, *174*(8): 832–837.
5   Steele, J. R. (1990). Biomechanical factors affecting performance in netball: Implications for improving performance and injury reduction. *Sports Medicine*, *10*(2): 88–102.
6   Butler, R. J., Crowell, H. P. 3rd, & Davis, I. M. (2003). Lower extremity stiffness: Implications for performance and injury. *Clinical Biomechanics*, *18*(6): 511–517.
7   Podraza, J. T., & White, S. C. (2010). Effect of knee flexion angle on ground reaction forces, knee moments and muscle co-contraction during an impact-like deceleration landing: Implications for the non-contact mechanism of ACL injury. *The Knee*, *17*(4): 291–295.
8   Pollard, C. D., Sigward, S. M., Ota, S., Langford, K., & Powers, C. M. (2006). The influence of in-season injury prevention training on lower-extremity kinematics during landing in female soccer players. *Clinical Journal of Sports Medicine*, *16*(3): 223–227.
9   Dempsey, A. R., Elliott, B. C., Munro, B. J., Steele, J. R., & Lloyd, D. G. (2012). Whole body kinematics and knee moments that occur during an overhead catch and landing task in sport. *Clinical Biomechanics*, *27*(5): 466–474.
10  Bisseling, R. W., Hof, A. L., Bredeweg, S. W., Zwerver, J., & Mulder T. (2008). Are the take-off and landing phase dynamics of the volleyball spike jump related to patellar tendinopathy? *British Journal of Sports Medicine*, *42*(6): 483–489.
11  Steele, J. R., & Brown, J.M.M. (1999). Effects of chronic anterior cruciate ligament deficiency on muscle activation patterns during an abrupt deceleration task. *Clinical Biomechanics*, *14*(1): 247–257.
12  Blackburn, J. T., & Padua, D. A. (2008). Influence of trunk flexion on hip and knee joint kinematics during a controlled drop landing. *Clinical Biomechanics*, *23*(3): 313–319.
13  Cowling, E. J., & Steele, J. R. (2001). Is lower limb muscle synchrony during landing affected by gender? Implications for variations in ACL injury rates. *Journal of Electromyography and Kinesiology*, *11*(4): 263–268.

14  Laughlin, W. A., Weinhandl, J. T., Kernoek, T. W., Cobb, S. C., Keenan, K. G., & O'Connor, K. M. (2011). The effects of single-leg landing technique on ACL loading. *Journal of Biomechanics*, *44*(10): 1845–1851.

15  Yoo, J. H., Lim, B. O., Ha, M.., Lee, S. W., Oh, S. J., Lee, Y. S., & Kim, J. G. (2010). A meta-analysis of the effect of neuromuscular training on the prevention of the anterior cruciate ligament injury in female athletes. *Knee Surgery, Sports Traumatology, Arthroscopy*, *18*(6): 824–830.

16  Cook, J. L., & Purdam, C. R. (2003). Rehabilitation of lower limb tendinopathies. *Clinical Journal of Sports Medicine*, *22*(4): 777–789.

17  Foster, C., Florhaug, J. A., Franklin, J., Gottschall, L., Hrovatin, L. A., Parker, S., Doleshal, P., & Dodge, C. (2001). A new approach to monitoring exercise training. *Journal of Strength & Conditioning Research*, *15*(1): 109–115.

# Chapter 11

# Throwing mechanics in injury prevention and performance rehabilitation

*Steve McCaig and Mark Young*

## Introduction

Shoulder and elbow pain associated with throwing is common in many sports and has collectively been termed throwing arm pain (TAP). These types of injuries are thought to occur due to three main factors:

1　Technical flaws
2　Insufficient physical competencies (e.g. shoulder mobility and strength)
3　Excessive or inadequate workload

Whilst most sports practitioners are involved in the physical preparation, injury management and workload monitoring of a throwing athlete, technique analysis is often the sole domain of the coach, or assumed to be a factor beyond modification. A detailed understanding of optimal throwing biomechanics and common technique errors will lead to more effective interventions and coordinated approaches to injury management for these athletes. This chapter will discuss TAP and provide the practitioner with valuable strategies to both prevent and manage these injuries in the throwing athlete.

## Throwing arm pain

A broad range of shoulder and elbow pathologies, as highlighted in Table 11.1, can cause TAP. Baseball has led the research into this condition, as 45 per cent to 58 per cent of all injuries occur in the upper limb, and the majority of these injuries relate to throwing. Cricketers

*Table 11.1* Shoulder and elbow injuries commonly associated with throwing

| Common shoulder conditions related to throwing | Common elbow conditions related to throwing |
| --- | --- |
| Rotator cuff tears | Ulnar collateral ligament strains |
| Rotator cuff tendinopathy | Elbow joint osteophytes |
| Capsular lesions | Medial epicondyle tendinopathy |
| Labral lesions (including SLAP tears) | Ulna neuropathy |
| Bicep tendon tears and tendinopathy | Loose bodies in the elbow joint |

also commonly report pain with throwing; however, it rarely causes missed games, as these players typically choose to field in alternative positions to avoid throwing.[1,2]

## Analysis of throwing biomechanics

Optimal throwing biomechanics maximise throwing performance whilst minimising injury risk. Whilst most biomechanical analysis has been completed on baseball pitchers, overhead throws in other sports are considered to be similar.[3] However, there remain some specific differences in throwing sports to consider, such as variations in the size of the ball or implement, time required to release the ball, distance thrown and base of support.

Whilst in reality, throwing should be considered one synchronous motion, for ease of analysis we typically divide the throw into six components:[4]

1 Preparation phase
2 Stride
3 Arm cocking
4 Acceleration
5 Deceleration
6 Follow through.

### 1. Preparation phase

This is the first phase of the throw, and analysis needs to consider:

- Footwork required to place athlete's momentum towards the target
- Feet positioned side-on to target
- Weight on back leg.

### 2. Stride

The stride phase starts when the front hip is maximally flexed to step towards the target, and finishes at front foot contact (FFC). Key points to note at FFC are:

- Front foot pointing to target
- Front knee flexed to around 45°
- Stride length is approximately 80 per cent of height
- Pelvis is slightly open to target
- Shoulder is abducted at 100°, externally rotated to 50° and 20° of horizontal abduction
- Elbow flexed to 90°.

### 3. Arm cocking

The third stage of the throw begins at FFC and terminates at maximal external rotation (MER) of the upper limb. Critical features of this stage include:

- Pelvic rotation towards the target, followed by trunk
- Front arm pulled in close to side
- Front knee stable
- Upper limb forced into MER, which is a combination of GHJ, scapula posterior tilt, trunk extension and elbow valgus.[5,6]

## 4. Acceleration

The acceleration phase starts after MER and ends at ball release. Features of this stage worth noting are:

- Shoulder rapidly internally rotates and horizontally adducts
- Scapula protracts
- Elbow extends
- Shoulder rotates up to 7,000° per second and elbow at 2,500° per second[4]
- Front knee extends, stopping pelvis rotation
- Trunk continues to flex and rotate.

## 5. Deceleration

Deceleration commences at ball release and terminates at maximal internal rotation of the upper limb. In this phase, the shoulder continues to internally rotate and horizontally adduct, whilst the elbow continues to extend and pronate. The front knee is extended and the trunk flexes and continues to rotate until the back leg lifts off the ground.

## 6. Follow-through

The follow-through completes the throwing motion and allows a continuation of deceleration (except for shoulder IR) until the next task begins. Completing the follow-through is critical to absorbing the high forces generated within the body.

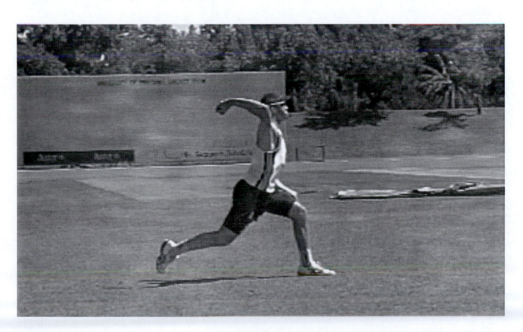

*Figure 11.1* Side-on view of arm cocking phase at maximal external rotation

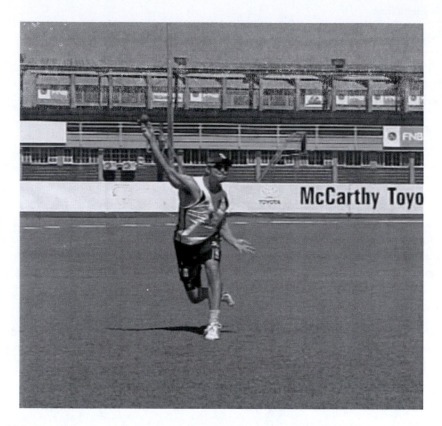

*Figure 11.2* Front-on view of end of acceleration phase at ball release

### Throwing biomechanics and injury

Now that we have detailed the main biomechanical features of the throw, this provides us with a better platform upon which to understand TAP.

## Shoulder injuries

The highest stresses to the upper limb occur during arm cocking, acceleration and deceleration,[7] and it is therefore no surprise that most injuries occur during these phases. During arm cocking and acceleration, the shoulder reaches extreme ranges of external rotation, and in this position two phenomena occur which are thought to cause shoulder injury – internal impingement and the 'peel back' phenomenon.[8,9]

### Internal impingement

During extremes of shoulder external rotation in abduction, the posterior aspect of the humeral head abuts on the posterior superior glenoid. This is known as internal impingement. During internal impingement, the labrum, supraspinatus and infraspinatus tendons are trapped between the glenoid and the humerus; due to high forces and repetitions, this can lead to labrum and rotator cuff lesions in elite throwers. These forces are increased with anterior instability, scapula protraction and horizontal abduction.[9]

### 'Peel back' phenomenon

During shoulder external rotation in , the long head (LH) of biceps tendon has been found to twist and this, combined with distraction forces on the shoulder increasing tension on the tendon, causes the superior labrum to 'peel back' from the glenoid. The combination of a tight posterior inferior capsule moving the humeral head superiorly and anterior forces at the shoulder causing instability can lead to superior labrum anterior-posterior (SLAP) lesions.[9]

### Deceleration stresses

During deceleration the LH of biceps works to decelerate elbow extension and pronation, as well as prevent distraction and anterior shear forces at the shoulder.[4,10] These excessive forces are thought to lead to the development of SLAP lesions and biceps tendon injuries, as labrum stress is at its greatest during deceleration.

The high eccentric stresses of the shoulder external rotators during this phase, as the shoulder horizontally adducts and internally rotates, can cause micro-trauma to the posterior cuff and capsule.[9] This can lead to posterior cuff tendinopathies and scarring of the posterior capsule, which can lead to posterior capsule tightness.[11]

## Elbow injuries

Elbow pain in throwers has been clearly linked to increased valgus stress. Valgus stress at the elbow is restrained by the ulna collateral ligament (UCL) medially and laterally by the radio-capitellum joint. During throwing, the valgus forces at the elbow can exceed the tensile strength of the UCL. This can create UCL strains and tears. This increases valgus laxity, which then leads to the radial head being compressed against the capitellum. This can cause osteochondritis of the radial head and capitellum and can lead to loose bodies forming in the elbow joint. Increased valgus motion causes the medial aspect of the olecranon to abut the olecranon fossa. This can lead to osteophyte formation and stress fractures of the olecranon. This collective process is known as valgus-extension overload.[12]

Throwers can also develop tendinopathy and tears in the muscles of the common flexor origin as these muscles act as secondary stabilisers to valgus stress. Ulnar neuropathy may also develop as the ulnar nerve is compressed in the ulnar groove with increased valgus laxity.

### Key factors in performance and injury prevention

Several key factors have been identified to improve throwing performance (velocity) and reduce injury risk:

### Stride length

Increased velocity occurs when stride length is between 85 and 90 per cent of body length.[14] This increases the time for forces to be developed[13] and is critical for velocity.

### Foot alignment at FFC

If the foot lands to the left of the target for a right-handed thrower this is called an 'open position'. This results in:

- Early pelvis rotation
- The shoulder lagging into horizontal abduction
- Reduced force transfer to the upper limb[4]
- Increased stress anteriorly at the shoulder and valgus stress at the elbow.

If the foot lands to the right of the target for a right-handed thrower this is called a 'closed position'. This results in:

- Reduced pelvis and trunk rotation
- Reduced force transfer to upper limb during acceleration
- Increased deceleration loads on upper limb due to reduced pelvis and trunk rotation in follow-through.

### Front knee position

At FFC the front knee must be stable and extend during acceleration. This transfers forces from the legs to the trunk and, ultimately, the upper limb. Any knee flexion results in reduced velocity.

### Pelvis and trunk rotation

Faster throwers have increased pelvis and trunk rotational velocities; however, the timing is critical.[15] Key points here are:

- Maximum pelvis velocity should occur in cocking, whilst maximum trunk rotation should occur in acceleration;
- This trunk-pelvis separation induces a stretch-shortening cycle on the abdominals that increases force production;
- Early rotation results in an 'open position' (see above);
- Delayed rotation results in a leading elbow (see below).

### Trunk flexion

Trunk flexion in acceleration transfers forces to the upper limb from the legs and trunk, while during deceleration it helps to decelerate the upper limb. Slower throwers have been found to be more upright, whilst increased contralateral trunk flexion increases elbow stress.[16]

### Shoulder abduction

Shoulder abduction should be between 90° and 110°, with 100° considered optimal to minimise upper-limb loads and maximise velocity:[17]

- Reduced abduction increases elbow valgus stress[17]
- Less abduction reduces shoulder distraction forces.[5]

(a)

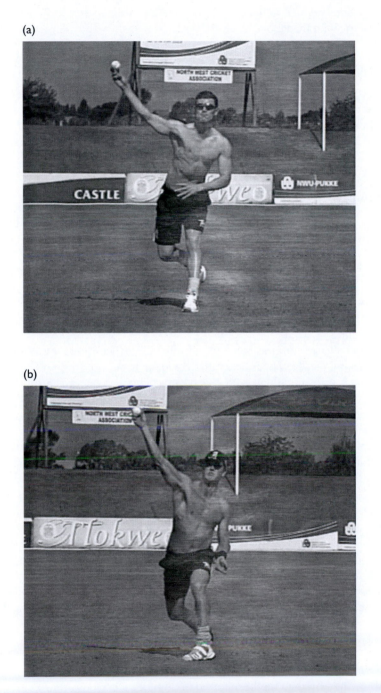

(b)

*Figure 11.3* Example of good and poor foot alignment at front foot contact. In (a), front foot is aligned with the target, while in (b), the front foot is in a 'closed' position

### Shoulder horizontal abduction

Excessive horizontal abduction in late cocking increases anterior stress at the shoulder, while increased horizontal adduction in acceleration increases valgus stress at the elbow,[5] which is known as 'leading with the elbow'.

### Shoulder external rotation

At FFC the external rotation should be approximately 50°. Increased external rotation increases anterior stress at the shoulder and valgus stress at the elbow.[18]

Increased external rotation range at end of acceleration (MER) is critical for throwing velocity, but this also increases stress at the shoulder and elbow.[19] A better indication of injury risk than MER is ratio of MER to passive external rotation range.[20]

### Elbow flexion

Increased elbow flexion during throwing results in reduced valgus stress at the elbow and distraction forces at the shoulder.[19]

### Assessing throwing technique

3D motion analysis is the gold standard of assessing throwing technique. However, as access to 3D motion analysis is limited, there is a need for a valid and reliable field test to assess throwing technique.

Despite the challenges around validity and reliability when designing a measuring tool for throwing technique, we have found that the benefit of assessing and discussing technique parameters with the athlete and coach outweighs the concerns around accuracy of the measurement tool. We have developed a throwing matrix, or 'checklist', as a simple method of assessing throwing technique for coaches, physiotherapists and trainers working within cricket (see Table 11.2). The matrix is designed to assess for injury risk and to aid performance improvement. High-speed video footage of the throwing motion is reviewed and evaluated compared to the scoring criteria. The athlete is filmed from the open side, front and behind. They are instructed to throw the ball as hard and as accurately as possible towards a target at a pre-determined distance. Due to natural variation between throws, it is important to assess a number of throws to get an overall feel for the athletes' throwing technique.[7] Athletes are then given an overall score as a percentage of 100.

Feedback is immediately given to the player, with specific throwing technique drills and targeted conditioning exercises prescribed by the coach and physiotherapist to improve throwing performance and reduce risk of injury. In a group of elite cricketers, we found an association between a poor score on the matrix and the incidence of TAP during a three-month competitive tour. More significantly, the tool provided a starting point to open dialogue with the coach and player around throwing technique, performance and injury risk.

## Throwing workloads

Increased throwing workload has been linked to shoulder and elbow injuries in baseball and cricket.[21,22] Based on these findings, throwing guidelines have been developed in adolescent baseball (www.usabaseball.com/medpositionstatement.html). Although higher workloads

*Table 11.2* The 'Throwing Matrix' assessment sheet

| Throwing matrix | Score | Comments |
|---|---|---|
| Stride length (>80%) | 2 | |
| Cocking phase – MER (>160) | 2 | |
| Front knee through release (50 to 30) | 2 | |
| Lag between hip and shoulder | 2 | |
| Weight transfer (at ball release) | 2 | |
| Shoulder rotation (Horizontal abduction) | 2 | |
| Front arm – Active pull through | 2 | |
| Armpit angle (>90) | 2 | |
| Stance – Front foot to target | 2 | |
| Follow through (line of arm & length) | 2 | |
| **Total Scrore** | 20 | |
| **Percentage** | 100% | |

Scores: 2 = desirable, 1 = restricted/less than ideal, 0 = poor/risk

| Action points |
|---|
| 1 |
| 2 |
| 3 |

increase risk of injury, a sufficient volume of throwing is required to improve technique and physically prepare the athlete to tolerate higher volumes of throwing. Close monitoring of throwing volume, frequency and intensity is important for the throwing athlete. Coaches must structure practice so that each throw counts, and avoid unnecessary throwing in practice. For example, in cricket, the regular use of throwing aids during batting practice has greatly reduced the volume of throwing players are required to complete during practice.

## Throwing and fatigue

Throwing when fatigued increases the risk of injury. Fatigue is manifested in a number of ways, most notably:[23]

- Reduced maximum external rotation
- Decreased knee extension during ball release
- Decreased horizontal adduction torque
- Decreased velocity.

Fatigued throwers increase their upper-limb use in order to maintain velocity, which creates even more stress on shoulder and elbow structures. This is why it is important to coach lower-body and force transference competencies and to emphasise to athletes that the throw begins at the feet.

## Physical adaptations in throwers

### Shoulder range of motion

A gain in shoulder external rotation range of motion (ERG) and a decrease in internal rotation range (GIRD) is found on the dominant side in overhead athletes and is due to a combination of bony and soft tissue adaptations.[24] Increased humeral retroversion is a bony adaptation that is common in throwers,[25,26,27] whilst the soft tissue changes which lead to ERG and GIRD are:

• Acquired laxity in the anterior capsule due to high anterior shear forces in throwing
• Tightness in the posterior capsule as a result of stress during deceleration.

Humeral retroversion is defined as the acute angle between the axis of the elbow joint and the centre of the humeral head. Throwers with increased humeral retroversion will present with ERG and GIRD, but their total range of motion may be similar on both the dominant and non-dominant sides. It is a protective adaptation to throwing, allowing for greater range of external rotation without stressing the anterior capsule. The proximal humeral epiphysis is open between the ages of 12 and 16, and throwing during these ages causes this adaptation. Throwers with increased humeral retroversion have been found to be less likely to sustain shoulder and elbow injuries.[25,26,27]

As humeral torsion influences shoulder rotation and horizontal flexion range of motion, it is important to account for this when screening throwers.[28] Humeral retroversion can be easily measured via ultrasound. If the athlete's ERG is equal to GIRD, when corrected for humeral retroversion, then they are considered to have normal shoulder rotation ROM. If GIRD is greater than ERG when corrected for humeral retroversion, they are considered to have a restriction in their posterior shoulder.

Changes in shoulder rotation have been found to occur immediately post throwing and over the course of a season, with GIRD found to increase.[29,30] It is therefore important to know a thrower's shoulder rotation range pre-season and monitor this in-season. Regular mobility exercises to maintain range, particularly IR and horizontal flexion, should be completed in-season.

**Shoulder strength** – Internal rotation strength has been found to increase, and external rotation strength decrease, in the dominant shoulder of throwers when measured both isokinetically and isometrically. As a consequence, the ratio of external rotation strength to internal rotation strength has been found to reduce.[31,32] These changes are thought to be contributing factors to throwing injuries.[33,34] It is therefore important to assess rotator cuff strength pre-season and regularly monitor in-season in throwers to reduce injury risk. Regular cuff conditioning exercises should be completed to prevent reduction in cuff strength and minimise the risk of injury.

## Lower-limb and trunk function in throwing

Rotation of the pelvis occurs due to a combination of bilateral hip rotation, back leg hip abduction and extension.[35] Adequate range of thoracic rotation is required so that trunk rotation can be delayed while the pelvis rotates. Any inadequacies in hip or thoracic rotation results in reduced force transfer to the upper limb.

To generate and overcome the large forces involved with throwing, high levels of strength in the hip abductors, hip extensors, quadriceps and hamstrings are required. High EMG activity in these muscles has been found to occur during the pitching motion.[36] Leg power in the frontal plane has been found to correlate well with throwing velocity.[37] This further highlights the need to both assess and develop the entire kinetic chain of the throwing athlete.

## Rehabilitation and return to throwing

During the rehabilitation of the throwing athlete it is critical to regain adequate mobility, strength and control of not only the upper limb, but also the trunk and hips. Manual therapy and mobility exercises should be directed at the posterior shoulder, pectoralis minor length, thoracic spine extension and rotation, as well as hip extension and rotation. Cross body adduction and sleeper stretch improve shoulder internal rotation range. Specific exercises to improve scapula and rotator cuff control and strength during shoulder motion are critical for glenohumeral joint stability. Upper-body exercises, such as push up, rowing and pull down variations with cables, dumbbells and suspension trainers, integrate scapula and rotator cuff function whilst developing strength in the muscles used to accelerate and decelerate the upper limb during throwing. Gripping and forearm exercises to improve strength in the common flexor origin group should be included to help with valgus stability at the elbow. In addition to isolation exercises, heavy rowing, pull down and deadlift exercises are useful.

Exercises directed at improving hip mobility, leg and trunk strength should be included and can be started immediately; lunges in multiple planes, single leg squats, balance drills and trunk exercises can be initiated even if the athlete is immobilised in a sling. Medicine ball throws have been found to replicate trunk activity when throwing[38] and are commonly used to improve transfer of forces from the lower limb and trunk as part of performance training and rehabilitation.

Return-to-throwing programmes should be started once the athlete is cleared clinically and has the underpinning physical capabilities required. However, it is possible to work on specific technical aspects of the throw, such as stride length and foot alignment during front foot contact, without throwing a ball. It is recommended that athletes begin throwing over shorter distances and progress to longer distances first prior to increasing intensity with a rest day in between each session. Focus should be on technique, and throwing should not be completed with fatigue initially. The athlete should be monitored post throwing for the presence of any signs or symptoms, such as reduced posterior shoulder range of motion or external rotation strength, which may indicate failure to tolerate loading or inadequate recovery.[39] The volume and type of throws completed should be based around the requirements of the sport, whilst greater task complexity can be added once they are able to achieve throwing at full intensity in closed environments.

---

Rehabilitation of throwing injuries must include:

- Mobility exercises & manual therapy to address any restrictions, particularly in the shoulder, thoracic cage or hip joint
- Rotator cuff exercises for strength, endurance and cuff balance
- Strength exercises for the muscles that decelerate the upper limb in throwing

- Lower-limb and trunk exercises to develop strength and power
- A graded return to throwing, increasing intensity then volume
- Monitoring of changes in range and strength in response to a return to throwing

## Summary

Throwing is a whole body motion that is initiated from the ground via the legs and transferred to the upper limb via the trunk. It is a complex task and injuries are common – they mostly occur due to technical faults, inadequate physical competency or workload errors. Assessment and development of the entire kinetic chain is therefore critical to both prevent and rehabilitate these injuries. Since throwers develop changes in shoulder mobility and strength, which can lead to injury, the physical preparation and rehabilitation of throwers must ensure they have the lower-limb, trunk and upper-limb mobility and strength required for throwing. Finally, it is vital to understand the technical components of the throw, and to this end, the 'Throwing Matrix' is useful, and specific coaching interventions can be guided by these findings.

## Notes

1 Dick, R., Sauers, E. L., Agel, J., Keuter, G., Marshall, S. W., McCarty, K., & McFarland, E. (2007). Descriptive epidemiology of collegiate men's baseball injuries: National Collegiate Athletic Association Injury Surveillance System, 1988–1989 through 2003–2004. *Journal of Athletic Training, 42*:183–193.

2 Ranson, C., & Gregory, P. (2008). Shoulder injury in professional cricket. *Physical Therapy in Sport, 9*:34–39.

3 Fleisig, G. S. (2010). Biomechanics of overhand throwing: Implications for injury and performance. In M. Portus (Ed.), *Conference of Science, Medicine & Coaching in Cricket: Conference Proceedings* (pp. 17–20). Queensland, Australia: Cricket Australia.

4 Fleisig, G. S., Andrews, J. R., Dillman, C. J., & Escamilla, R. F. (1995). Kinetics of baseball pitching with implications for injury mechanisms. *American Journal of Sports Medicine, 23*: 233–239.

5 Werner, S. L., Fleisig, G. S., Dillman, C. J., & Andrews, J. R. (1993). Biomechanics of the elbow during baseball pitching. *Journal of Orthopaedic and Sports Physical Therapy, 17*: 274–278.

6 Mihata, T., McGarry, M. H., Kinoshita, M., & Lee, T. Q. (2010). Excessive glenohumeral horizontal abduction as occurs during the late cocking phase of the throwing motion can be critical for internal impingement. *American Journal of Sports Medicine, 38*: 369–74.

7 Oyama, S. (2012). Baseball pitching kinematics, joint loads, and injury prevention. *Journal of Sport and Health Science, 1*:80–91.

8 Jobe, C. M. (1995). Posterior superior glenoid impingement: expanded spectrum. *Arthroscopy, 11*: 530–536.

9 Burkhardt, S. S., Morgan, C. D., & Kibler, W. B. (2003). The disabled shoulder; spectrum of pathology Part 1; Pathoanaotmy and biomechanics. *Arthroscopy, 19*: 404–420.

10 Escamilla, R. F., & Andrews, J. R. (2009). Shoulder muscle recruitment patterns and related biomechanics during upper extremity sports. *Sports Medicine, 39*: 569–590.

11 Tyler, T. F., Nicholas, S. J., Roy, T., & Gleim, G. W. (2000). Quantification of posterior capsule tightness and motion loss in patients with shoulder impingement. *American Journal of Sports Medicine, 28*:668–673.

12 Wilson, F. D., Andrews, J. R., Blackburn, T. A., & McClusky, G. (1983). Valgus extension overload in the pitching elbow. *American Journal of Sports Medicine, 11*:83–88.

13 Stodden, D., Fleisig, G. S., Mclean, S. R., Lyman, S. L., & Andrews, J. R. (2001). Relationship of pelvis and upper torso kinematics to pitched baseball velocity. *Journal of Applied Biomechanics, 17*:164–172.

14 Montgomery, J., & Knudson, D. (2002). A method to determine stride length for baseball pitching. *Applied Research in Coaching and Athletics Annual, 17*:75–84

15 Escamilla, R. F., Fleisig, G. S., Barrentine, S., Andrews, J., & Morrman, C. 3rd. (2002). Kinematic and kinetic comparisons between American and Korean professional baseball pitchers. *Sports Biomechanics, 1*:213–228.

16 Aguinaldo, A. L., & Chambers, H. (2009). Correlation of throwing mechanics with elbow valgus load in adult baseball pitchers. *American Journal of Sports Medicine, 37*:2043–2048.

17 Matsuo, T., Flesig, G. S., Zheng, N. Q., & Andrews, J. R. (2006). Influence of shoulder abduction and lateral trunk on peak elbow varus torque for college baseball pitchers during simulated pitching. *Journal of Applied Biomechanics, 22*:93–102.

18 Matsuo, T., Escamilla, R. F., Fleisig, G. S., Barrentine, S. W., & Andrews, J. R. (2001). Comparison of kinematic and temporal parameters between different pitch velocity groups. *Journal of Applied Biomechanics, 17*:1–13.

19 Werner, S .L., Gill, T. J., Murray, T. A., Cook, T. D., & Hawkins, R. J. (2001). Relationships between throwing mechanics and shoulder distraction in professional baseball pitchers. *American Journal of Sports Medicine, 29*:354–358.

20 Miyashita, K., Urabe, Y., Kobayashi, H., Yokoe, K., & Koshida, S. (2008). The role of shoulder maximum external rotation during throwing for elbow injury prevention in baseball players. *Journal of Sports Science and Medicine, 7*:223–28.

21 Olsen, S. J. 2nd, Fleisig, G. S., Dun, S., Loftice, J., & Andrews, J. R. (2006). Risk factors for shoulder and elbow injuries in adolescent baseball pitchers. *American Journal of Sports Medicine, 34*:905–912.

22 Saw, R., Dennis, R., Bentley, D., & Farhart, P. (2011). Throwing workload and injury risk in elite cricketers. *British Journal of Sports Medicine, 45*:805–808.

23 Escamilla, R. F., Fleisig, G. S., Barrentine, S. W., Andrews, J. R., & Morrman, C. (2007). Pitching biomechanics as a pitcher approaches muscular fatigue during a simulated baseball game. *American Journal of Sports Medicine, 35*:23–33.

24 Borsa, P. A., Laudner, K. G., & Sauers, E. L. (2008). Mobility and stability adaptations of the shoulder of the overhead athlete: A theoretical and evidence-based perspective. *Sports Medicine, 38*:17–36.

25 Pieper, H. G. (1998). Humeral torsion in the throwing arm of handball players. *American Journal of Sports Medicine, 26*:247–253.

26 Whiteley, R. J., Adams, R. D., Nicholson, L. L., & Ginn, K. A. (2010). Reduced humeral torsion predicts throwing-related injury in adolescent baseballers. *Journal of Science and Medicine in Sport, 13*:392–396

27 Myers, J. B., Oyama, S., Rucinski, T. J., & Creighton, R. A. (2011). Humeral retrotorsion in collegiate baseball pitchers with throwing-related upper extremity injury history. *Sports Health, 3*:383–389.

28 Myers, J. B., Oyama, S., Goerger, B. M., Rucinski, T. J., Blackburn, J. T., & Creighton, R. A. (2009). Influence of humeral torsion on interpretation of posterior shoulder tightness measures in overhead athletes. *Clinical Journal of Sports Medicine, 19*:366–71.

29 Kibler, W. B., Sciascia, A., & Thomas, S. J. (2012). Glenohumeral internal rotation deficit: Pathogenesis and response to acute throwing. *Sports Medicine Arthroscopy Review, 20*:34–38.

30 Reinold, M. M., Wilk, K. E., Macrina, L. C., Shehame, C., Dun, S., Fleisig, G. S., Crenshaw, K., & Andrews J. R. (2008). Changes in shoulder and elbow passive range of motion after pitching in professional baseball players. *American Journal of Sports Medicine, 36*:523–527.

31 Wilk, K. E., Andrews, J. R., Arrigo, C. A., Keirns, M. A., & Erber, D. J. (1993). The strength characteristics of internal and external rotator muscles in professional baseball pitchers. *American Journal of Sports Medicine, 21*:61–66.

32 Magnusson, S. P., Gleim, G. W., & Nicholas, J. A. (1994). Shoulder weakness in professional baseball pitchers. *Medicine and Science in Sports and Exercise, 26*:5–9.

33 Trakis, J. E., McHugh, M. P., Caracciolo, P. A., Busciacco, L., Mullaney, M., & Nicholas, S. J. (2008). Muscle strength and range of motion in adolescent pitchers with throwing-related pain: Implications for injury prevention. *American Journal of Sports Medicine, 36*:2173–2178.

34 Byram, I. R., Bushnell, B. D., Dugger, K., Charron, K., Harrell, F. E., & Noonan, T. J. (2010). Pre-season shoulder strength measurements in professional baseball pitchers: Identifying players at risk for injury. *American Journal of Sports Medicine, 38*:1375–1382.

35 Robb, A. J., Fleisig, G. S., Wilk, K., Macrina, L., Bolt, B., & Pajaczkowski, J. (2010). Passive ranges of motion of the hips and their relationship with pitching biomechanics and ball velocity in professional baseball pitchers. *American Journal of Sports Medicine, 38*:2487–2493.

36 Campbell, B. M., Stodden, D. F., & Nixon, M. K. (2010). Lower extremity muscle activation during baseball pitching. *Journal of Strength & Conditioning Research, 24*:964–971.

37 Lehman, G., Drinkwater, E. J., & Behm, D. G. (2013). Correlation of throwing velocity to the results of lower body field tests in male college baseball players. *Journal of Strength & Conditioning Research, 27*:902–908.

38 Stodden, D. F., Campbell, B. M., & Moyer, T. M. (2008). Comparison of trunk kinematics in trunk training exercises and throwing. *Journal of Strength & Conditioning Research, 22*:112–118.

39 Whiteley, R. J. (2010). Throwing mechanics, load monitoring and injury: Perspectives from physiotherapy and baseball as they relate to cricket. Cricket Australia. Conference of Science and Medicine in Coaching in Cricket, 21–24.

Key factors for assessing throwing performance and injury risk are:

stride length
Foot alignment at front foot contact
Front knee positon
Pelvic and trunk rotation
Shoulder horizontal abduction & external rotation
Elbow flexion

Chapter 12

# Core stability in injury prevention and performance

*Lee Burton and Gray Cook*

## Introduction

In recent years, increased emphasis has been placed on training the 'core' musculature in both personal fitness and sports conditioning programmes.[1] The general public often associates effective core muscle training with well-defined abdominals and small waistlines. In sport, though, the emphasis should undoubtedly be placed on training for function rather than aesthetics. Therefore, testing and training practices should reflect the total capacity and function of the core muscles, rather than performing tests or exercises such as the sit-up, which often has little application to daily activities and sports performance.

Focused strengthening of the core muscles surrounding the torso, hips and shoulder girdles will not guarantee appropriate timing, coordination and motor control for effective functioning during both static and dynamic muscle actions. Dysfunctions in timing, coordination and motor control have been linked to factors associated with increased injury risk, which makes identifying and eliminating them a priority for any clinician or strength and conditioning professional.

Deficits in coordination of the core musculature have been associated with injuries local to the core, lumbar spine and sacroiliac joint.[2,3,4,5] As a result, it is relevant to target strategies to normalize changes in core coordination in order to reduce future injury risk, as well as normalize the effect of any prior injury.

Deficits in core motor control do not only predispose us to low back pain, however. These coordination changes have also been related to lower extremity injuries.[6,7] For instance, it has been observed that a combination of trunk proprioception, trunk displacement following perturbation and a history of low back pain provided the strongest model for identifying athletes at risk for knee ligament injury.[8,9] Interestingly, all of these variables were relevant in identifying female athletes at risk for anterior cruciate ligament (ACL) injuries, specifically while a history of low back pain was the only predictor for ACL injuries in males. Previous work has suggested that increases in trunk displacement following perturbation are associated with deficits in core timing.[10] The results of this study highlight the importance of the core to spine and lower extremity injury, and thus normalizing core function is an integral part of programming for injury prevention and performance.

## What is the core?

The core is literally the centre of all function, from relaxed breathing to explosive sports skills and movement performance. Accordingly, the tests performed to gauge core function should reflect this diversity.

The deeper core muscles can be likened to a supportive canister around the vital organs. The diaphragm creates the roof of the canister and the pelvic floor musculature creates the floor. The transversus abdominis and lumbodorsal fasciae form the walls of the canister.[11] The diaphragm assists with inspiration and the pelvic floor musculature performs a supportive role for the internal organs.[12] The transversus abdominis functions as a stabilizing muscle, maintaining spinal stability during upright posture while also assisting with expiration. The paraspinals (e.g. interspinalis, intertransversalis, rotatores and multifidus) that link together vertebral segments function to stabilize each vertebra and also fine-tune the sensory information about spinal movement to improve the proprioception necessary for reflex stabilization.[13,14]

The more superficial core muscles include the erector spinae, rectus abdominis, internal/external oblique abdominis and supportive musculature around the pelvic and shoulder girdles. These muscles function to reinforce posture and spinal stability, and in more dynamic activities, to transfer energy to the upper and lower extremities, depending on the activity. The deeper core muscles maintain tonic activation for nearly all activities, while the more superficial core muscles are increasingly recruited as physical demands escalate.[14,16,15]

Activities that are quick, forceful and explosive require stabilization and motion control throughout the torso. When the core musculature becomes dysfunctional, neural control errors can result in excessive recruitment of the more superficial core muscles during relatively low intensity activities (e.g. bending over to pick up a dropped object).[5,14,16] This high threshold recruitment strategy overwhelms the capacity of the deeper core muscles to maintain spinal stability, which places potentially injurious forces on passive spinal ligaments and discs.

We can see, therefore, that core muscle testing should precede core muscle training to determine whether lower intensity rehabilitation-type exercises that emphasize recruitment of the deeper core muscles should occur as the first step before progressing to higher-intensity exercises (if needed) that integrate both the deeper and more superficial core muscles. Neurological tuning of the core muscles is critical. This is analogous to a race car, which is built to be very fast, powerful and durable, but without consistent fine-tuning and testing, small issues can be overlooked and create significant problems.

## Assessment of core competency

The anatomical structure of the core muscles makes them best suited for stabilization. The flat-layered muscles efficiently transfer energy and control motion. Conversely, the long spindle-shaped muscles of the extremities have anatomical and neuromuscular affinity for the production of movement. The tendons of extremity muscles are designed to store energy, and the long sections of contractile tissue are designed to lengthen and shorten far beyond resting length. The muscles of the extremities respond favourably to full-range concentric exercise, and their tendons develop with plyometric training. However, the core muscles cannot be appropriately tested or trained in the same way as extremity musculature. The core muscles possess a full range of movement, but peak muscle activity is needed in the midranges of function. Timing and alignment are more important than peak force, and reflex stabilization is more important for function than conscious activation.

Testing and training of the core muscles should be based on anatomical structure and function while considering basic ranges of motion, low-level core function and high-level core function for activities requiring extra support. In order to assess and set baselines for the numerous levels of core muscle functioning, wide arrays of tests are needed. There cannot simply be one test to establish generalized function of the core muscles; numerous tests can and should be utilized, depending on the goal of the exercise professional and athlete being tested.

The effectiveness of core muscle training strategies should be demonstrated with objective testing. Both the deep and superficial core musculature must be given adequate attention during testing so as not to perpetuate recurrent problems in core muscle training and rehabilitation following injury. In this chapter, three phases or levels of core muscle testing will be presented, with examples of tests which can be utilized to set baselines for the different levels of core muscle function.

## Phase 1

The first level of core muscle testing involves movement pattern screening. This approach to testing starts with motor control and demonstrates the natural reflex behaviour of the core musculature. Isolated core muscle testing may not reveal higher-level deficits in core muscle functioning. For example isolated testing of the core muscles may indicate normal levels of isometric and concentric strength, but when applied to *real world* movement scenarios, the core muscles may not effectively maintain spinal stability. Movement screening allows the exercise professional to check for initial risk factors, which may predispose the client to injury. The Functional Movement Systems (FMS) screening is an example of a tool designed to assess movement competencies.[17,16,18] Injury prevention has to be the priority for any professional working in sport, and screening techniques can be a way of identifying specific risk factors. This is discussed in greater detail in chapter 6.

## Phases 2 and 3

The second phase of testing occurs once movement pattern competency has been established. Core muscle performance can be looked at on both a global and local platform. The second level of testing takes a global view of how well energy transfer takes place throughout the body, as well as identifies right and left side asymmetries. Energy transfer from the upper body to the lower body and vice versa is assessed during this level of testing. A global platform is demonstrated by movements, such as a tall or half-kneeling medicine ball chop pass, Y-balance test, hop and stop, standing long jump and standing medicine ball throw to the left and to the right. The third level is designed to test the function of the local core. This level of testing is less dynamic and attempts to determine the muscle function and stabilization ability of the muscles of the torso. The local platform of tests would include the double leg lowering and side-bridge or plank.

Performance information relative to core muscle function helps the exercise professional discern the existence of core muscle dysfunction. If local core muscle testing demonstrates adequate strength (within normal parameters), then isolated training of the core musculature is not necessary. However, movement pattern exercises might be necessary to integrate normally functioning core muscles into patterns that might be awkward or uncoordinated. It should be noted that all global core muscle tests are done to assess left-right symmetry (except for the standing long jump). The standing long jump assesses the productivity and energy transfer between links in the kinetic chain. The tests performed in this level and the previous levels will allow a baseline of core function to be established which will help direct the best training option.

The outline of tests is as follows:

1   Movement Pattern Screening: The Functional Movement Screen;
2   Global Core Muscle Performance: tall and half-kneeling medicine ball throw, standing long jump, standing left and right baseline throw, y-balance test and hop-and-stop;
3   Local Core Muscle Performance: double-leg lowering and side bridge/plank.
      Skill testing with respect to the core musculature is most effectively discussed at a sports-specific level, once movement patterns and local and global core muscle tests are within acceptable ranges.

### First phase: Movement pattern screening

Movement pattern screening tests are designed to capture movement pattern quality and can be assessed by using the Functional Movement Screen.[17,18] The results are intended to rank an individual's movement patterns into a hierarchy, to easily identify the most deficient movement pattern. The test is comprised of seven fundamental movement patterns that require mobility and stability. The movement patterns include: deep squatting, stepping, lunging, reaching, leg raising, push-up and rotary stability. These movements are utilized and designed to identify compensatory movement patterns in the kinetic chain by observing right- and left-side imbalances and mobility and stability weaknesses.

These seven movements challenge the body's ability to facilitate movement through the proximal-to-distal sequence. This course of movement in the kinetic chain allows the body to produce movement patterns more efficiently. However, weaknesses in the kinetic linking system result in progressively inefficient movement patterns over time. Once an inefficient movement pattern has been isolated, exercise strategies can be instituted to avoid further deterioration and injury.

Once the movement pattern screening has been performed the score can be utilized to determine the most significant movement pattern dysfunction. Recent research has indicated that, in certain populations, lower scores can place individuals at higher risk for injury. This criteria can be utilized as a general rule until more research can be obtained.[19] More importantly, this screen can be used to set a baseline of movement efficiency for the individual, which will assist in directing the next level of testing.

### Second phase: Global core muscle performance

The results of the movement pattern screening will help to identify areas of weakness. Based on these weaknesses you can better determine which tests are the most appropriate for the individual. The movement pattern screening challenges the core muscles in different positions and stances; the dysfunctions observed during the screening can then be further assessed during the third level testing. It should be noted that if significant movement or mobility dysfunctions exist, those should be addressed prior to higher-level core muscle testing. The global core muscle tests are both qualitative and quantitative in nature. The tests assess energy transfer, symmetry and productivity in different positions and movements.

The Y-balance test measures the ability of each lower extremity to stabilize the spine during multi-planar movements.[20] It can be performed by simply standing on one foot and reaching out as far as possible with the toes with the opposite limb. It is performed by having the client stand on one leg on the centre of a foot-plate with the most distal aspect of the toes at the starting line. While maintaining a single-leg stance, the individual client is asked to reach the toes out as far as possible and touch down with the free limb in the anterior (see Figure 12.1), postero-medial (back toward the midline of the body; 45-degrees [see Figure 12.2]), and posterolateral (back away from the body; 45-degrees [see Figure 12.3]) directions in relation to the stance foot.

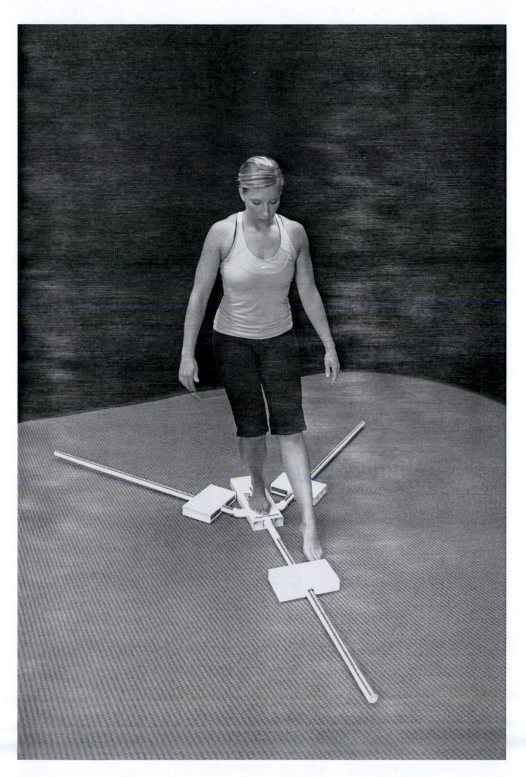

*Figure 12.1* Y-balance test: anterior

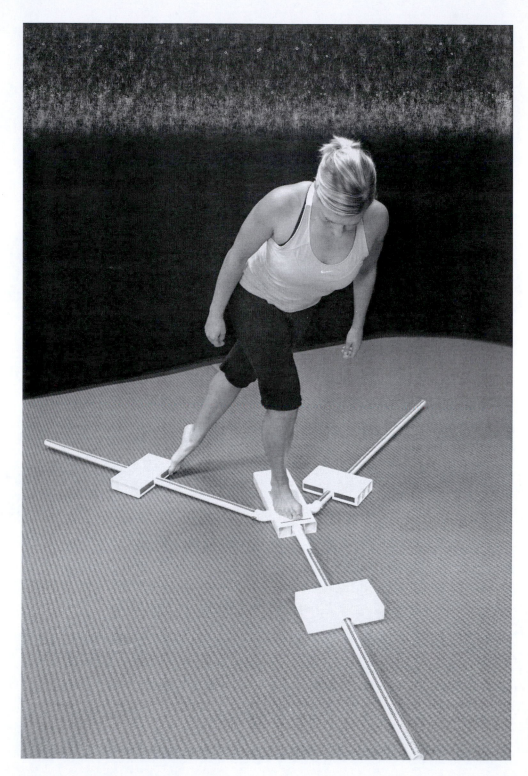

*Figure 12.2* Y-balance test: posteromedial

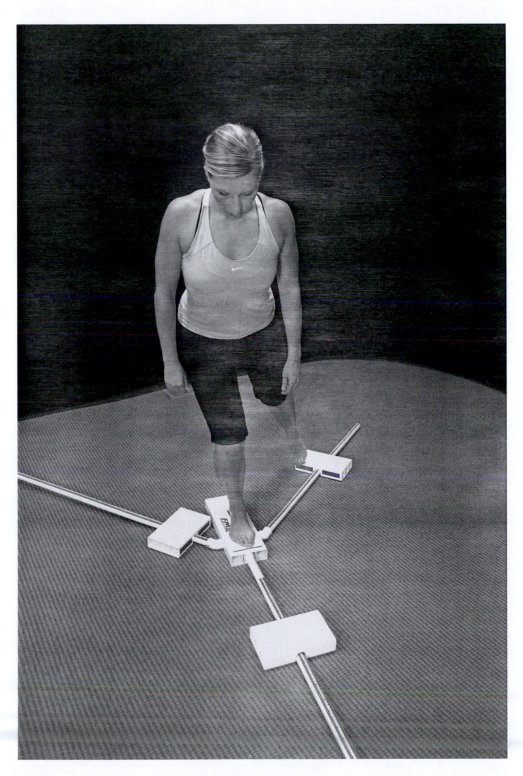

*Figure 12.3* Y-balance test: posterolateral

A medicine ball bounce chop pass can be performed to gauge force production and symmetry of the core muscles. This test can be performed in a half-kneeling or split-stance and tall-kneeling or squat-stance; the core muscles will respond differently in these two positions, so it is important to test both positions. The kneeling position will assist in eliminating compensatory motions in the lower extremities, thus allowing more emphasis to be placed on the core muscles.

The half-kneeling chop pass begins by having the athlete assume a half-kneeling position with the down knee placed under the hip; the opposite ankle is then positioned under the knee so that the knee is at a 90-degree angle. The ankle on the down knee remains dorsiflexed with the toes extended. The base width between the down knee and ankle should be approximately four inches; a board can be placed between the knee and foot to ensure positioning (see Figure 12.4a–b). The tall-kneeling chop pass begins by having the individual

(a)

(b)

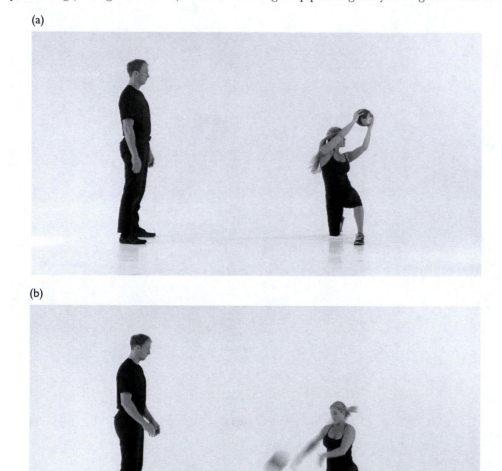

*Figure 12.4* (a) Starting position for downward right diagonal throw; (b) Release position for downward right diagonal throw

get into kneeling position, with their knees under the hips and feet pulled toward their shins so that the soles are vertical to the floor. In both positions, the client is instructed to maintain an upright posture throughout the test, allowing little to no torso movement during the test.

The medicine ball used for each of the medicine ball throw tests should be approximately 3 per cent of body weight.[17] The client should perform a two-handed throw downward to the floor and at a 45-degree angle (to the right and left), attempting to make the ball bounce as high as possible with little to no torso motion. The quality of the throw should be judged subjectively by the height of the bounce and the amount of stability maintained through the torso. The client should perform five repetitions throwing to the right and left sides. The key for this test is to observe torso stability and asymmetry between throws to the right and left sides. The baseline can be set by the height of the bounce, using a wall as a back-drop to determine the bounce height of each throw.

A standing left- and right-side two-handed medicine ball throw for distance can also be performed to demonstrate energy transfer from the lower to the upper extremities. The athlete is positioned with feet slightly wider than shoulder width and then asked to throw a medicine ball as far as possible, without allowing either foot to lose contact with the floor. The medicine ball should be approximately 3 per cent of body weight. The distance the ball travels is then measured. The client can perform up to five repetitions to the right and left sides in order to gauge symmetry and distance.

Research for the medicine ball tests is very limited, so normative data and reliability has not been established. Therefore, the focus should remain on quality and symmetry for the client being tested and comparing results with similar population groups or team members. This consistency is important until more research is gathered and normative data established.

The standing long jump is a global core muscle test demonstrating the ability to transfer energy from the upper extremities and torso to the lower extremities. This test is performed by having the athlete place their toes just behind a mark; the athlete then performs a countermovement and jumps horizontally with maximal effort. The distance is then measured from starting mark to the nearest point of contact. The client must land on both feet for the score to count. The best of three trials is recorded. The baseline measurement can then be compared to normative data[21] (see Table 12.1).

While the standing long jump is a global core muscle test that demonstrates energy transfer from a symmetrical stance position, the hop-and-stop test demonstrates energy transfer from

Table 12.1 Percentile ranks for standing broad jump in elite male and female athletes (8)

| Percentile | Male | Female |
|---|---|---|
| 90 | 375cm | 315cm |
| 80 | 339cm | 293cm |
| 70 | 309cm | 279cm |
| 60 | 294cm | 264cm |
| 50 | 279cm | 249cm |
| 40 | 264cm | 234cm |
| 30 | 249cm | 219cm |
| 20 | 234cm | 204cm |
| 10 | 219cm | 189cm |

an asymmetrical and single-leg stance position. This test attempts to measure the force production, absorption and energy transfer, while performing a lower-body plyometric activity. The hop-and-stop test utilizes two bilateral leg functions, a maximal hop for distance and a maximal controlled leap.[22]

The maximal hop for distance is performed by having the athlete place their toe on a starting mark with the hip and knee of the suspended limb at 90-degree angles and the hands placed on the hips. A single maximal hop is performed without swinging the suspended leg or removing the hands from the hips. The objective is to achieve maximal horizontal distance while landing on the same take-off foot and without placing the opposite foot down for support. The horizontal distance is measured to the closer mark of the landing foot.

Poor performance in the standing broad jump and hop-and-stop tests may indicate inefficiency in transferring energy through the torso into the extremities in a dynamic fashion. This inefficiency can be due to multiple factors, including poor mobility and stability, a decrease in strength or flexibility or a combination of each factor listed.

### Third phase: Local core muscle performance

The local core muscle performance is measured by performing specific activities, which attempt to isolate abdominal muscle function. These muscles are designed to stabilize the spine and pelvis during movement, which is why it is important to perform tests that are designed to challenge these actions. The tests utilized in this level of measurement provide additional feedback on muscle dysfunction. The tests performed in the previous levels were more dynamic in nature, focusing on entire movement patterns and energy transfer. In this section we will describe two tests that are commonly utilized, which provide both qualitative and quantitative information regarding local core muscle functioning for isometric strength and endurance.

The first test is the side bridge as described by McGill.[23] This test is performed by having the athlete lie on their side with the legs extended. The time is measured from when the athlete lifts their hips and gets into the proper alignment until the hips return to the floor. The side bridge is tested bilaterally in order to determine if there is a significant asymmetry noted between the right and left side bridge.

The required endurance times for the side bridge that may be used as a guide when testing are 81 seconds for the right and 85 seconds for the left.[23] Poor performance in this test indicates endurance weakness in the quadratus lumborum and abdominal wall musculature.[15]

The next test, which assesses local core muscle strength, is the double-leg lowering test.[24] This test specifically assesses the ability of the abdominal musculature to control the pelvis while the legs are lowered from a vertical position. The double-leg lowering test uses a sphygmomanometer to monitor pelvic tilt with pressure changes. The test is performed by placing the sphygmomanometer under the lumbar spine and inflated to 40mmHg. The athlete's hips are then passively flexed to 90 degrees while maintaining full knee extension. Should the athlete not be able to achieve this position, the limitation is more one of mobility, and this should be addressed separately. Both legs are then slowly lowered while attempting to maintain a posterior pelvic tilt. The angle of the legs (relative to the floor) is measured when the posterior pelvic tilt is lost (see Figure 12.5a–b). When using the sphygmomanometer, a loss of posterior pelvic tilt is determined by a decrease of 10mmHg of pressure.[24] The angle should be approximately 40 to 50 degrees before losing the posterior pelvic tilt. An inability to maintain the posterior pelvic tilt while lowering the legs indicates weakness in the abdominal musculature.

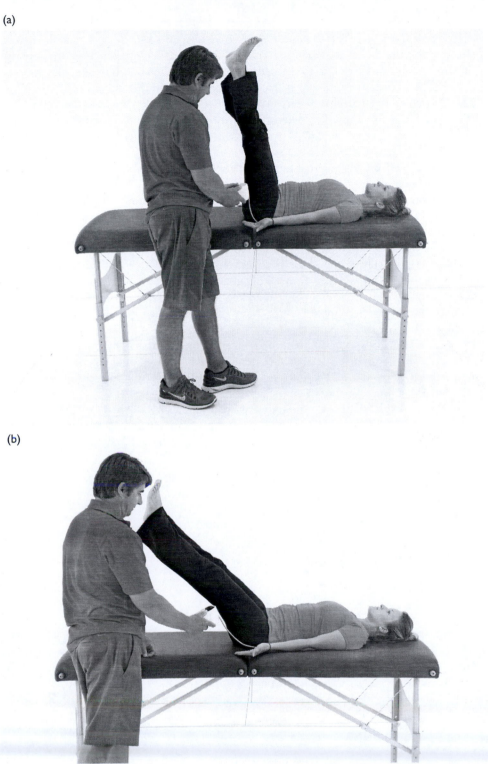

*Figure 12.5* (a) Starting position for the double-leg lowering test; (b) Lower the legs until pelvic control
is lost

The side bridge and double-leg lowering are two local core muscle tests that specifically isolate abdominal muscle function. The local core muscles are designed to stabilize the torso during movement; these tests provide baseline data on how the abdominal muscles perform this action. The two tests described challenge the local core muscles isometrically.

There is one other factor that can significantly alter core stabilization and that is the presence of pain with movement. Pain alters movement in unpredictable and inconsistent ways so the painful movement or area must be properly addressed in order to create effective core training.

Once it has been established that the individual does not have pain with movement, the results from the screening and testing must be properly assessed. Therefore, any movement patterns and test results that are considered dysfunctional or below the baseline of accepted movement competency must be prioritized and managed through corrective strategies.

The most efficient path to regaining core stabilization and performance does not necessarily look like clean compartments of flexibility training followed by core stabilization techniques. It is actually a progression back into a movement pattern, utilizing mobility and flexibility techniques to gain proper range of motion followed by motor control activities to enhance stability. This type of progression will allow more efficient movement patterning to occur. Once proper movement patterns have been established, strengthening and power activities for the core can be introduced.

Employing mobility and flexibility techniques takes priority when improving core performance. There are a variety of flexibility techniques that can and should be utilized, from soft tissue methods to partner and self-stretches. Often, individuals should focus on improving mobility in and around the thoracic spine, ankles and hips.

Common mobility techniques to improve thoracic spine mobility can include side-lying rotations and quadruped reaches (see Figure 12.6). Mobility techniques for the hips can be addressed through stride stretches, as well as half-kneeling activities (see Figure 12.7). In the

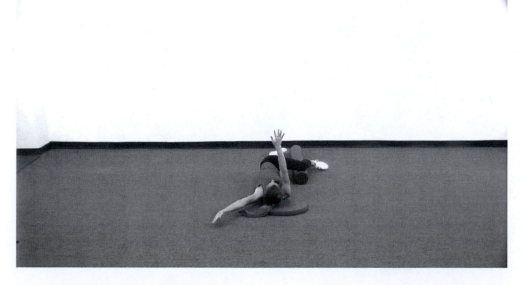

*Figure 12.6* Thoracic spine mobility stretches

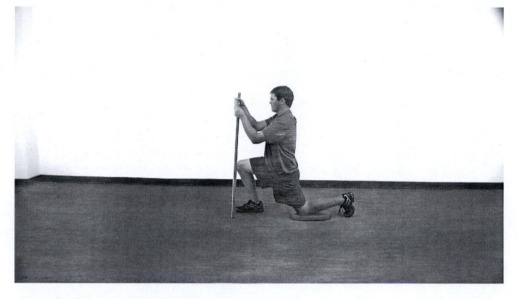

*Figure 12.7* Half-kneeling hip mobility stretch

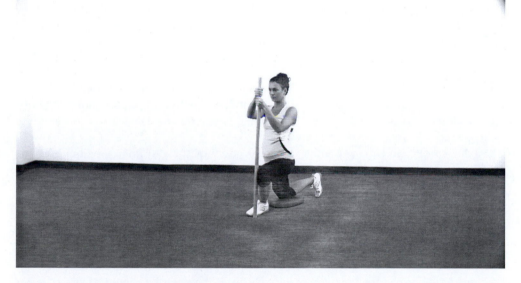

*Figure 12.8* Half-kneeling position for ankle mobility

half-kneeling position, the ankle mobility can be addressed by having the person move into dorsiflexion (see Figure 12.8). These will allow improvement in mobility as well as expose asymmetries in the area.

Once mobility has been properly addressed, motor control activities must be utilized to improve movement pattern efficiency. Techniques focused on enhancing proper coordination and motor control through reflex stabilization should be incorporated. In order for effective reflex stabilization and proper coordination to occur, the emphasis on proper set-up and technique are of the utmost importance. The athlete must place their focus on maintaining proper posture and positioning with less emphasis on resistance, sets and reps. We must choose a position as well as an exercise that will force the athlete to stabilize and coordinate effectively without compensating in order to perform the exercise. We should work to find the right balance between making the position and resistance too difficult where technique is lost, and placing the athlete against their weakness where they must utilize effective muscle recruitment and coordination to perform the technique.

The resistance, sets and reps should be manipulated based on the athlete's ability to maintain the proper position and posture while performing the exercise. Often, we can challenge the core by manipulating the position prior to increasing the resistance, sets and reps. For example, while performing a half-kneeling chop technique, we can increase the difficulty of the exercise by narrowing the base of the support (placing the foot more in line with the back knee). This simple change in position would force more stabilization in the core and lower extremities without manipulating the resistance, sets and reps. The resistance, sets and reps can be manipulated once proper positioning and posture are established. The emphasis must be placed on the quality of the movement throughout the exercise. This emphasis should ensure that once the movement pattern has been established it will be maintained.

Chop-and-lift techniques are very effective in improving reflex core stabilization. There are many variations of chopping and lifting. First, identify whether tall-kneeling or half-kneeling positioning will provide the best outcomes; reviewing the test results can do this. The focus should be on what was identified as the biggest dysfunction and asymmetry. The type of chop-and-lift exercises can range from simply holding the position to medicine ball chops. The most important factor is to ensure that proper technique is emphasized and maintained throughout in order to allow for the most effective motor control and coordination during the activities.

Once mobility, motor control and asymmetries have been addressed, movement pattern training should be introduced. Activities that first focus on proper techniques that utilize fundamental patterns such as deep squatting, lunging and single-leg stance should be incorporated.

Initially, movement pattern training can focus on establishing or improving hip-hinge or deadlift mechanics. The deadlift is a very fundamental movement that will provide a solid foundation for fundamental movements to be improved and strengthened, since proper hip-hinging is needed.

There are many variations on deadlifting; it is most important to first establish proper mechanics in the hip-hinge and focus on technique. Single-leg or double-leg deadlifting should be utilized based on what was identified during testing and previous mobility and motor control activities. The type of resistance (bar, bands, kettlebells, dumbbells, etc.) will vary depending on the goals you are trying to achieve. The deadlift should be viewed as an integral and fundamental part of core stability. Strengthening and power activities that utilize proper fundamental movements will ensure that the core continues to perform efficiently.

## Summary

The most holistic approach to any type of training should begin with a systematic approach to movement screening, testing and assessing. This will allow proper baselines, weaknesses and goals to be identified and established. It is extremely important when the focus is on core training to not only begin but also periodically monitor movements, because athletes are commonly injured and also have inappropriate training practices in some cases.

There are four keys to effectively improve core stabilization within programming for athletes:

1   Periodic screening, investigating critical biomarkers such as pain or dysfunction;
2   Using a hierarchy of movement to find the weakest link. This creates more efficient corrective strategy because only the most fundamental pattern is attacked at any given time, following a more neurodevelopmental progression;
3   Employing corrective strategy to create quick and efficient feedback;
4   Emphasizing and demanding proper technique when training strength and power movements.

Most training is done to create a positive adaptation, but physical adaptation with regard to strength and conditioning can take weeks. However, attacking inefficient movement patterns is largely dependent on motor control and stabilization. This can change in a short amount of time, especially with improved mobility and opportunities to use that new mobility at the appropriate level of stress.

Thus, the assignment of two to three key correctives is more important than an entire programme focused on core stabilization. These strategies can be done as a movement prep cool-down but can also be done within the workout as a superset to make sure that movement pattern quality is maintained throughout the exercise session.

## Notes

1   Akuthota, V., & Nadler, S. F. (2004). Core strengthening. *Arch Phys Med Rehabil*, *85*:86–92.
2   Nelson-Wong, E., Alex, B., Csepe, D., Lancaster, D., & Callaghan, J. P. (2012). Altered muscle recruitment during extension from trunk flexion in low back pain developers. *Clin Biomech*, *27*(10):994–998.
3   Shadmehr, A., Jafarian. Z., & Talebian, S. (2012). Changes in recruitment of pelvic stabilizer muscles in people with and without sacroiliac joint pain during the active straight-leg-raise test. *J Back Musculoskelet Rehabil*, *25*(1):27–32.
4   Mehta, R., Cannella, M., Smith, S. S., & Silfies, S. P. (2010). Altered trunk motor planning in patients with nonspecific low back pain. *J Mot Behav*, *42*(2):135–44.
5   Cholewicki, J., Greene, H. S., Polzhofer, G. K., Galloway, M. T., Shah, R. A., & Radebold, A. (2002). Neuromuscular function in athletes following recovery from a recent acute low back injury. *J Orthop Sports Phys Ther*, *32*(11):568–575.
6   Boling, M. C., Padua, D. A., Marshall, S. W., Guskiewicz, K., Pyne, S., & Beutler, A. (2009). A prospective investigation of biomechanical risk factors for patellofemoral pain syndrome: The joint undertaking to monitor and prevent ACL injury (JUMP-ACL) cohort. *Am J Sports Med*, *37*(11):2108–2116.
7   Plisky, P. J., Rauh, M. R., Kaminski, T. W., & Underwood, F. B. (2006). Star excursion balance test as a predictor of lower extremity injury in high school basketball players. *J Orthop Sports Phys Ther*, *36*:911–919.
8   Zazulak, B. T., Hewett, T. E., Reeves, N. P., Goldberg, B., & Cholewicki, J. (2007). Deficits in neuromuscular control of the trunk predict knee injury risk: A prospective biomechanical-epidemiologic study. *Am J Sports Med*, *35*(7):1123–30.
9   Renkawitz, T., Boluki, D., & Grifka, J. (2006). The association of low back pain, neuromuscular imbalance, and trunk extension strength in athletes. *Spine*, *6*(6):673–683.

10 Vera-Garcia, F. J., Elvira, J. L., Brown, S. H., & McGill, S. M. (2007). Effects of abdominal stabilization maneuvers on the control of spine motion and stability against sudden trunk perturbations. *J Electromyogr Kinesiol, 17*(5):556–67.

11 Hides, J., Wilson, S., & Stanton, W. (2006). An MRI investigation into the function of the transversus abdominis muscle during 'drawing-in' of the abdominal wall. *Spine, 31*(6): 175–178.

12 Hodges, P. W., Sapsford, R., & Pengel, L. H. (2007). Postural and respiratory functions of the pelvic floor muscles. *Neuro and Urodyn, 26*(3):362–371.

13 Stokes, M., Hides, J., Elliott, J., Kiesel, K., & Hodges, P. (2007). Rehabilitative ultrasound imaging of the posterior paraspinal muscles. *J Ortho Sports Physical Ther, 37*(10):581–595.

14 Cholewicki, J., van Dieen, J. H., & Arsenault, A. B. (2003). Muscle function and dysfunction in the spine. *J Electromyogr Kinesiol, 13*(4):303–304.

15 McGill, S. M., Juker, D., & Kropf, P. (1996). Quantitative instramuscular myoelectric activity of quadratus lumborum during a wide variety of tasks. *Clin Biomech, 11*:170–172.

16 Reeves, N. P., Cholewicki, J., & Silfies, S. P. (2006). Muscle activation imbalance and low-back injury in varsity athletes. *J Electromyogr Kinesiol, 16*(3):264–272.

17 Cook, G. (2001). Baseline Sports Fitness Testing. In *High-Performance Sports Conditioning* (pp. 19–48), B. Foran (Ed.), Champaign, IL: Human Kinetics.

18 Cook, G., & Burton, L. (2007). Impaired Patterns of Posture and Function. In *Musculoskeletal Interventions: Techniques for Therapeutic Exercise* (pp. 379–399), M. L. Voight, B. J. Hoogenboom & W. E. Prentice (Eds.), New York: McGaw-Hill.

19 Kiesel, K., Plisky, P. J., & Voight, M. L. (2007). Can serious injury in professional football be predicted by a preseason Functional Movement Screen? *North Am J Sports Phy Ther, 2*(3):147–158.

20 Juris, P. M., Phillips, E. M., Dalpe, C., Ewards, C., Gotlin, R. S., & Kane, D. J. (1997). A dynamic test of lower extremity function following anterior cruciate ligament reconstruction and rehabilitation. *J Ortho Sports Phys Ther, 26*(4):184–191.

21 Harman, E., & Garhammer, F. Administration, scoring and interpretation of selected tests. In T. R. Baechle & R. W. Earle (Eds.), *Essentials of Strength Training and Conditioning* (pp. 249–294). Colorado Springs, CO: National Strength and Conditioning Association.

22 Plisky, P. J., Gorman, P. P., Butler, R. J., et al. (2009). The reliability of an instrumented device for measuring components of the star excursion balance test. *N Am J Sports Phys Ther, 4*(2):92–99.

23 McGill, S. M., Childs, A., & Liebenson, C. (1999). Edurance times for low back stabilization exercises: Clinical targets for testing and training from a normal database. *Arch Phys Med Rehabil, 80*:941–944.

24 Krause, D. A., Youdas, J. W., Hollman, J. H., & Smith, J. (2005). Abdominal muscle performance as measured by the double leg–lowering test. *Arch Phys Med Rehabil, 86*:1345–1348.

# Chapter 13

# Flexibility in injury prevention and performance

*Anthony Blazevich*

## Introduction

Flexibility training is considered to be an integral part of most athletic training programmes, yet in some sports there is much debate as to the importance of flexibility training and how it should be structured within a programme. The purpose of this chapter is to discuss issues surrounding the use of muscle stretching in the context of the athletic performance program design for athletes. The term 'flexibility' will be used in this chapter to encapsulate both range-of-motion (ROM) and muscle-tendon extensibility (i.e. stiffness) aspects simultaneously.

## Why stretch?

While much is known about the neuromuscular and soft tissue adaptations to strength, endurance and other forms of training, very little is known about the adaptive process elicited by stretching training, despite what is often written in textbooks and articles. It is well known that increases in ROM and, sometimes, reductions in resistance to stretch (i.e. increased tissue extensibility) result from both acute and chronic stretch training; however, the changes in muscle fibre (or fascicle) and tendon properties predicted to occur, and often discussed in book chapters and on websites, have not been found by researchers. Nonetheless, it is known that even short (e.g. 5s) bouts of stretching can increase the energy stored within a muscle or muscle-tendon unit for a given load application (although longer bouts of stretching of up to an hour are required to prolong the effect). Alterations in force production, as well as increases in both the stretch length and force handled before injury (failure), are known to occur under these conditions. However, to best program the stretching training, it is also important to consider the following:

1   Increases in ROM, a shift in the torque-angle relation about a joint (i.e. the force-length relation for a muscle-tendon unit) toward longer muscle lengths,[1] and an increase in eccentric muscle strength,[2] can result from stretch training and may influence force production and assist with injury minimisation.
2   Chronic static-passive stretching regimes have been shown to reduce injury rates, and particularly reduce the incidence of soft tissue (muscle, ligament, tendon) injury;[3,4] less flexible athletes are often found to have a greater rate of injury.[5,6] Stretching is probably more effective for injury prevention when other forms of training (e.g. strength and balance training) are simultaneously added to a conditioning program[7,8] – a varied injury prevention strategy is clearly ideal.

3   Stretching training after exercise may reduce general soreness (e.g. in joints, muscles and the lower back) and thus improve feelings of recovery and well-being.[3]

4   Acute stretching done in preparation for exercise has rarely been shown to reduce all-cause injury rates.[9] However, a number of common injuries (e.g. ankle sprains, bone fractures, contact injuries) are not associated with ROM deficits or excessive tissue stiffness, and most are influenced by other factors (e.g. compartment syndromes, inflammatory conditions); there is reasonable evidence that pre-exercise stretching reduces soft tissue injury rates,[10] and this reduction should theoretically be greater when athletes are required to move through large ROMs.

5   Stretching may confer self-confidence, preparedness and other perceptual benefits. Many athletes use pre- or post-exercise stretching in order to feel 'prepared' for the rigors of exercise and to check for signs of muscle tightness, soreness or injury, and/or to detect between- or within-limb imbalances in stiffness.

## Stretching, flexibility and sporting performance

The forces generated by muscle fibres are transferred laterally between fibres, between fibre bundles (fascicles) and between muscles within a muscle group before reaching the tendon and skeleton. Therefore, any change in the mechanical (e.g. stiffness or energy storage efficiency) properties of the muscle or tendon induced by stretching training can affect the transfer of force and, ultimately, performance.

Stiffer muscle-tendon units are thought to allow a more rapid and efficient transfer of force from the muscle to the skeleton, so stiffer individuals may have an advantage in tasks requiring high levels of force production in isometric or concentric contractions.[11] Also, the passive elastic component significantly contributes to total muscle force, especially at longer muscle-tendon lengths (see Figure 13.1), so variations in stiffness will directly influence force production. Stiffer muscle-tendon units should also recoil faster after being stretched while loaded,

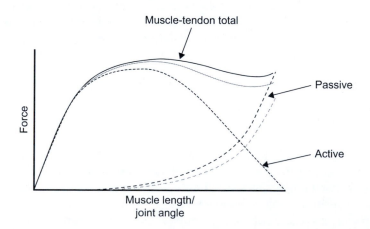

*Figure 13.1* Effect of changing passive muscle-tendon stiffness on muscle force production. The total force output (solid line) is equal to the sum of active (dashed line) and passive (dotted line) forces. Changes in stiffness with the inclusion or exclusion of stretching (e.g. grey lines show a reduction in passive and total force, especially at longer muscle lengths) should theoretically impact on muscle force production

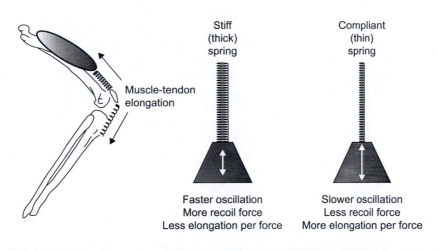

*Figure 13.2* Limbs flex and extend much like a spring (left image). Stiffer muscle-tendon units tend to provide a faster oscillation frequency (ideal for fast SSC movements) with greater recoil force but less elongation for a given muscle force (middle image). The opposite is true for more compliant muscle tendon units (right image)

as they act as a spring during stretch-shorten cycle (SSC) movements (see Figure 13.2). By contrast, more compliant (i.e. less stiff) muscle-tendon units may be of benefit when SSC movements are performed at a slower frequency or through a larger ROM (e.g. countermovement jump) because the natural speed of stretch and shortening (i.e. the natural frequency of the system) matches more precisely the speed of the movement. Greater compliance might also be important when large forces are applied rapidly to the body, such as when landing from significant height (>80 cm) in drop jumps, because of the significant energy absorption that is required during deceleration of the body. Thus, changes in tissue stiffness elicited by stretching training may influence athletic performance under specific conditions, and therefore optimising tissue stiffness is an important strength and conditioning goal.

Interestingly, despite the theoretical assumptions and anecdotal evidence that chronic stretching training might reduce performance in high-force or faster stretch-shorten cycle-type activities, stretching training lasting several weeks or months has not been associated with reductions in isometric or concentric force production,[12] has been associated with increases in strength in well-trained weightlifters due to an improved ability to store elastic energy (or a reduction in inhibitory reflex involvement),[13] can improve performance in SSC movements,[14] and was shown not to affect running economy in well-trained endurance runners.[15] These findings provide some evidence that stretching training might be implemented without negatively affecting performance, and may improve it in some instances. As discussed below, a clear testing/monitoring programme is therefore required in order to determine the best use of stretching training for each athlete.

## Periodisation of stretching training

It may be beneficial to periodise stretching training in order to improve joint ROM, with the aim of reducing injury risk and/or allowing athletes to achieve a sufficient ROM to employ a specific movement technique whilst achieving a high level of stiffness. The goal of such periodisation is to train effectively in a preparation period with lower injury risk by increasing flexibility, and then to achieve an optimum level of muscle-tendon stiffness at a specific point in the training year (i.e. to peak) by reducing flexibility training. Such a strategy can be referred to as macrocycle-based stretching periodisation, because stretching regimes during each training phase are targeted to a specific purpose. Unfortunately, no studies have examined the efficacy of this strategy, although it appears to be in common usage and can be trialled on an athlete-to-athlete basis to assess its effectiveness.

> Stretch training may be periodised in order to most effectively improve joint ROM, with the aim of reducing injury risk and/or allowing athletes to achieve a sufficient ROM to adopt the correct sporting techniques whilst achieving the desired level of muscle-tendon stiffness.

Microcycle-based periodisation is also possible (see simplified example in Table 13.1). For example athletes who compete on a weekly basis may perform a greater volume of static stretching after competition and for the few days following in order to retain or improve flexibility, reduce soreness or muscle ache and potentially minimise injury risk during training. However, the stretch volume can be reduced in the days preceding the next competition in order for an increase in muscle-tendon stiffness to be achieved; in particular, negligible

Table 13.1 Example (deliberately simplified) weekly stretch programme for a sprint runner showing microcycle-based periodisation. As with other training programs (e.g. strength, endurance, plyometrics), weekly stretch programs should vary between athletes, depending on their current flexibility requirements and their functional responses to the training.

| | Monday | Tuesday | Wednesday | Thursday | Friday | Saturday (comp) | Sunday |
|---|---|---|---|---|---|---|---|
| **a.m.** | Warm-up and drills | 6 × run-throughs (60–100 m) | | 6 × run-throughs (60–100 m) | | | Recovery session |
| | Full stretch | Short stretch | | Choice: Short stretch or dynamic stretch | | | Full stretch |
| **p.m.** | Max velocity (3 × 80–150 m) + over-speed (2 × 60 m tows) | Drills Starts × 10 | Ramped speed – 6 × 80 m, last run at max.) | Starts × 6 if perfect | 3 × 60 m run-throughs | Comp | |
| | Half stretch | Half stretch | | | | Half stretch | |
| | | | Dynamic stretch | Dynamic stretch | Dynamic stretch | | |

**Full stretch** = 2 × 15 s per stretch – passive (PNF if required): Foot inversion/eversion, ankle dorsiflexion/plantarflexion, calf stretch (straight and bent knee), quad stretch, hamstrings (straight and bent knee), adductor, glut/hip flexion, upper body stretches.
**Half stretch** = 1 × 15 s per stretch – passive: Foot inversion/eversion, ankle dorsi-/plantarflexion, calf stretch (straight and bent knee), quad stretch, hamstrings (straight and bent knee), adductor, glut/hip flexion, upper body stretches.
**Short stretch** = 1 × 5–10 s stretch – passive: Ankle dorsiflexion/plantarflexion, calf stretch (straight and bent knee), quad stretch, hamstrings (straight and bent knee), glut/hip flexion, upper body stretches.
**Dynamic stretch** = Leg swings (front-to-back and across body) with or without brief static hold, dynamic glut/hip flexion with brief hold, arm vertical extension with brief hold.

stretching may be done after the final training session prior to competition. Noticeable changes in ROM and extensibility (i.e. stiffness) can be achieved within these several-day blocks after one competition and before the next. It is also important to note that muscle-tendon (and joint) stiffness might need to vary between joints, between muscle groups and between individual athletes, and so a periodised plan needs to account for this.

## Stretching as part of a complex training program

Within a complex training programme, muscle stretching may be done before or after training or competitions, or in separate sessions. There are benefits and costs associated with each.

> Muscle stretching may be done before or after training or competitions, or in separate sessions. There are benefits and costs associated with each, so an understanding of these is necessary.

### Stretching before exercise or sport participation

#### Potential benefits

Acute improvements in ROM should allow for easier movement through the potentially large ROMs required during exercise or sports participation. Possible reductions in tissue stiffness (i.e. increases in extensibility) are also thought to allow for greater energy storage before injury, and thus the likelihood of soft-tissue injury might be reduced. Importantly, acute improvements in ROM and reductions in stiffness have been shown after as little as 5 s of stretching,[16] so long stretch durations may not be necessary in order to have the desired effects.

Pre-exercise stretching may also be performed in order to test for areas of high joint/ muscle stiffness, soreness or injury, and it may increase subjective feelings of athlete preparedness. There is also some evidence that chronic stretching routines (pre- and post-exercise) can reduce the general soreness that accompanies sports and exercise.[3]

Active forms of stretching, and dynamic-ballistic stretching in particular, are often associated with improvements in muscle force production and movement capacity. A selection of dynamic-ballistic stretches that target important body parts that are relevant to sporting performance should thus be an integral part of a pre-exercise preparatory routine. Also, roller massage (e.g. use of a foam roller) may be beneficial, as it may reduce muscle stiffness and increase ROM without affecting muscle force production. The muscle areas (calf, anterior or lateral thigh, hamstrings, lateral hip and gluteal areas in the lower limbs) are typically rolled with firm pressure for 5–30 s, with either fast (one full up-and-back roll per second) or slow (4–5 s per roll) strokes; less pressure is often applied during fast rolling.

#### Potential costs

Static-passive (and PNF) forms of stretching can impair muscle force (and power) production in the period immediately after stretching, although activities performed some time (e.g. 15 min) after stretch are unlikely to be affected, since the recovery of the stretch-induced force loss is rapid. The time taken to stretch may also be long enough for a drop in body temperature to occur, which can impair subsequent exercise performance. Importantly, however, the post-stretch strength loss appears to occur at shorter, rather than longer, muscle lengths[17] and does not appear to affect eccentric muscle force;[18] most injuries occur at longer muscle lengths (acute joint angles) and during eccentric actions. Given these issues, static-passive stretches should: (1) be done relatively early in a pre-exercise preparation routine to allow for possible force reductions to resolve, (2) be held only briefly (unless substantive increases in ROM are required) in order to minimise the likelihood of force losses, and (3) be followed by a complete warm-up and sports-specific practice. When following these guidelines, and stretches are performed as part of a comprehensive routine, impairments in performance are rarely seen.

### Pre-exercise stretch programme design

There are a number of ways in which a pre-exercise preparation routine can be organised, and thus many ways in which stretching can be incorporated (see Table 13.2). Three general programmes are:

1   Single-block design: active or passive stretching techniques are performed sequentially within a single block over (usually) a 10–30 min period, typically after a low-intensity warm-up. A progressive and complete warm-up routine is then completed after the static-passive stretching block. This design is used by athletes who have a requirement to significantly improve their ROM prior to exercise participation, or who use the stretch block for psychological preparation or to monitor for stiffness imbalances and soreness.
2   Multiple-block design: different body regions are conditioned separately and in a deliberate order, and thus the stretching of a muscle group is performed in conjunction with specific exercise drills or movements. This allows an athlete to focus on a particular body region independently in order to detect stiffness or injury problems and to maintain body temperature throughout the warm-up period.
3   Mixed design: active or passive stretches are done (or repeated) at any point within a warm-up program. Typically, the stretches are done in conjunction with specific exercise drills or movements that utilise the particular muscle group, similar to the multiple-block design. However, this design allows for single stretches to be done between each warm-up drill according to the subjective feeling of 'tightness' of each muscle group; stiffness in a muscle or joint can be treated with (usually) brief active or passive stretches between drills, or a prolonged period of stretching can be imposed. This design may allow for maintenance of both body temperature and motivation throughout a warm-up period.

> Pre-exercise stretching routines can be organised in several ways, including (1) single block design, (2) multiple block design, and (3) mixed design.

## Stretching after exercise or sport participation, or in a separate session

### Potential benefits

Post-exercise or 'out-of-training' stretching is usually employed for the purpose of improving ROM. The use of longer-duration (e.g. >15s) static or PNF stretches performed for 2–4 repetitions is ideal. The incorporation of such stretching in sporting populations is often associated with a reduced total rate of injury, and soft-tissue injury in particular. Younger and female athletes typically have greater flexibility, so they will likely need a lower volume of post-exercise stretching for the purpose of increasing joint ROM when compared to older or male athletes.

With respect to post-exercise stretching for recovery, it is hypothesised that stretching can reduce intramuscular pressure by reducing tissue stiffness, which allows for (1) an improved blood perfusion and thus tissue recovery, and (2) an accelerated metabolite clearance to minimise the activation of pain and pressure receptors and, thus, to minimise muscle ache and pain. The reduction in intramuscular pressure can also directly reduce perceptions of muscle pain and fatigue. Nonetheless, although stretching training appears to reduce 'bothersome soreness',[3] further research is required to substantiate these claims, and athletes should determine for themselves whether they perceive such benefits. Post-exercise stretching also provides an opportunity to assess injury and tightness, which can then be treated appropriately.

## Potential costs

Stretching of injured tissues can aggravate injury, and should be done only when advised by a medical practitioner or physiotherapist. Also, chronic stretching training may exacerbate hypermobility in some athletes, which may further increase injury risk during sports training or competition; extreme flexibility is also a risk factor for injury.

*Table 13.2* Simplified example of a pre-exercise stretch programme for a sprint runner with different program designs.

| Single-block design | Multiple-block design | Mixed design |
|---|---|---|
| Jog warm-up (5min) | Jog warm-up (5min) | Jog warm-up (5min) |
| Static stretches (2 x 5s) | Static stretches (2 x 5s) | *Straight-leg calf (1 x 5s)* |
| *Straight-leg calf* | *Straight-leg calf* | (*Bent-knee calf not needed*) |
| *Bent-knee calf* | *Bent-knee calf* | Ankling drill x 2 |
| *Bent-knee hamstring* | Ankling drill x 2 | *Bent-knee hamstring (1 x 5s)* |
| *Straight-knee hamstring* | *Bent-knee hamstring* | Clawing drill x 2 |
| *Hip flexor* | *Straight-knee hamstring* | *Bent-knee hamstring (1 x 5s)* |
| *Glut/hip flexion* | Clawing drill x 2 | (*Straight-knee not needed*) |
| *Quadriceps (with hip ext.)* | *Hip flexor* | *Hip flexor (1 x 5s)* |
| *Adductor* | *Glut/hip flexion* | Knee lift drill x 1 |
| *Anterior shoulder* | *Quadriceps (with hip ext.)* | *Glut/hip flexion (1 x 5s)* |
| Jog warm-up (2 min) | Knee lift drill x 2 | Knee lift drill x 1 |
| Ankling drill x 2 | *Adductor* | *Glut/hip flexion (1 x 5s)* |
| Clawing drill x 2 | Side crab | (*Quadriceps not needed*) |
| Knee lift drill x 2 | Carioca (left and right) | *Adductor (1 x 5s)* |
| Side crab | *Anterior shoulder* | Side crab |
| Carioca (left and right) | Full sprint-specific warm-up … | Carioca (left and right) |
| Full sprint-specific warm-up | | *Anterior shoulder* |
| | | Full sprint-specific warm-up |

## When to avoid stretching

Although there are many potential benefits of stretching, there are also some instances in which muscle stretching should not be performed. These include:

- Hypermobility
- Joint ankylosis (i.e. abnormal stiffness of a joint, often associated with inflammation)
- Clinical osteoporosis
- Recent surgery
- Painful or stiff joints
- Joint inflammation
- Nerve compression
- Angiopathy or other blood vessel disorder.

These conditions should be assessed by a trained practitioner before stretching is performed.

## Flexibility testing: An essential feedback tool

Given our limited knowledge of the neuromuscular and performance adaptations that result from acute or chronic stretching training and our incomplete understanding of the effects of stretching training on muscle-tendon stiffness, it is not possible to draft specific guidelines as far as optimum stretching programme design or degrees of flexibility are concerned. Thus, there is a need for continuous monitoring of stretching practices and flexibility scores in athletes. Whilst we tend to assess multiple dimensions of athletic competency, assessment of flexibility and muscle-tendon stiffness and their relationship with performance outcomes is seldom explored. It is therefore rarely possible to track the relationship between flexibility and performance, either for a given athlete over time or within a group of athletes. This ensures that the opportunity to set an optimum range of joint flexibility scores or to design an appropriate stretching programme is lost and a major part of the overall athlete training programme can never be optimised. Thus, a muscle stretching and flexibility monitoring programme should be implemented with a view to optimising performance whilst reducing injury risk.

> Muscle stretching and flexibility monitoring programmes should be implemented with a view to optimising performance whilst reducing injury risk.

## Summary

Muscle stretching training is commonly used by athletes. However, the neuromuscular adaptations resulting from acute (e.g. pre-exercise) and longer-term training are not well understood. Therefore, it is not possible to draft guidelines for individual athletes with different ROM, muscle-tendon stiffness or force production requirements. Nonetheless, there are numerous potential injury prevention and performance improvement benefits associated with well-implemented stretching programs. Consideration should be given to the types of stretching performed (e.g. static, passive, active, dynamic, PNF) and its macro- and micro-level periodisation. When used prior to exercise, potential improvements in ROM, performance and feelings of preparedness need to be set against possible performance losses, so stretching should be performed early in a warm-up routine, its volume (and the types of stretch used) should be sufficient for the requirements of the athlete and its organisation within the warm-up should be considered. Importantly, a dedicated performance monitoring programme is essential in optimising the use of stretching in the context of a broader athletic training programme.

## Notes

1 Alonso, J., McHugh, M. P., Mullaney, M. J., & Tyler, T. F. (2009). Effect of hamstring flexibility on isometric knee flexion angle-torque relationship. *Scandinavian Journal of Medicine and Science in Sports, 19*(2), 252–6.

2 Handel, M., Horstmann, T., Dickhuth, H. H., & Gulch, R. W. (1997). Effects of contract-relax stretching training on muscle performance in athletes. *European Journal of Applied Physiology and Occupational Physiology, 76*(5), 400–8.

3 Jamtvedt, G., Herbert, R. D., Flottorp, S., Odgaard-Jensen, J., Havelsrud, K., Barratt, A., . . . Oxman, A. D. (2010). A pragmatic randomised trial of stretching before and after physical activity to prevent injury and soreness. *British Journal of Sports Medicine, 44*(14), 1002–9.

4 McKay, G. D., Goldie, P. A., Payne, W. R., & Oakes, B. W. (2001). Ankle injuries in basketball: injury rate and risk factors. *British Journal of Sports Medicine, 35*(2), 103–8.

5 Arnason, A., Sigurdsson, S. B., Gudmundsson, A., Holme, I., Engebretsen, L., & Bahr, R. (2004). Risk factors for injuries in football. *American Journal of Sports Medicine, 32*(1 Suppl), 5S–16S.

6 Witvrouw, E., Danneels, L., Asselman, P., D'Have, T., & Cambier, D. (2003). Muscle flexibility as a risk factor for developing muscle injuries in male professional soccer players: A prospective study. *American Journal of Sports Medicine, 31*(1), 41–6.

7 Mandelbaum, B. R., Silvers, H. J., Watanabe, D. S., Knarr, J. F., Thomas, S. D., Griffin, L. Y., . . . Garrett, W., Jr. (2005). Effectiveness of a neuromuscular and proprioceptive training program in preventing anterior cruciate ligament injuries in female athletes: 2-year follow-up. *American Journal of Sports Medicine, 33*(7), 1003–10.

8 Olsen, O. E., Myklebust, G., Engebretsen, L., Holme, I., & Bahr, R. (2005). Exercises to prevent lower limb injuries in youth sports: Cluster randomised controlled trial. *British Medical Journal, 330*(7489), 449.

9 Thacker, S. B., Gilchrist, J., Stroup, D. F., & Kimsey, C. D., Jr. (2004). The impact of stretching on sports injury risk: A systematic review of the literature. *Medicine and Science in Sports and Exercise, 36*(3), 371–8.

10 McHugh, M. P., & Cosgrave, C. H. (2010). To stretch or not to stretch: The role of stretching in injury prevention and performance. *Scandinavian Journal of Medicine and Science in Sports, 20*(2), 169–81.

11 Wilson, G. J., Murphy, A. J., & Pryor, J. F. (1994). Musculotendinous stiffness: Its relationship to eccentric, isometric, and concentric performance. *Journal of Applied Physiology, 76*(6), 2714–9.

12 Kroll, P. G., Goodwin, M. E., Nelson, T. L., Ranelli, D. M., & Roos, K. (2001). The effect of increased hamstring flexibility on peak torque, work, and power production in subjects with seventy degrees or greater of straight leg raise. *Physical Therapy, 81*:A27.

13 Wilson, G. J., Elliott, B. C., & Wood, G. A. (1992). Stretch shorten cycle performance enhancement through flexibility training. *Medicine and Science in Sports and Exercise, 24*(1), 116–123.

14 Kallerud, H., & Gleeson, N. (2013). Effects of stretching on performances involving stretch-shortening cycles. *Sports Medicine, 43*(8), 733–50.

15 Nelson, A. G., Kokkonen, J., Eldredge, C., Cornwell, A., & Glickman-Weiss, E. (2001). Chronic stretching and running economy. *Scandinavian Journal of Medicine and Science in Sports, 11*(5), 260–5.

16 Kay, A. D., & Blazevich, A. J. (2008). Reductions in active plantarflexor moment are significantly correlated with static stretch duration. *European Journal of Sport Science, 8*(1), 41–46.

17 Herda, T. J., Cramer, J. T., Ryan, E. D., McHugh, M. P., & Stout, J. R. (2008). Acute effects of static versus dynamic stretching on isometric peak torque, electromyography, and mechanomyography of the biceps femoris muscle. *Journal of Strength and Conditioning Research, 22*(3), 809–17.

18 Ayala, F., De Ste Croix, M., Sainz De Baranda, P., & Santonja, F. (2013). Acute effects of static and dynamic stretching on hamstring eccentric isokinetic strength and unilateral hamstring to quadriceps strength ratios. *Journal of Sports Sciences, 31*(8), 831–9.

# Part 3

# Injury processes, prevention and return to performance

# Chapter 14

# Muscle injuries

*Dan Lewindon and Justin Lee*

## Introduction

Muscle injuries occur frequently in all sports and at every level of participation.

As we continue to strive for greater athletic performance and our competition schedule continues to expand, it is perhaps understandable that our muscles may fail to tolerate the intensity, volume or frequency of our efforts. Re-injury rates are also common, in part due to the pressure to return our athletes to sport as soon as possible and also perhaps due to our limited understanding of modifiable risk factors and rehabilitation. To compound this, re-injury recovery time will often be significantly longer than for a first-time injury.[1]

Whilst pressures in sport will always remain, and the use of a risk management approach to returning an athlete will frequently be adopted, as a profession, we must continue to aspire to a better understanding of both the prevention and reconditioning of soft-tissue injury.

There has been a surge of good, quality research targeting aspects of rehabilitation and reconditioning over the last decade, resulting in a better understanding of muscle function and injury cause and effect, and providing us with clues and strategies that may add meaningful value to our programming. The merging of the medical and strength and conditioning spheres has given both sides a greater appreciation of the specialism and impact that both professions can have in the prevention and management of soft tissue injuries.

The purpose of this chapter is to:

1 Briefly summarise normal muscle function and the mechanical and pathophysiological processes that occur with injury;
2 Present the current role of imaging with respect to injury grade, prognosis and return to play;
3 Discuss the science behind key aspects of our rehabilitation, specifically the influence of exercise on tissue repair and, ultimately, functional recovery, reconditioning and return to sport;
4 Review current concepts in the prevention of muscle injuries.

The chapter will focus on soft-tissue injuries in the lower limb, with a biased attention to the hamstring group (as this is the most prevalent soft-tissue injury seen in running-based sports), but with the aim that the concepts discussed can be applied across all muscles.

## Specific muscle function

Successful rehabilitation requires an understanding of the requirements of the injured muscle in the context of the whole kinetic chain function and the demands of sport and life. That said, a greater knowledge of specific muscle function and structure could influence some of the priorities during this process and allow us to be more specific in our exercise selection.

In broad terms, the muscle tendon unit (MTU) is composed of contractile 'machinery' encased in a three-layered connective tissue support, anchored at either end through a tendon-bone connection. The sliding filament mechanism of muscle contraction has been embedded in our consciousness for decades and remains the principle model referred to in all basic human physiology texts. This involves a ratcheting system of shortening and lengthening to produce limb motion. Whilst thought to be accurate in characterizing the action of the contractile machinery, it cannot be the whole story in high force/speed lengthening or shortening movements. It is neither metabolically nor time efficient and negates the important roles of the free tendon and non-contractile tissue (collagen within the muscle unit) of the whole muscle unit.

Performance in high-speed and high-force activities is heavily dependent on the free tendon and non-contractile tissue within the muscle to either **amplify** or **absorb** force depending on the situation.[2] This is discussed in chapter 15 but is a crucial concept in muscle injury and rehabilitation. Inefficient elastic tissue or poor neuromuscular timing will increase the burden to the system and may increase the risk of injury.

## The MTU as a force amplifier

Under plyometric conditions, the tendon portion of the MTU acts like a spring, harnessing energy for use. In this situation (often termed the stretch-shorten cycle – SSC), where contact times may be incredibly short, it has been proposed that active lengthening and shortening occurs in the free tendon and intra-muscular elastic tissues, while the muscle itself contracts maximally and isometrically.[2]

## The MTU as a shock absorber

In conditions of absorption (for example landing from height, downhill walking, catching a ball or resisting a weight or opponent), the tendon provides the initial lengthening of the MTU, absorbing the force at high speed whilst the contractile portion of the muscle again contracts.[3] Once joint motion (ankle dorsiflexion in the case of landing) is completed and the MTU length reaches its maximal point of elongation, the tendon recoils, returning some energy to the muscle and dispersing the rest as heat. Simultaneously, the muscle relaxes its contraction and lengthens, absorbing the tendon force but, crucially, at a much slower rate, reducing the risk of injury. The tendon in this case is acting as a *buffer*, delaying the rate of absorption of force.[2]

These eccentric actions are critical in protecting the muscle and improving force production and efficiency. They require a finely tuned nervous system with a unique 'neuro-signature' to work both at a central and peripheral nervous system level.[4] They also require the appropriate tendon and series mechanical properties to deliver this performance and injury protection. It is little wonder, therefore, that eccentric training is consistently highlighted as a key component of successful muscle rehabilitation.[5]

> High-force/high-speed movements involve distinct mechanisms and neural pathways – our rehabilitation must reflect these differing functions.

# Muscle structure

Large variations are observed in skeletal muscle size, fibre composition, architecture, orientation and tendon size and length. This variation gives us clues regarding the likely functional characteristics of the muscle and therefore, perhaps, begins to demonstrate the specificity that may be applied to our exercise selection.

## Architecture

Muscle architecture (defined as the arrangement of fibres in a muscle relative to the axis of force production) is a very good indicator of muscle function.[6] To illustrate this in broad terms, a fusiform muscle where longer myofibres are arranged in parallel with the direction of limb motion is more suitably designed to produce limb motion. Conversely a pennate muscle, characterized by muscle fibres arranged at an angle to a central tendon slip, gives the potential for greater packing of contractile fibres within the same space to produce limb stiffness/higher resistance to motion, rather than joint excursion.[6]

There is now some emerging evidence utilizing ultrasound measurement in athletes with a history of hamstring strain that demonstrates a significant reduction in fascicle length in athletes with a history of hamstring strain, suggesting this as a primary risk factor for future injury if left uncorrected.[7]

The length of the free tendon will also clearly go some way to revealing the muscle's function as discussed above – a longer tendon infers greater energy storage and release.

An additional architectural variant, which has also recently been proposed as a risk factor for hamstring strains, is the ratio between tendon/aponeurosis size and muscle size at the muscle tendon junction (MTJ). In the long head of *biceps femoris*, it has been demonstrated that the larger the tendon/aponeurosis relative to the muscle, the lower the relative stress at the MTJ, as the load can be spread over a larger relative surface area.[8]

## Fibre type

Muscle is composed of slow and faster twitching fibres, which differ in size, energy demand and force potential.[9] An understanding of the relative blend of fibres in a target muscle through understanding its normal/desired function will also impact on the rehabilitation process by guiding the prescription of exercise duration, intensity, load and speed of limb movement as rehab progresses.

## Practical examples

1. Although both are considered medial hamstrings and immediate neighbours, the designs of *semitendinosus* and *semimembranosus* differ considerably. *Semitendinosus* demonstrates significantly greater relative muscle fibre length, a lower cross-sectional area with a more parallel arrangement of fibres and a longer distal free tendon.[6] Mechanically, therefore, it has the architecture to contract through a greater range of motion and potentially harness a greater degree of tendon buffering/elastic energy.

*Semimembranosus*, on the other hand, with its shorter fibre length, increased cross-sectional area and shorter tendon, has perhaps a greater role in stabilizing the knee through stiffening the medial joint and resisting rotational forces. This selectivity of muscle activation within neighbouring muscles has been demonstrated in EMG studies both in the lower and upper limb.[9]

2. Soleus has been demonstrated to have a relatively high concentration of type I/slower-twitch fibres, with a very large relative cross-sectional area and short fibre length. It is therefore considered to be able to produce high force over narrow joint ranges and have a high resistance to fatigue.[11]

3. Triceps brachii has a very high relative cross-sectional area *and* relative fibre length. It therefore needs to be trained through large ranges and with a bias towards high-force movements.[11]

## Plasticity of muscle

Muscle tissue demonstrates a high degree of plasticity and can adapt with structural changes within a few training sessions or within a few days of immobilization.[12] Poor exercise choices or prolonged and unnecessary immobilization following injury can quickly lead to changes to both architecture and muscle fibre type that may predispose the athlete to future injury.

Architecturally, this is clearly seen in hamstring rehabilitation, where the use of a concentric-only seated loading following injury is believed to have a negative impact on resilience by maintaining/shifting the angle of peak force of the muscle towards inner available range, where in contrast it needs to be strong in outer range and in eccentric movements.[13]

> An understanding of the target muscles' architecture and specific function will help guide exercise selection within the retraining programme. Muscle is plastic and adapts quickly and selectively to different types of stimuli (and lack thereof).

## The injury process

Muscle injuries can be broadly subdivided into strains, contusions and lacerations.[14] Recovery from these distinct injury mechanisms occurs in broad terms through a blend of regeneration and repair, with repair the dominant pathway. This is characterized by the formation and maturation of a collagen-based scar. For the purposes of this chapter, we will concentrate on muscle strain mechanisms and pathophysiology.

### Mechanisms

The typical mechanism reported in muscle strain injuries involves a **rapid eccentric/active lengthening contraction** that exceeds the strain tolerance of the MTU and results in damage to muscle and neurovascular tissues.[14] This most commonly occurs at the MTJ, although injuries also occur more superficially to myofascial tissue and can occasionally involve the free tendon or a combination of all three.[15]

> It is worth noting that recovery time of myofascial injuries can be significantly quicker than those involving the MTJ or, particularly, the free tendon.

A less common but potentially more troublesome mechanism of injury described particularly in hamstrings is an **over-stretching**, beyond the absolute range of the muscle. This has been reported in ballet dancers, water-skiers and in specific mechanisms in rugby (competing over a ball), football and tennis (splits).[16] Over-stretch injuries are often associated with significantly increased recovery time despite an apparently less severe initial presentation.[17] Interestingly, this mechanism seems to predominantly affect the semimebranosus (SM) tendon (> 80% cases).[16,17] When we consider the unique architecture of the SM described previously, perhaps this renders it more vulnerable to extremes of joint range.

Neuromuscular **fatigue** is heavily implicated in muscle injury risk with epidemiological studies consistently demonstrating an increase in injury frequency in the third and fourth quarters of matches.[18,19,20] Adding to this, recent electromyographical (EMG) studies have demonstrated significant reduction in both eccentric neural activity of long head *biceps femoris* and eccentric knee flexor strength following a bout of repeated sprints,[18] with the authors suggesting this exposes the muscle to increased strain and injury risk.

## Pathophysiology

Once injured, the tissue undergoes a four-stage reparative process, which is broadly summarized in Table 14.1.

There is an immediate 'depowering' of the muscle due to the failure of the excitation-contraction coupling mechanism, which serves to protect the muscle from further damage while the initial inflammatory stage is in full flow and typically resolves after five to seven days.[21]

The timeline for each repair phase is highly variable and highly overlapping, but the general consensus is that care should be taken for the first two to three days to minimize any stress to the injury site but should then begin in earnest thereafter with pain-free isometric loading.[14]

The repair and maturation process can take many months to complete and has been consistently demonstrated not to follow a linear relationship with functional restoration in the individual. Athletes often demonstrate apparent full-functional recovery long before radiological recovery is seen.[14,22]

Therefore, an understanding of the pathophysiological process will certainly guide us in our acute-management decision making but cannot form the basis for a timescale-driven management strategy. Early respect for physiology and directions of stress must be married with sensitive, objective and functional markers to enable progression through rehabilitation. As always it is essential we place the athlete at the *centre* of this process, not least because their opinion on the injury, its severity and convalescence time may be a very good indicator of return timescale.[23]

*Table 14.1* Injury Repair

| Phase | Major events | Timeline |
|-------|--------------|----------|
| Bleeding | Stabilisation of haemorrhage | *Hours* |
| Inflammatory phase | Inflammatory cascade (cell migration to injury site to clear debris and begin repair) | *A few days* |
| Repair & remodel phase | Concomitant repair and regeneration, characterized by development of collagenous scar and new vessels | *1–3 weeks* |
| Maturation phase | Progressive strengthening of scar and new myofibres | *Months* |

> Injury results in a predictable repair process, which is not always aligned with functional recovery.[22]

## The role of imaging in muscle injury

Our understanding of muscle injury has come a long way with the development and greater use of imaging techniques. This has allowed clinicians to evolve from the simple 1–3 grading description of proportion of muscle damage, to a delineation of where the injury occurs within the MTU and a more accurate understanding of the proportion of damage seen. A large part of this evolution is thanks to the ever more sophisticated imaging techniques at our disposal.

The role of imaging acute muscle injuries in sport has changed significantly over the last 20 years, from merely confirming a clinical diagnosis to defining the exact location of the injury within the MTU, the size of disruption at the tear site and the longitudinal length and cross-sectional area of muscle oedema. These factors have all been used to assist with predicting outcome following muscle strain injury.

Magnetic resonance imaging (MRI) is the imaging technique of choice in the assessment of indirect muscle injury. It is more sensitive than ultrasound (US) in the detection of grade I injuries and aids in defining the prognosis following indirect muscle injury. Whilst perhaps not as sensitive a tool and certainly more user-dependent, diagnostic US is becoming increasingly popular in the assessment of acute muscle injury. It has several important advantages over MRI, including superior spatial resolution, lower cost, convenience, portability and dynamic evaluation of the injury.

## Grading muscle injuries

The following table lists the radiological grading system used within European football's Champions league.[24]

Whilst Table 14.2 provides us with a sound basis to make broad predictions on recovery time in footballing populations, we must remember that no two injuries are exactly the same,

Table 14.2 Characteristics of hamstring muscle strain grades using MRI[23]

| Grade | Appearance on MRI | Average recovery time |
|-------|-------------------|------------------------|
| 0 | No visible muscle oedema or macroscopic architectural distortion. It is possible that these subtle muscle injuries are present but are below the sensitivity of current MRI detection. | 8 days |
| I | Feather-type pattern increased signal is seen within the muscle at the injury site on fluid-sensitive fat-suppressed sequences, but there is *no* macroscopic architectural distortion of the muscle. | 17 days |
| II | 'Feathery' muscle oedema and macroscopic distortion of normal muscle architecture at the injury site. Frequently, perifascial fluid is extensive and spreads in a dependent (gravity assisted) fashion from the injury site. | 22 days |
| III | Complete disruption of the musculotendinous unit, with haematoma filling the space between the two. Grade III injuries are most frequently seen at the tendon proximal origin, rather than the distal insertion. | 73 days |

and the recovery time will be influenced by a multitude of both extrinsic and intrinsic risk factors that may be un-modifiable, such as age, previous history and muscle fibre type, or may be modifiable, such as strength, flexibility or training programme. The average times listed must be taken with caution, and their application to other muscle groups as a predictive template would be unwise.

## Managing muscle injuries

Successful rehabilitation of all injuries requires a carefully blended mix of science and art. The focus of this section is on the *science* of muscle strain rehabilitation. The *art* component of rehabilitation is less tangible, as it rests heavily on practitioner experience and factors including the relationship with the athlete and knowledge of the sport. It certainly should not be discounted or devalued as a less important consideration, however. Intuition, communication and empathy are highly valuable skills in rehabilitation.

For the purposes of this section, rehabilitation is sub-divided into three broad and commonly used phases:

1    Acute rehabilitation
2    Progressive loading
3    Return to performance.

### *Phase 1: Acute rehabilitation*

The immediate post-injury period involves the stabilization of bleeding and the beginnings of a repair/regeneration cascade. Typically, from a therapeutic perspective, both pain and inflammation are mediated through the application of ice and compression. A brief period of immobilization may also be warranted, where active lengthening and loading is avoided again to provide an environment of recovery and limit excessive scar tissue formation.[6] This may include the use of crutches or heel raises for an acute hamstring strain, a sling for a biceps strain or an abdominal brace for an acute obliques strain.

---

The decision to unload is taken predominantly on clinical grounds but should only be used until normal loading is pain-free. As already described, muscle atrophy can occur very rapidly, particularly in weight-bearing muscles.

---

### *Ice*

'Ice-ice-ice' is ingrained into every sports medicine practitioner as a method of limiting secondary injury and mediating the inflammatory response, although the reality here is that there remains a distinct lack of clarity and, crucially, evidence regarding its best use.[25] Consideration of the depth of lesion to determine time of application would clearly make sense but is complicated by adipose tissue. A more pragmatic standpoint currently is that its primary use is to mediate pain and therefore restore/better maintain function.

> When it comes to ice, a standardized approach of 10–20 minutes every two hours, titrated to athlete response, remains our best strategy, and further work is needed in this area.

### Pills, potions and diet

Use of anti-inflammatory medications in this acute period may be best avoided, since acting to blunt the normal inflammatory response cannot be considered best practice and has in some studies been associated with poorer outcomes.[26]

The use of novel injection therapy to expedite this phase has been discussed more recently in the literature but will not be included in this chapter, as it is not, in the experience of the authors, a meaningful adjunct to the recovery timeline. Attention to good dietary habits through this period, however, is considered important, and significant detail can be found regarding this in chapter 4.

### Loading

Following an initial short period of relative rest, we need to begin to apply a very low level of load to the injured tissue, as this will help enhance the recovery process and minimize preventable atrophy. We do, however, need to carefully monitor the response (pain, inflammatory signs, range of motion) to ensure the load applied is not excessive.

Introductory loading may involve a simple return to full weight-bearing through the use of pool therapy or weight-assistance treadmills, or carefully applied low-level isometric contractions in mid-range joint positions, stressing a slow build-up of contraction and low sense of effort. Mid-range isometric activation minimizes the strain to the injury while placing it in an advantageous position to generate force.

> *'Protecting the lines of stress'* is a key concept here. We need to respect the fragility of the injury and create an environment where healing can be optimized, without forgetting that the athlete cannot detrain in all areas.

As discussed in chapter 1, injury is an opportunity to improve, and this model of what we *can* do rather than stressing what we *cannot* do is a better mindset to adopt. Whether athletic improvements at this point can be physical, psychological, technical or tactical will be governed by the injury and its severity, but it is essential that we take the athlete's 'eyes' away from focusing excessively or exclusively on their injury.

Within this phase, we need to find novel methods of maintaining general fitness and strength levels without applying undue stress to the injury. In simple terms, it is important to steer clear from any training that will stress the injured tissue and detract from the recovery. This may mean an upper-body conditioning block, single-leg training or perhaps recumbent training.

## Electrical stimulation and occlusion training

To achieve more 'bang for our buck', we could consider novel adjuncts to muscle activation, through electrical stimulation (perhaps away from the lesion site but to the target muscle group) or low-intensity occlusion of the affected limb.

Acute and protracted changes to neural tissue have been shown following hamstring strain; thus an externally applied electrical stimulus to encourage better neural synchronisation might be advantageous.

Occlusion has been demonstrated in the literature and in practice to produce improvements in muscle strength and architecture under much lower loads than traditional modes of strength training,[27] although its use following soft-tissue injury both at a cellular level and in terms of return to training time is currently unknown.

Examples of early loading exercises are seen below:

Progression through this phase is dependent on functional signs and symptoms, although clearly, injury severity should play a role in our thought process. We must be satisfied that the athlete has earned the right to add load to the tissue with minimal risk.

Risk validation can be achieved in all phases of rehab using considered exit criteria. As an example, potential criteria to exit from phase 1 of a rehabilitation program for a hamstring injury can be seen in Table 14.6. Clearly the first row indicates a tolerance of low-level weight-bearing function, whilst the second gives an indication of stabilization in the acute inflammatory signs. The final two criteria are designed to give an indication of a safe return to low-level jogging, where the hamstring is comfortable in two-joint stretch or mid-swing

Table 14.3 Examples for use of electrical stimulation and occlusion in acute rehab

| Quads Strain Acute Rehabilitation | | | |
| --- | --- | --- | --- |
| Adjunct | Placement | Settings | Exercise |
| Electrical Stimulation | Overlying proximal and distal target muscle | 30–40Hz intermittent program 3 x 15 repetitions (pause unit in rest) | Seated knee extensions |
| Occlusion | Upper thigh | 100mmHg constant pressure 3 x 15 repetitions (de-pressurise in rest) | |

Table 14.4 Examples of acute phase exercise

| Calf Muscle Loading | | | |
| --- | --- | --- | --- |
| Exercise | Sets | Reps | Pace |
| Seated calf raise | 5 | 6-second hold | isometric |

Table 14.5 Examples of acute phase exercise

| Infraspinatus Muscle Loading | | | |
| --- | --- | --- | --- |
| Exercise | Sets | Reps | Pace |
| Wall external rotations | 5 | 6-second hold | isometric |

*Table 14.6* Acute exit criteria following hamstring strain

*Acute Hamstring Exit Criteria*

1. Pain-free gait, stair use, body-weight squat
2. Reduction in morning stiffness/irritability
3. Pain-free seated active knee extension > 75% limb symmetry
4. Pain-free single-leg bridge hold in 90, 45 and < 30 degrees knee flexion

phase, and comfortable loading isometrically in mid- to end-swing and stance phase (but at a much lower intensity). Ticks in these boxes give confidence to all concerned that the athlete can progress safely into a loading phase.

> To allow progression to phase 2 of rehabilitation, the following exit criteria should be passed:
>
> 1  Resolution of pain during activities of daily living
> 2  Pain-free ROM to >75% of contralateral side
> 3  Demonstrable pain-free isometric contractile function in mid-, inner and outer range
> 4  Resolution of inflammatory signs

## Phase 2: Progressive loading

Once the athlete is comfortable using the affected tissue in simple activities of daily living, we can start to develop the capacity of the tissue to tolerate stress, through progressive manipulation of load, volume, speed and movement complexity.

Monitoring through this period is again critical to ensure that we do not exceed tissue tolerance and regress into an inflammatory cycle or re-injure the athlete. It is also important to carefully plan all elements within the programme and avoid the temptation to mindlessly flog an injured athlete. We need to organize and periodize our reconditioning program to allow time for adaptation and, ultimately, to ensure best outcomes.

## 'You cannot fire a cannon from a canoe'

Whether dealing with lower- or upper-limb muscle injury, rehabilitation should involve attention to the functional interaction of the trunk and periphery in our exercise selection. This can be simply achieved through ensuring the trunk remains stable and well positioned when the limb is in motion/generating force and selecting exercises that will expose deficits in trunk strength and control in sport-relevant movements.

> When considering muscles acting on the hip specifically, appropriate stability of the trunk is clearly a crucial consideration in rehab to minimize unnecessary strain and has been demonstrated to result in favourable outcomes following hamstring strains.[28] The same argument can be extended to the other end of the chain at the foot and ankle, which sets the tone for the interactions occurring proximally.

## Specific loading

As discussed, exercises need to represent the desired function of the muscle wherever possible to ensure that architecture, morphology and neuromuscular function are rehabilitated appropriately. Always also consider the planes of movement that the muscle works and joint(s) it spans. We need to consider and manipulate all factors to ensure we are being thorough.

## Practical example

A seated, concentrically biased program in hamstring rehabilitation may result in adaptive changes to length/tension and neuromuscular properties that may increase risk of future injury.[12] A far better model sees the progression of loading, maintaining the isometric theme from the acute phase with progressive manipulation of moment arm, load, speed of activation, asymmetry and a perhaps reduction in predictability. This must then be progressed further with the inclusion of active lengthening/eccentric movements, targeting the muscle first as a 'buffer' then as an 'amplifier' as per our description of muscle function above.

Examples of this progressive model in both hamstring and adductor rehabilitation are demonstrated in Figures 14.1 and 14.2.

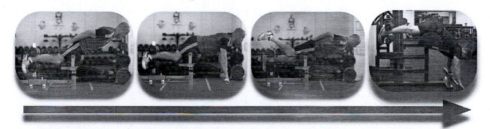

Progressive increase in isometric load. Further development possible through:
1. Increasing external load
2. Applying asymmetrical load
3. Introducing eccentric movement about hip

Figure 14.1

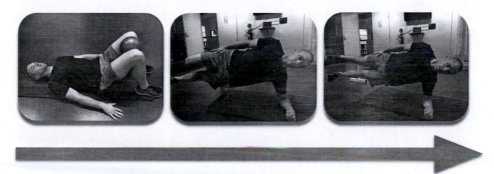

Progressive increase in isometric load. Further development possible through:

1. Increasing external load
2. Introducing eccentric movement (lateral lunge, sliding lunge)
3. Increasing speed and movement complexity

Figure 14.2

---

**Eccentric bias essential**

The use of eccentric loading in rehabilitation is essential. As described throughout this chapter, it is the most likely mechanism of injury in muscle strains and requires unique neural and structural qualities that need to be regained to reduce risk of recurrence and regain functional performance.[5,12,29]

There is a significant body of research highlighting the protective effects of Nordic hamstring training, and it would be remiss not to mention this specific drill in this chapter.[28] This 'buffer' drill should always be included in hamstring rehabilitation.

---

## Dynamic correspondence

In addition to specifically loading the muscle, rehabilitation needs to use functionally relevant movements to ensure we are reconditioning the athlete as a whole, not just honing in on the area of damage. Simple examples here might include squats, step-ups, prowler pushes and multi-plane sled tows for lower limb injuries in pushing/running athletes, or unstable press-ups, single-arm rope pulls and wrestling movements for upper-body injuries in contact athletes.

---

It is critically important to keep the athlete's focus away from their injury by targeting familiar movements and attention to skill-based tasks, thereby engaging brain and body in equal measure.

---

## Return to running

Following a lower-limb muscle injury, an early return to running can be very successful, providing the entry criteria are accurate and the athlete is monitored closely. Such is the lure of this milestone to athlete and coach, however, that we can be tempted to rush to achieve it. We therefore need to be clear how we integrate running and justify its introduction and progression. A good understanding of the role and demands of the muscle in running is essential to ensure we regain the strength, rate of force production and capacity needed to tolerate running with minimal risk.

This is usually achieved by a combination of the graded exposure model of increasing running load, pace and volume very gradually, and monitoring response[30] while continuing to strengthen the muscle appropriately. Additional progressions in the demand of linear running can also be achieved with surface manipulation (e.g. sand or soft track with intermittent hard matting).

## Practical example

The accelerated running program provides a nice example of this model, where the athlete accelerates, maintains a specific pace and decelerates a specific distance. These variables are then manipulated either through speed in the middle phase or through a reduction in the acceleration/deceleration distances.[30]

Initially, it is wise to commence with a one day on : one day off split to allow for adequate recovery before reloading. Once the athlete demonstrates that they are able to withstand this, we can graduate to a 2-on : 1-off ratio. Usually, in field sports, this represents a typical training week schedule, but in athletics, progression to a 3-on : 1-off schedule can be made once the athlete has shown their ability to tolerate the loading. This tolerance can be assessed in a number of ways, ranging from subjective scoring of soreness and fatigue, to objective measures of ROM and contractile function. Further detail on running mechanics and rehabilitation running can be found in chapter 9.

## Build complexity of reconditioning

Many sports require athletes to perform a huge variety of contrasting movement tasks within a single phase of play. An example might be a rugby union winger who, when chasing a kick, needs to:

- Maximally accelerate 30m
- Decelerate rapidly while avoiding the opposition
- Jump vertically to compete/regain possession of the ball
- Drive forward against resistance from opponents
- Run at tempo pace 40m in an arc back into offensive line for the next play.

If we focus on the demand this places on the muscles, it is clear that progressively increasing training complexity through incorporating multiple blocks of contrasting movements and demand might be an important component of rehabilitation. In practical terms, this might mean organizing one of the rehabilitation sessions into sets as follows:

As this model progresses, the use of pre-fatiguing the athlete to further stress the muscle and the neuromuscular system will give further confidence to all concerned that they are functionally ready to progress beyond this phase and be re-integrated into training.

Table 14.7 Incorporation of multiple movements into rehabilitation

| Transition Training (Rectus Femoris Strain in Rugby Player) |
| --- |
| 1. Specific loading: 8 repetitions eccentric sit-up + 10kg plate |
| 2. Function drill 1: Down/up, accelerate 5m and tackle a shield |
| 3. Function drill 2: 10m forward sled tow in bear crawl (heavy) |
| 4. Function drill 3: 30m recovery run at ¾ pace + ball skills/target pass |
| 60 seconds rest |

*Table 14.8* Exit criteria progressive rehabilitation phase

| *Progressive Rehab Hamstring Exit Criteria* |
| --- |
| 10 x 50m running at 80% maximum pace with 10m acceleration/deceleration and predictable direction changes |
| 20 minutes light skills training: non-contact drills (partial session content < 70% max pace) |
| > 80% limb symmetry in single-leg prone isometric hold + prone pull load |
| > 80% limb symmetry in single-leg dead-lift strength, capacity and form |
| > 80% limb symmetry in single-leg step-up strength, capacity and form |
| No reaction to rehabilitation |

### Exit criteria

Below are four key exit criteria for a rugby player to enter a return-to-training phase:

> To allow progression to phase 3 of rehabilitation, the following exit criteria should be passed:
>
> 1    No reaction to rehabilitation
> 2    Full pain-free ROM
> 3    Demonstrable pain-free contractile function/strength to >85% of contralateral side
> 4    Commencement of lower-velocity sports-relevant tasks (e.g. running, light kicking, groundstrokes, throws).

### Phase 3: Return to training and performance

Once the injured muscle demonstrates comparable strength properties and functional capacity to pre-injury, the athlete will be looking to return to a competitive state in their training. Clearly, the 'functional' performance of the athlete will rightly go a long way to governing return to competition. Accurate measurement tools under 'live' conditions, coach-led assessment of technique and form in key movements and player confidence in training, collisions and under duress can give real confidence to all stakeholders that they are ready to perform. The functional components of this phase are described in detail in chapter 18.

### Specific muscle testing

In terms of assessing muscle function, any testing should look to quantify the strength and capacity of the rehabilitated tissue as thoroughly as possible. This is a process that may involve isolated muscle testing, functional performance of the whole limb or, indeed, a mixture of both. Key areas to consider here include:

1    Tissue strength and angle of peak strength (does angle relate to the needs of the muscle in function?)
2    Muscle capacity
3    Rate of force development (RFD)
4    Neuromuscular timing and coordination.

Clearly, gaining an accurate understanding of these parameters may require equipment not readily available outside a laboratory setting (such as isokinetic dynamometry, force platforms or jump mat systems). Nonetheless, every effort must be made to ensure the muscle is fully prepared to return to performance. The following examples provide the reader with a variety of solutions.

*Practical examples*

1   The endurance capacity of the infraspinatus muscle can be assessed using a side-lying external rotation capacity test with a 5kg weight;
2   An isokinetic dynamometer can be used to accurately assess strength, RFD, angle of peak force and agonist/antagonist ratios following a hamstring strain;
3   A force platform can be used to determine single-leg reactivity/stiffness (20cm single-leg drop jump) following a gastrocnemius strain;
4   A three-hop for distance can be used to assess single leg explosive power following a quadriceps strain.

---

To allow progression to competition, the following exit criteria should be passed:

1   Completion of match/event intensity training with pre-injury performance. Wherever possible, this should be demonstrable using objective RTP markers, such as running speed, throwing velocity, jumping height or kicking distance;
2   Return of baseline or > 90 per cent limb symmetry strength, power and capacity;
3   The athlete is confident in the resilience of the previously injured site and is not shielding it from full ballistic contractions.

---

## Prevention of re-injury: Current concepts

It is widely accepted that athletes will return to sport successfully before their injuries have resolved radiologically, operating with a diminishing but elevated risk of re-injury for a sustained period. Even in cases where isolated tissue characteristics and functional measures of athletic performance have demonstrably returned to normal, re-injuries still occur and ongoing prevention should be considered an essential component of rehabilitation. Recent work has demonstrated ongoing electromyographical delays in efferent firing long after functional restoration of muscle strength has been achieved.[31]

In terms of basic ongoing prevention, we should consider several key areas, namely:

1   Range of motion restoration/maintenance
2   Adequate tissue preparation for sport
3   Eccentrically biased strength development
4   Synergist assessment and development
5   Sport-relevant movement conditioning.

## Prevention milestone angle of motion

A typical feature of muscle injury concerns the loss of apparent tissue range of motion. Whether this is truly a reflection of a change in tissue organisation/scarring or simply a neurally mediated reflex to guard against positions of vulnerability (i.e. outer range), once identified it should be addressed. A detailed understanding of the role of stretching and its application is beyond the scope of this chapter and can be found in greater detail in chapter 13. Whilst there is little to no evidence within the literature that a pre-emptive stretching program will mitigate injury risk, injury that results in a functional loss of range below the range engaged in sport clearly presents a risk to the athlete.

## Prevention milestone issue preparation

By extension, warm-ups are a fundamental component of all training sessions. The benefits of increasing muscle temperature include an increase in tissue compliance and neuromuscular activation. Protracted warm-up times are often applied to previously injured muscles to allow ample time to ensure muscle-tendon unit warmth and optimal neuromuscular activation.

## Prevention milestone-centric training

Eccentric strengthening has been demonstrated to increase tissue range and even myofibril length (sarcomeregenesis) and result in improvements in outer-range strength, which will reduce injury risk.[32] As described previously, training muscles according to their function will ensure that our nervous system is tuned properly. The protective effect of eccentric exercise has been demonstrated to occur quickly, with authors proposing this is due to enhancement of nervous system function in the first instance.[33] From an isolated tissue perspective, eccentric training should therefore be a considered part of any muscle injury prevention and rehabilitation program.

## Prevention milestone 4 – synergists

No muscle works in isolation and assessment of causation, and, indeed, tenuously initial risk may include an understanding of synergists capacity and strength. A simple example here might be attention to gluteus maximus (with squat > 90 degrees or hip thrusters) and adductor magnus (with high-box step-ups) as additional hip extensors when dealing with hamstring strain.

## Prevention milestone movement conditioning

Wherever possible we should use our strength and conditioning to re-enforce sport relevant performance and injury resilience. The sole use of concentric-only double leg squats (whilst an excellent exercise to develop strength qualities in the lower limb) is clearly completely insufficient to maintain posterior chain function in a running athlete in isolation. We must all be students of our sport and apply our conditioning accordingly. This means that if a muscle is a high-velocity muscle (quadriceps, gastrocnemius, for example), the programme must contain elements of high-velocity–based training. We cannot expect a muscle to be ready to tolerate high speeds if we have only trained it to move slowly.

## Summary

Muscle injuries continue to account for a significant proportion for all injuries reported across all sports. Effective rehabilitation requires a clear understanding of the target muscles' architecture and specific functional characteristics to best inform exercise prescription. It requires a bias towards eccentric strengthening and clear and well-reasoned exit criteria. Crucially, reconditioning does not finish once the athlete has returned to sport but must continue for an extended period to minimize future injury risk.

## Notes

1 Fyfe, J., Opar, D., Williams, M. et al. (2013). The role of neuromuscular inhibition in hamstring injury recurrence. *Journal of Electromyography and Kinesiology 23*, 523–530.
2 Roberts, T. J., & Konow, N. (2013). How tendons buffer energy dissipation by muscle. *Exercise Sport Science Review, 41*(4), 186–193.
3 Ishikawa, M., Pakaslahti, J., & Komi, P. (2007). Medial gastrocnemius muscle behavior during human running and walking. *Gait Posture 25*(3), 380–384.
4 Hoppeler, H., & Hertz, W. (2014). Eccentric exercise: Many questions unanswered. *Journal of Applied Physiology, 116*, 1405–1406.
5 LaStayo, P., Woolf, J., Lewek, M. et al. (2003). Eccentric muscle contractions: Their contribution to injury, prevention, rehabilitation, and sports. *Journal of Orthopaedics and Sports Physical Therapy, 33*, 557–571.
6 Ward, S., Eng, C., Smallwood, L. et al. (2009). Current measurements of lower extremity muscle architecture accurate? *Clinical Orthopaedic Related Research, 467*, 1074–1082.
7 Timmins, R. et al. Differences exist in the architectural characteristics of the biceps femoris long head in previously injured individuals. *Journal of Science and Medicine in Sport, 18*, e143-e144.
8 Fiorentino, N. M., & Blemker, S. S. (2014). Musculotendon variability influences tissue strains experienced by the bicepsfFemoris long head muscle during high-speed running. *Journal of Biomechanics, 47*(13), 3325–3333.
9 Schiaffino, S., & Reggiani, C. (2011). Fiber types in mammalian skeletal muscles. *Physiological Reviews, 91*, 1447–1531.
10 McAllister, M., Hammond, K., Schilling, B. et al. (2014). Muscle activation during various hamstring exercises. *Journal of Strength & Conditioning Research, 28*(6), 1573–1580.
11 Wickiewicz, T., Roy, R., Powell, P. et al. (1983). Muscle architecture of the human lower limb. *Clinical Orthopaedics and Related Research, 179*, 275–283.
12 Lieber, R. L. (2009). *Skeletal muscle structure, function, and plasticity*. Baltimore, MD: Lippincott Williams & Wilkins.
13 Brockett, C. L., Morgan, D. L., & Proske, U. (2004). Predicting hamstring strain injury in elite athletes. *Medicine & Science in Sports & Exercise, 36*(3), 379–387.
14 Järvinen, T. A., Järvinen, T. L., Kääriäinen, M. et al. (2005). Muscle injuries: Biology and treatment. *American Journal of Sports Medicine, 33*, 745.
15 Pollock, N., James, S. L., Lee, J. C., & Chakraverty, R. (2014). British athletics muscle injury classification: A new grading system. *British Journal of Sports Medicine, 48*(18), 1347–1351.
16 Askling, C. (2011). Types of hamstring injuries in sports. *British Journal of Sports Medicine, 45*(2), e2-e2.
17 Askling, C. M., Tengvar, M., Saartok, T., & Thorstensson, A. (2008). Proximal hamstring strains of stretching type in different sports injury situations, clinical and magnetic resonance imaging characteristics, and return to sport. *The American Journal of Sports Medicine, 36*(9), 1799–1804.
18 Timmins, R. G., Opar, D. A., Williams, M. D., Schache, A. G. et al. (2014). Reduced biceps femoris myoelectrical activity influences eccentric knee flexor weakness after repeat sprint running. *Scandinavian Journal of Medicine & Science in Sports, 24*, 299–305.

19 Brooks, J. H., Fuller, C. W., Kemp, S.P.T., & Reddin, D. B. (2005). Epidemiology of injuries in English professional rugby union: Part 1 match injuries. *British Journal of Sports Medicine*, *39*(10), 757–766.

20 Brooks, J. H., Fuller, C. W., Kemp, S. P., & Reddin, D. B. (2006). Incidence, risk, and prevention of hamstring muscle injuries in professional rugby union. *The American Journal of Sports Medicine*, *34*(8), 1297–1306.

21 Warren, G. L., Ingalls, C. P., Lowe, D. A. et al. (2001). Excitation-contraction uncoupling: Major role in contraction-induced muscle injury. *Exercise and Sport Sciences Reviews*, *29*(2), 82–87.

22 Orchard, J., & Best, T. (2002). The management of muscle strain injuries: An early return versus the risk of recurrence. *Clinical Journal of Sport Medicine*, *12*(1), 3–5.

23 Moen, M., Reurink, G., Weir, A. et al. (2014). Predicting return to play after hamstring injuries. *British Journal of Sports Medicine*, *48*, 1358–1363. doi:10.1136/bjsports-2014–093860

24 Ekstrand, J., Healy, J.C., Waldén, M., Lee, J.C., English, B., & Hägglund, M. (2012). Hamstring muscle injuries in professional football: The correlation of MRI findings with return to play. *British Journal of Sports Medicine*, *46*(2), 112–117.

25 Bleakley, C., Glasgow, P., Webb, M. (2012). Cooling an acute muscle injury: Can basic scientific theory translate into the clinical setting? *British Journal of Sports Medicine*, *46*, 296–298.

26 Orchard, J., Best, T., Mueller-Wohlfahrt, H. et al. (2008). The early management of muscle strains in the elite athlete: best practice in a world with a limited evidence basis. *British Journal of Sports Medicine*, *42*(3), 158–159.

27 Wernbom, M., Augustsson, J., & Raastad, T. (2008). Ischemic strength training: A low-load alternative to heavy resistance exercise? *Scandinavian Journal of Medicine & Science in Sports*, *18*, 401–416.

28 Sherry, M.A., & Best, T.M. (2004). A comparison of 2 rehabilitation programs in the treatment of acute hamstring strains. *Journal of Orthopaedic & Sports Physical Therapy*, *34*(3), 116–125.

29 Thorborg, K. (2012). Why hamstring eccentrics are hamstring essentials. *British Journal of Sports Medicine*, *46*(7), 463–465.

30 Brukner, P., & Khan, K. (2001). *Clinical sports medicine*. New South Wales, Australia: McGraw-Hill.

31 Fyfe, J.J., Opar, D.A., Williams, M.D., & Shield, A.J. (2013). The role of neuromuscular inhibition in hamstring strain injury recurrence. *Journal of Electromyography and Kinesiology*, *23*(3), 523–530.

32 O'Sullivan, K., McAuliffe, S., & DeBurca, N. (2012). The effects of eccentric training on lower limb flexibility: A systematic review. *British Journal of Sports Medicine*, *46*(12), 838–45.

33 LaStayo, P., Marcus, R., Dibble, L., Frajacomo, F., & Lindstedt, S. (2014). Eccentric exercise in rehabilitation: Safety, feasibility, and application. *Journal of Applied Physiology*, *116*(11), 1426–1434.

# Chapter 15

# Tendon injuries

*Craig Ranson, David Joyce and Polly McGuiggan*

## Introduction

The management of tendinopathy is one of the most challenging aspects of sports medicine. Reports of new medications, injections, surgery, physical and exercise therapies for tendinopathy are constantly appearing, and this vast spectrum of tendon treatments indicates that universally successful methods are yet to be established.

Almost any tendon of the body can become painful. In the lower limbs, the Achilles and patellar tendons of running and jumping athletes are commonly afflicted and have garnered the most research and clinical attention. However, pain and pathology are also frequently encountered in the tendons of, for example, the hip adductors, hamstrings, tibialis posterior and peroneal muscles. Although not strictly a tendon, the plantar fascia is also sometimes considered part of this often-dysfunctional family. The upper limb is also not without its problem tendons, including those of the common extensor origin of the elbow (particularly *extensor carpi radialis brevis* – 'tennis elbow'), the rotator cuff of the shoulder, and the *abductor pollicus brevis* and *extensor pollicus longus* tendons of the thumb (de Quervain's disease). The tie that binds all these tendinopathies together is load. Essentially, tendons become deranged when they are subjected to loads beyond which they are capable of accommodating in the short-term, or adapting to over the longer term. This is why hip adductor tendinopathies are frequently seen in kicking sports,[1] and shoulder tendinopathies have a high incidence within throwing sports.[2]

The aim of this chapter is to review and explore tendon injury assessment and management. The most important and clinically useful information related to the likely pathological continuum, as well as risk factors for tendon injury, will be presented. However, the primary emphasis of the chapter is the within-season management of tendinopathy, focusing on facilitating the return to and preservation of high-level function.

## The role of tendons within the musculoskeletal system

In the simplest terms, tendons transfer force from muscles to bone. This force is a combination of that generated by the muscle to which the tendon belongs, and the external forces acting on the kinetic chain. When a force is applied to a tendon, it initially stretches and then transfers the force to the structure to which the tendon attaches. The degree to which it stretches before the force is transferred is governed by the stiffness of the tendon, which itself is determined by a combination of the type of collagen fibrils and the cross-sectional area of the tendon (i.e. the number and size of parallel collagen fibrils).

As well as transferring force, tendons play an essential role in the storage and return of elastic energy during movement. A tendon can recoil at twice the speed of a muscle and so pre-loading it through stretch means that the muscle-tendon unit can propel the limb with a velocity and efficiency far in excess of isolated muscle eccentric-concentric coupling. An obvious example of this is in running: when the limb is loaded during the early part of the stance phase, dorsiflexion of the ankle results in stretching of the Achilles tendon. The calf muscles maintain an isometric contraction during ankle dorsiflexion,[3] with the joint movement being afforded by stretch of the tendon. When the limb is unloaded during the second half of the stance phase, the tendon recoils, helping to power the runner into the flight phase. It is estimated that this utilisation of elastic energy reduces the metabolic cost of running by around 30 per cent.[4]

> These biomechanical principles provide a basis for utilising isometric muscle training within tendon rehabilitation programmes.

The more a tendon stretches for a given force, the more energy it will store. How much it will deform for a given force is determined by its stiffness. Thus a compliant tendon will strain more and store more energy when a force is applied to it, whilst a stiff tendon will store less energy (for a given force) but be able to transfer that force more quickly and is likely to withstand a greater force before failure. In association with these respective mechanical properties, an overly compliant (floppy) tendon might be at increased injury risk because of the relatively high levels of energy storage and strain, whereas an overly stiff tendon may also be at risk due to its reduced energy storage capacity. Indeed, it is possible that reduced tendon elasticity or excursion may shift the burden of power production to the muscle fascicles. The fatigue and strain associated with repeated and inefficient changes in muscle fascicle length may be a key factor in both tendinopathy and muscle strain injury.

## Under the microscope: The role of the tenocyte in tendon function

Similar to muscle that atrophies in response to immobilisation, or hypertrophies in response to load, tendons also adapt their structure according to the demands placed upon them. Cells known as *tenocytes* conduct this process by producing the collagen that makes up tendon tissue. Tenocyte activity is strain-dependent, which means that increasing tendon load increases tenocyte productivity. This 'mechanotransduction' effect[5] provides the basis for 'heavy-load' exercise-based tendinopathy rehabilitation programmes.[6,7] However, although load up-regulates tenocyte activity, this process does not occur instantly, and after a high-tendon-load (HTL) competition or training session, the 'clean-up operation' of tendon tissue regeneration can take two to three days.[8] Repeated sessions of HTL activities on the same day or on consecutive days are therefore likely to be destructive to tendons, as they will not have sufficient regeneration time. However, quantifying what constitutes 'high load' is difficult and varies greatly between and within individuals. For example low load for a jumping athlete in training may be extremely high load for a middle-aged squash player, and low load during a competitive long jump season may represent very high load for the same athlete returning to training after the off-season. Clearly, setting programmes with tendon load in mind is no easy task and must be individualised.

## The progression to tendinopathy

Essentially, tendinopathy represents a maladaptive response to overload. A causative spike in training load over days or weeks, particularly after a period of time off or low load, can often be identified. Examples of this might be plyometric sessions undertaken in the first day of pre-season, or three badminton games in a row after two weeks of no training due to illness. A change in one or, more usually, a combination of the factors in Tables 15.1 and 15.2 can often be linked to the development of tendon pain.

Unlike sudden-onset sports injuries – for example hamstring strains – the pathology of tendinopathy is often elusive, and the symptoms can initially be mild, allowing the athlete to continue to train and compete, albeit often not as well as they would like. Whilst athletes, coaches and medical staff are usually happy to allow an athlete with a strained hamstring several weeks of rehabilitation time, this is not often the case with tendinopathy.

> Not affording early stage tendinopathy a sufficient reduction in load, followed by a graduated return to full training and play, often leads this injury down the rocky road to chronicity.

Table 15.1 Potential tendinopathy risk factors and their mitigation

|  | Risk Factor | Example | Management |
|---|---|---|---|
| Extrinsic | Rapid change of training volume, frequency and/or intensity | Training camps<br>Resuming training after long-term injury | Appropriate spacing of HTL activities, particularly in athletes with a history of tendon pain |
|  | Change in footwear | Control to cushion or vice versa<br>Brand/model<br>Worn out/not worn in<br>Sole type (studs, cleats, blades) | Obtain a stock of footwear models that suit the athlete<br>Rotate two to three pairs<br>Optimise shoe-surface interface |
|  | Change in terrain | Cambers/hills/sand/tarmac | Introduce gradually |
|  | Equipment change | Racket grip size, string tension or weight | Alter gradually |
|  | Increased external resistance | Weighted jumps (jacket, squat jumps) | Introduce gradually and use only in very robust athletes, even then with caution |
|  |  | Parachute or bungee resisted runs | Introduce gradually and use only in very robust athletes, even then with caution |

(Continued)

*Table 15.1* (Continued)

|  | Risk Factor | Example | Management |
|---|---|---|---|
| Intrinsic | Age | Young athlete growth related enthesopathy | Reduce HTL activities in periods of rapid growth |
|  |  | Older athlete tendon degradation | Substitute all but essential high-tendon load activities |
|  | Body weight | Increased fat mass | Use diet and exercise strategies to optimise body composition |
|  |  | Increased lean mass may be desirable for the sport, e.g. rugby, but stressful for lower body tendons | Consider negative effects in athletes predisposed to tendon pain |
|  | Anatomical | Plantaris causing friction on medial Achilles | Carefully manage other, modifiable, risk factors |
|  |  | Short free Achilles tendon may affect deep portion of soleus – muscle fascicles strip off | May require surgical management |
|  |  | Short free tibialis posterior tendon causing tarsal tunnel stenosis |  |
|  |  | Unstable (subluxing/dislocating) or high (alta) patella may stress shield some parts of the patellar tendon and over-load others | Taping/bracing<br>Exercise rehabilitation |
|  | Genetics | Genetic predisposition likely to be a factor in tendinopathy | Carefully manage other, modifiable, risk factors |
|  | Various musculoskeletal (mobility &) strength characteristics | See Table 16.2 | See Table 16.2 |
|  | Technique | Forefoot jumper or lander results in high patellar tendon load | Difficult to change so may need to modify other risk factors |
|  |  | Over- or rapid pronation (medial bow of Achilles tendon) | Appropriate footwear |
|  |  | Slice serve in tennis – compressive stress on rotator cuff | Introduce technique change gradually |
|  |  | Curveball in baseball – medial elbow epicondylalgia |  |

Table 15.2 Musculoskeletal mobility and strength risk factors for common tendinopathies

| Tendinopathy | Limited Mobility | Excessive Mobility | Weakness |
|---|---|---|---|
| Plantar fasciaopathy | 1st MTP DF<br>Ankle DF | 1st MTP DF<br>Ankle DF<br>Subtalar pronation<br>Intertarsal motion<br>Tarso-metarsal motion | Tibialis posterior<br>Plantar-flexors<br>Foot intrinsics |
| Tibialis posterior tenosynovitis | Subtalar pronation<br>1st MTP DF<br>Ankle DF | Ankle DF<br>Subtalar pronation | Tibialis posterior<br>Plantar-flexors<br>Foot intrinsics<br>Soleus |
| Achilles tendinopathy | 1st MTP DF<br>Ankle DF | 1st MTP DF<br>Ankle DF<br>Subtalar pronation | Tibialis posterior<br>Plantar-flexors<br>Foot intrinsics |
| Patellar tendinopathy | Ankle DF<br>Quadriceps/knee flexion<br>Hamstrings<br>Subtalar pronation | Patella medial & lateral<br>Patella alta | Quadriceps |
| Popliteus tendinopathy | | Knee external rotation | Popliteus<br>Medial Hamstrings |
| Adductor enthesopathy | Hip internal rotation<br>Hip extension<br>FABER | Hip external rotation<br>Hip extension<br>FABER (bent knee fallout)<br>Pubic symphysis/SIJ | Hip adductors<br>Hip abductors<br>Hip extensors |
| Iliopsoas tendinopathy | Hip internal rotation<br>Hip extension | Hip internal rotation<br>Hip extension | Lower abdominals<br>(excessive anterior pelvic tilt) |
| Rotator cuff/ long head biceps tendinopathy | Shoulder internal rotation (GIRD)<br>Thoracic Extension/ rotation/side-flexion | Shoulder external rotation<br>Shoulder elevation<br>Acromio-claviclar joint | Rotator cuff/long head biceps<br>Scapulo-humeral musculature<br>Scapulo-thoracic musculature<br>Lower body & trunk kinetic chain |
| Lateral epicondylagia | Wrist flexion/extension | Forearm pronation | Supinator<br>Wrist extensors |
| de Quervain's disease | | Wrist ulnar deviation<br>Forearm pronation | EPL & APB<br>Grip<br>Elbow flexors |

Just as appropriate loading is required for healthy tendon structure, insufficient loading has also been proposed as a potential cause of tendinopathy. This is the 'stress-shielding' theory of tendon breakdown, whereby portions of tendons, such as the deep patellar tendon, or areas of the adductor origin, may become deranged due to insufficient tensile loading.[9]

Compression may also be a factor in tendon injury, particularly at attachment sites (entheses) where tendon tissue might be squashed against structures such as bone, bursae or fat pads. Insertional Achilles tendinopathy is a prime example. Compression and friction may also precipitate pathology where tendons run alongside or cross over each other. Examples include medial Achilles tendinopathy associated with *plantaris* compression and invagination,[10] and tenosynovitis of the *extensor pollicis longus* and *abductor pollicis brevis* tendons in de Quervain's disease. It is for this reason that interventions that increase tendon compression, such as aggressive or ballistic groin stretching in adductor tendinopathy, or heel drops over a step for insertional Achilles tendon pain, often exacerbate symptoms and should be avoided.

## Diagnosing tendinopathy

Most tendinopathies are not difficult to diagnose, as they tend to be characterised by a well-localised pain and have a distinctive gradual onset, although the time period can vary from increasing discomfort within a single session to slowly worsening symptoms over a period of weeks or months. Increasing morning stiffness and decreased functioning (for example reduced running speed, jumping ability or grip strength) are other common features. Nonetheless, a thorough clinical assessment to stage the injury, exclude associated pathologies and characterise the risk factors are crucial to devising appropriate management strategies.

### Diagnostic imaging

Diagnostic imaging can be helpful in determining the extent of tendon abnormality. The most useful first-line investigation is often ultrasound scan (USS). USS can demonstrate a variety of abnormalities that may be associated with tendon pain and pathology. Moreover, the machines are relatively inexpensive and portable and allow dynamic images of moving tendons. Ultrasound imaging can also be used to help localise treatment, e.g. guided injections and surgery. However, USS does have its limitations in that skilled operators are required, and deep tissue, joints and bone are not readily visualised.

Magnetic resonance imaging (MRI) is occasionally helpful as a secondary modality and is useful for providing high-resolution images of deep tendons, tendon tears and ruptures, and associated joints and bones, e.g. the patello-femoral joint, as osteophytes of the patellar-apex may be implicated in patellar tendinopathy.

The mechanical properties of some tendons (specifically the Achilles and patellar tendons) can be determined in vivo using a combination of ultrasound and a dynamometer, or in more dynamic and functional activities such as hopping, running and jumping using ultrasound, 3D motion analysis and a force-plate. From these measurements it is possible to determine the force and length change in the tendon during loading, and from this calculate tendon stiffness. Excessively compliant tendons will strain more for a given force and are therefore more likely to experience overload than a stiffer tendon. There is large inter-individual variability in tendon stiffness,[11] which may explain why some athletes develop tendinopathy whilst others experiencing similar loads do not.

## What causes tendon pain?

By and large, the exact tendon pain mechanisms remain very poorly understood, providing obvious challenges with regards to targeting them therapeutically. However, a recent review article by Rio and colleagues provides an excellent overview of many potential physiological and pathophysiological sources of tendon pain.[12]

It is important to note that not all pathological tendons are painful. Tendons can often exhibit structural abnormalities yet remain relatively pain-free. In fact, individuals who have suffered a complete tendon rupture often report that they had no preceding pain. This is not to say that abnormal tendon structure, imaged via ultrasound or MRI, for example, should be ignored, as there is some evidence that even if asymptomatic, tendons may be at greater risk of becoming painful (or rupturing) if subjected to high loads.[13]

## Staging of tendinopathies

Classifying the stage of tendinopathy can provide a useful guide to management. Table 15.3 below provides a summary of the stages of tendinopathy according to a popular model.[14]

In the *reactive phase*, tenocyte activity is dramatically up-regulated as it attempts to respond to increased load by stiffening the tendon. It does this by increasing the concentration of hydrophilic proteins, causing fluid to flood into the tendon (creating that familiar fusiform swelling that can be seen on ultrasound). Persistent intratendinous swelling can begin to cleave apart the collagen framework.

This next stage along the tendinopathy continuum is the *dys-repair phase*, where the tenocytes are trying very hard to keep up with further increases in load, but excessive demand leads to areas of tissue breakdown. Finally, the *degenerative phase* is evidenced by large-scale tenocyte death (apoptosis) with major disorganisation of the collagen framework. USS reveals large areas of hypo-echoic structure-less, almost 'moth-eaten' tendon. Chronic abnormal tendon load may lead to permanent 'degenerative'[14] or 'degradative'[15] tendinopathathic change often characterised by extensive abnormal neo-vascularisation and intratendinous calcification (Figure 15.1).

Table 15.3  Tendinopathy stages[14] (adapted)

|  | Reactive | Dys-repair | Degenerative/degradative |
|---|---|---|---|
| **Onset** | Acute | Sub-acute | Chronic, or acute on chronic |
| **Irritability\*** | High | Moderate | Moderate-low |
| **Age/load** | Young (15–25yrs) | Young adult (20–35yrs) | Older (30–60yrs) or many years of plyometric-type sports |
| **Tendon response** | Active, to adapt to short-term increase in load. Possible inflammatory component | Active and attempting to heal, but some structural breakdown | Passive Evidence of apoptosis |
| **Capacity to repair potential** | Full | Reduced/limited | Limited/none |

\* Irritability is related to the amount of activity required to produce pain, the pain level and how long it takes to settle.

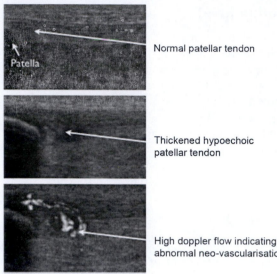

*Figure 15.1* Staging of tendinopathies

It is important to note that, although this process is thought of as a continuum, not every stage is necessarily symptomatic. For example it is likely that the newly painful patellar tendon in a 45-year-old runner will have traversed the reactive and dys-repair phases. It should also be noted that the stage of the tendinopathy is not necessarily consistent throughout an injured tendon. For example, whilst the central tendon may be in dys-repair, the area closer to the enthesis may already be degenerative. Moreover, the stages themselves can overlap. For example a degenerative tendon can, in response to an acute increase in loading, become intermittently reactive.

Although the degenerative continuum is plausible and potentially allows therapeutic modalities to be appropriately aligned to staging of tendon breakdown, inflammation has recently re-emerged as a possible contributor to tendinopathy. Rees and colleagues[15] opined that many of the typical features of athletic tendinopathy, such as tissue degradation and neo-vascularisation, are also seen in inflammatory conditions such as osteo- and rheumatoid arthritis. Though controversial, developing and harnessing pharmacological anti-inflammatory therapies might therefore become beneficial in the treatment of painful sporting tendons.

## Management of tendon pain

Given that tendon pain is likely to have multifactorial genesis (Tables 15.1 and 15.2), several factors are likely to require management within successful rehabilitation. Determining the most important factors that are contributing to the disorder and assessing their relative contributions is vital. In addition to addressing the tendon itself, the sporting or occupational load applied, the load attenuating factors (e.g. muscle strength, biomechanics), as well as the individual factors, such as central adiposity and attitudes to pain, may all need to be recognised and influenced. In saying that, identifying and managing the risk factors that are most easily modifiable (such as workload, footwear, equipment and strength) will often be more rewarding than chasing less modifiable risk factors, such as technique and bio mechanical deficiencies.

It is vital to understand that long-standing pathology produces muscle atrophy, and this must be addressed as increasing muscular cross-section area may have a sparing effect on the associated tendon.[16] Choosing exercises that will develop muscle strength and size without further over-loading the tendon is vital. It is therefore important to note that the tendon needs to be over-loaded compared to its current capacity in order to trigger adaptation, but that the over-load must be controlled. In this case, exercises that utilise the stretch-shortening cycle are not usually introduced until the end stage of rehabilitation. Slow, low-impact loading, particularly in the acute proliferative stages, can be implemented to avoid aggravating the tendon and should be structured so that high tendon loading occurs every 3–4 days.

What constitutes an HTL day will vary according to the individual, and as previously discussed, it is paramount that structured training/exercise programmes should ensure that HTL days are fitted around medium tendon load (MTL) days, as well as low tendon load (LTL) days. The aim is to progress the athlete's tendon strength over the course of the rehabilitation, such that what was once HTL can be re-classified as MTL and eventually LTL.

An example of this concept is as follows:

In the early stages of rehabilitation, HTL for Achilles tendinopathy may be performing $6 \times 5$ sec loaded isometric heel raises. As the tendon begins to adapt and cope with this (and increasing dosages), it can be reclassified as an MTL exercise, and skipping might provide HTL. As time goes on and the tendon strengthens further, heel raises would then become LTL, skipping MTL, and repeated hops for distance might become HTL.

## Principles of exercise prescription in tendinopathy management

There cannot be a recipe-based exercise programme for all people who present with tendon pain. The management strategy must take into account the staging of the disorder (as described above) whilst considering the athlete's circumstances. The principles of this can be seen in Table 15.4.

*Table 15.4* Load management basics for painful tendons

| | Reactive | Dys-repair | Degenerative/Degradative |
|---|---|---|---|
| **Restrict aggravating activity** | Until pain & any swelling subside, e.g. with reactive Achilles, able to hop pain free. May take 1 – 3wks | Until rehabilitation is completed. May take 8 – 12wks | For short period, e.g. 7 days, but then re-introduce load |
| **Other risk factors to address** | Relevant modifiable risk factors | Muscle atrophy & modifiable biomechanical issues | Relevant muscle atrophy & modifiable biomechanical issues |
| **Return to training/ competition** | Very slowly progress volume, load and speed, closely monitoring irritability | Only after rehabilitation is complete. Thereafter, graduate load in 3-day cycles | Graduate load in 3–4-day cycles |
| **Exercise rehabilitation** | Often poor response to heavy loading. If loading exercise is indicated – isometric only | Heavy load may be valuable but caution with 24–48-hour response | Heavy load valuable as long as associated (aggravating) loads are managed |

Of the many tendon treatment modalities, heavy-load exercise rehabilitation is widely touted as the most evidence-based tendinopathy management tool.[17,18] Whilst this may be the case for some types of tendinopathy (primarily those in the dys-repair phase), applying the programmes described in the scientific literature is often challenging in the sporting sphere. For instance, reactive and some compressive tendinopathies don't usually respond well to heavy-load application, and even if heavy loading is indicated, agreeing on the necessary time and commitment to complete a very demanding three-month programme with coaches and athletes is extremely difficult.

As discussed previously, appropriate strain application is likely to be very important in maintaining and improving tendon health. However, frequent, high repetition, heavy-load eccentric[6] and concentric-eccentric[7] programmes are not appropriate for use whilst an athlete continues to train and compete.[19] Isometric loading, on the other hand, may provide crucial in-season 'mechanotransduction' without the same propensity to provoke muscle and tendon pain.

The most effective dose of isometric exercise is not yet known; however, sample in-season programmes for a painful (dys-repair or degenerative) mid-portion Achilles tendon and patellar tendinopathies are provided in Table 15.5.

For each exercise, the load should be heavy, that is, the maximum that can be held for the duration of the repetition. Unless there are identified yet asymptomatic abnormalities in the contralateral tendon, then it may be beneficial to exercise both sides. Alternating sides between repetitions then governs the work-to-rest ratio, along with one-to-two–minute rest periods between sets. The frequency and timing of isometric loading sessions is an important consideration. A maximum of four sessions per week (back-to-back days only once), completed immediately after HTL activities (thereby 24–48hrs before the next HTL activity) is recommended so that adequate adaptation time is allowed.

Of course, exercise rehabilitation options are not limited to these relatively simple single joint/tendon loading exercises, and improving strength, control and mobility of synergists and related body areas is likely to benefit the affected tendon. For example exercises aimed at developing 'posterior chain' trunk and lower-limb function may help offload an injured patella tendon, just as improving foot and ankle control might be a big help to a diseased Achilles.

*Table 15.5* Sample Achilles and patellar tendinopathy exercise rehabilitation prescriptions

| Tendinopathy | Exercise | Isometric exercise | Position | Hold | Reps | Sets |
|---|---|---|---|---|---|---|
| Mid-portion Achilles 1 | 1 | Smith machine heel raise | Straight knee | 5secs | 6 | 3–5 |
| | 2 | | Bent knee | 5secs | 6 | 3–5 |
| Mid-portion Achilles 2 | 1 | Leg press heel raise | Straight knee | 30secs | 1 | 3–5 |
| | 2 | | Bent knee | 30secs | 1 | 3–5 |
| Patella tendinopathy 1 | 1 | Low foot leg press knee extensions | 20, 40, 60 deg knee flexion | 30secs | 1 | 3–5 |
| | 2 | | 0, 30, 60 deg knee flexion | 30secs | 1 | 3–5 |
| Patella tendinopathy 2 | 1 | Smith machine decline single-leg squat | 20, 40, 60 deg knee flexion | 5secs | 6 | 3–5 |

## In-season tendon load management

Given that athletes with lower-limb tendinopathy may not be able to complete as many sport-specific (HTL) training sessions as their teammates or competitors, creative conditioning strategies are essential to maintaining musculotendinous and cardiovascular robustness, along with obtaining optimal body weight for both the athlete's sport and their vulnerable tendon. To minimise aggravation of chronic Achilles pain, a professional footballer might complete much of each team warm-up via stationary bike intervals interspersed with low-amplitude skipping and lunge walk patterns, rather than joining in with running and jumping team-based warm-ups. Given that elite teams will have football-based sessions several days per week, over the course of a season, type of strategy might save many hours of HTL.

Other ways to appropriately modify training schedules to save tendons is via a 7–4–2 in-season training programme, whereby the same footballer with a history of tendinopathy completes, on average, per week (seven days), a maximum of four matches or football training sessions, with only two of these being back-to-back. Seven–three–one or 7–2–1 schedules (three, or even two HTL sessions a week with no back-to-back days) might also be instituted when athletes are returning from, or managing, acute or chronic reactive episodes.

Invariably, athletes with tendinopathy will have in-season flare-ups, and in addition to managing HTL and appropriately incorporating strain-based rehabilitative or prophylactic loading, other modalities can be considered. Completely off-loading severely reactive tendons can help them to settle more quickly. A walking boot and crutches might be worn to offload an acutely painful and swollen Achilles (Figure 15.3), and bilateral heel wedges worn in shoes for a few days can also be helpful. High-volume and blood-product (autologous whole blood or platelet-rich plasma) injections are controversial but can be beneficial[20] and at worst may provide a window of rehabilitation opportunity.[17] Certain oral medications such as the 'polypill' described by Fallon and colleagues can also be a useful adjunct.[21]

Surgery is rarely required but should be considered when high-quality conservative management is no longer effective, particularly in cases where anatomical abnormalities are likely to be causing tendon pain, for example when there is decompression of calcification of the proximal patellar tendon impinging on the tendon and underlying fat pad, or an invaginated plantaris tendon that is irritating the medial Achilles.[10]

## When should athletes recovering from tendon pain return to sport?

How and when return to sport-specific training and competition is accomplished will depend on the demands of the sport. If the sport requires high-intensity and high-volume running and this activity was previously provocative, it seems obvious yet necessary to stress that the athlete must walk before they can run. Initially, reasonably fast-paced 'striding' every three days should precede gradually progressing speed and then distance. Accelerations, decelerations and changes of direction can then be gradually incorporated. If track running is required, it is advisable to start in lane eight before progressing inward towards lane one. Progression to and management of other HTL activities should occur in line with the principles discussed earlier.

When resuming a jumping/landing sport (for example, basketball, volleyball, mogul skiing or gymnastics), it is sensible to progress from controlled double-leg jumping to single-leg, progressively adjusting the intensity, frequency and direction of tendon load. Deceleration is often as or more stressful for tendons than acceleration. Excessive braking loads can occur when slowing down sprints, and taking off and landing from jumps. Coaching to reduce braking loads can be effective. For example, jumping-off and landing-on the forefoot increases patellar tendon load,[22] whilst completing these activities in a more dorsiflexed ankle position may overload the Achilles tendon. With this in mind, patellar tendon loads can be modulated by initial running sessions consisting of runs up flights of stairs. Similarly, jumping from the ground up onto a step is a good way to re-introduce jumps, because the descent from peak jump height is shorter, meaning less force. This can be progressed to jumping on the ground, and then finally landing from a height. Obviously, each of these tasks can be increased in load by 50 per cent by moving from landing on two feet to landing on one.

## Summary

Given the difficulties of managing tendinopathy and the insidious effect tendon pain has on athlete performance and well-being, definitive early management is essential. It may seem like overkill at the time, but regardless of how important the upcoming training or competition seems, convincing coaches and athletes to take the necessary time and measures to resolve a first-time reactive tendinopathy will almost always be preferable to a career of recalcitrant tendon pain.

## Notes

1 Sheen, A.J., Stephenson, B.M., Lloyd, D.M., et al. (2013). 'Treatment of the sportsman's groin': British Hernia Society's 2014 position statement based on the Manchester Consensus Conference. *Br J Sports Med, 48*(14), 1079–1087.

2 Kibler, W.B., Kuhn, J.E., Wilk, K., et al. (2013). The disabled throwing shoulder: Spectrum of pathology – 10-year update. *Arthroscopy, 29*(1), 141–161, e126.

3 Lichtwark, G.A., & Wilson, A.M. (2007). Is Achilles tendon compliance optimised for maximum muscle efficiency during locomotion? *J Biomech, 40*(8), 1768–1775.

4 Sawicki, G.S., Lewis, C.L., & Ferris, D.P. (2009). It pays to have a spring in your step. *Exerc Sport Sci Rev, 37*(3), 130–138.

5 Khan, K.M., & Scott, A. (2009). Mechanotherapy: How physical therapists' prescription of exercise promotes tissue repair. *Br J Sports Med, 43*(4), 247–252.

6 Alfredson, H., Pietila, T., Jonsson, P., & Lorentzon, R. (1998). Heavy-load eccentric calf muscle training for the treatment of chronic achilles tendinosis. *Am J Sports Med, 26*(3), 360–366.

7 Kongsgaard, M., Kovanen, V., Aagaard, P., Doessing, S., Hansen, P., Laursen, A.H., . . . & Magnusson, S.P. (2009). Corticosteroid injections, eccentric decline squat training and heavy slow resistance training in patellar tendinopathy. *Scandinavian J of Med & Sci in Sports, 19*(6), 790–802.

8 Magnusson, S.P., Langberg, H., & Kjaer, M. (2010). The pathogenesis of tendinopathy: Balancing the response to loading. *Nat Rev Rheumatol, 6*(5), 262–268.

9 Orchard, J.W., Cook, J.L., & Halpin, N. (2004). Stress-shielding as a cause of insertional tendinopathy: The operative technique of limited adductor tenotomy supports this theory. *J Sci Med Sport, 7*(4), 424–428.

10 Alfredson, H. (2011). Midportion Achilles tendinosis and the plantaris tendon. *Br J Sports Med, 45*(13), 1023–1025.

11 Farris, D.J., Trewartha, G., & McGuigan, M.P. (2011). Could intra-tendinous hyperthermia during running explain chronic injury of the human Achilles tendon? *J Biomech, 44*(5), 822–826.

12 Rio, E., Moseley, L., Purdam, C., Samiric, T., Kidgell, D., Pearce, A.J., . . . & Cook, J. (2013). The pain of tendinopathy: Physiological or pathophysiological? *Sports Med, 44*(1), 9–23.

13  Fredberg, U., Bolvig, L., & Andersen, N. T. (2008). Prophylactic training in asymptomatic soccer play-ers with ultrasonographic abnormalities in Achilles and patellar tendons: The Danish Super League Study. *Am J Sports Med, 36*(3), 451–460.

14  Cook, J. L., & Purdam, C. R. (2009). Is tendon pathology a continuum? A pathology model to explain the clinical presentation of load-induced tendinopathy. *Br J Sports Med, 43*(6), 409–416.

15  Rees, J. D., Stride, M., & Scott, A. (2013). Tendons – time to revisit inflammation. *Br J Sports Med, 48*, 1553–1557.

16  Popp, K. L., Hughes, J. M., Smock, A. J., Novotny, S. A., Stovitz, S. D., Kochler, S. M., & Petit, M. A. (2009). Bone geometry, strength, and muscle size in runners with a history of stress fracture. *Med Sci Sports Exerc, 41*(12), 2145–2150.

17  Cook, J. (2010). Funky treatments in elite sports people: Do they just buy rehabilitation time? *Br J Sports Med, 44*, 221.

18  Magnussen, R. A., Dunn, W. R., & Thomson, A. B. (2009). Nonoperative treatment of midportion Achilles tendinopathy: A systematic review. *Clin J Sport Med, 19*(1), 54–64.

19  Visnes, H., Hoksrud, A., Cook, J., & Bahr, R. (2005). No effect of eccentric training on jumper's knee in volleyball players during the competitive season: A randomized clinical trial. *Clinical Journal of Sport Medicine, 15*(4), 227.

20  Charousset, C., Zaoui, A., Bellaiche, L., & Bouyer, B. (2014). Are multiple platelet-rich plasma injec-tions useful for treatment of chronic patellar tendinopathy in athletes? A prospective study. *Am J Sports Med, 42*(4), 906–911.

21  Fallon, K., Purdam, C., Cook, J., & Lovell, G. (2008). A 'polypill' for acute tendon pain in athletes with tendinopathy? *J Sci Med Sport, 11*(3), 235–238.

22  Zwerver, J., Bredeweg, S. W., & Hof, A. L. (2007). Biomechanical analysis of the single-leg decline squat. *Br J Sports Med, 41*(4), 264–268.

# Chapter 16

# Bone injuries

*Henry Wajswelner and Sophia Nimphius*

## Introduction

Bone is the most resilient tissue in the human body and under normal conditions remains highly resistant to injury. It is extremely adaptable to athletic loads, and with an understanding of how it adapts, and the mechanical underpinnings of how loading magnitude and frequency affects it, we can begin to understand the mechanisms of bone injury and rehabilitation.

Bone tissue is continuously being broken down and renewed, and when the delicate balance of bone breakdown and bone synthesis is upset, it can start to fail under a seemingly normal load. This type of bone failure is in contrast to those that result from acute high-load impacts.

The bone breakdown-synthesis balance is particularly susceptible to large increases in the volume of mechanical loads without appropriate periods of rest, resulting in bone stress that can progress to failure. This is just one example of how the bone balance can be upset. The complex nature of chronic bone stress and injury will be the focus of this chapter.

## Structure of bone

The structure and composition of bone gives it resistance to both high-impact and repetitive mechanical loads and strains. These qualities are critical to the skeletal system's role of motion and vital organ protection. Further, the tissue composition, microarchitecture and geometry of the bone give it both rigidity and flexibility, dictating its resilience to the magnitude, volume and direction of mechanical load applied to the system.

The direction of loading also influences bone's resiliency. Bone is most resistant to compression. Further, as a viscoelastic tissue, it is even stronger when the application of loading is at a higher rate. This is a highly beneficial property with respect to repetitive loading activities such as running and jumping. Furthermore, muscle contraction augments this compression, highlighting the close relationships between all aspects of the musculoskeletal system.

The anatomical terms *cortical bone* (compact bone) and *trabecular bone* (spongy bone) describe the substance and thus mechanical characteristics of each part of the bone, as shown in Figure 16.1.

Cortical bone is 'stiffer' and capable of handling great amounts of stress (force per unit area) but not large amounts of strain (relative amount deformation per unit length) prior

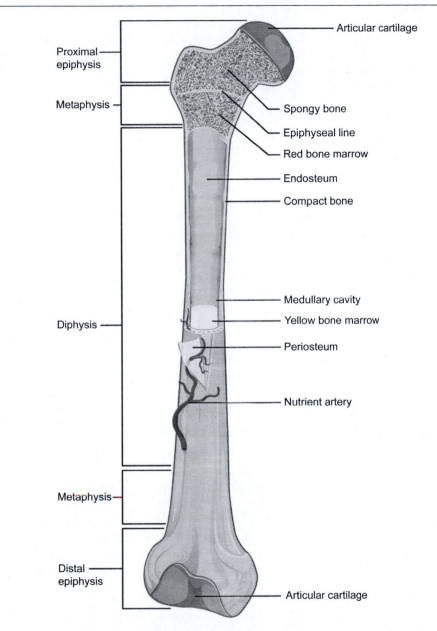

Proximal epiphysis

Metaphysis

Diphysis

Metaphysis

Distal epiphysis

Articular cartilage

Spongy bone

Epiphyseal line

Red bone marrow

Endosteum

Compact bone

Medullary cavity

Yellow bone marrow

Periosteum

Nutrient artery

Articular cartilage

*Figure 16.1* Diagram of a long bone with labelling of the basic anatomical structures. *Anatomy & Physiology*, Connexions Web site, http://cnx.org/content/col11496/1.6/

to tissue failure. On the other hand, trabecular bone has greater capacity to handle greater amounts of strain yet cannot handle a high magnitude of stress. From a practical perspective, we should therefore understand that cortical bone is potentially susceptible to injury during repeated higher-strain activities such as running. This concept is particularly important to monitor during the recovery from bone injury as discussed later in the chapter.

On the other hand, trabecular bone can become susceptible to injury during a high stress (or load) that is not effectively absorbed by the musculoskeletal system. Further, due to the greater metabolic turnover rate of trabecular bone in comparison to cortical bone, it becomes more susceptible to high stress when the breakdown rate of bone increases due to inadequate rest, recovery or nutrition aspects, also discussed later in the chapter.

## Bone strength

Bone strength is a function of many aspects of 'bone quality' that is derived from the following characteristics:

- whole bone geometry
- microarchitecture (such as characteristics of trabecular and cortical tissue)
- tissue properties (such as collagen cross-linking, cellular density and hydration).[1]

Many non-mechanical factors can accelerate or hinder the adaptation of the bone characteristics described above, such as hormones, nutrition, genes and age.[6] This provides an indication of the extrinsic and intrinsic factors that will ultimately influence risk to fracture, as described later in the chapter.

Bone mass is a fundamentally large determinant of bone strength. However, it has been noted that 70–85 per cent of peak bone mass is accounted for by genetic factors.[12] It is therefore important to maximize the remaining modifiable 20–25 per cent of bone mass, which is influenced by body mass index, lean mass, fat mass, physical activity, nutritional factors, thiazide diuretics, statins, Vitamin D and parathyroid hormone.[3]

## Common methods of bone health assessment

To assess the health of the skeletal system, it is common practice to measure whole body bone mineral density (BMD) using *dual energy X-ray absorptiometry* (DXA). Low BMD is characteristic of osteopenia and osteoporosis,[3] and so measurement of BMD provides profiling information for athlete development[4] and may allow for identification of 'at risk' athletes involved in repeated high-mechanical efforts, such as endurance running.[3] However, as bone health is determined by a variety of factors, the risk assessment for osteoporosis (or bone injury) should reflect the multi-factorial aspect of bone strength, and therefore other measures than just BMD should be considered.[1]

The use of another type of bone assessment method, *peripheral quantitative computed tomography* (pQCT) is gaining more widespread acceptance. A pQCT scan provides a measure of bone volume as well as an assessment of bone geometry. Bone morphology or, specifically, bone slenderness is associated with stress fracture risk,[8,11] and so the use of both BMD and bone geometry may function as a better predictor of bone strength.[5]

Of particular interest is the calculation of the stress-strain index (SSI) using the pQCT assessment. The SSI incorporates measures of bone geometry (cortical thickness and radius of bone) and cortical volumetric density to derive a theoretically more comprehensive indicator of bone strength (represented as the SSI). The volumetric density of the bone is indicated in Figure 16.2 by colour, with white representing the highest density. Overall greater bone strength or fracture resilience is indicated by the magnitude of the calculated SSI.

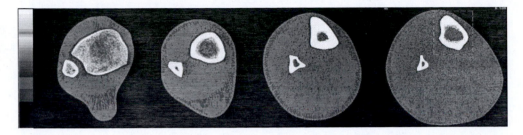

*Figure 16.2* pQCT images of the tibia representing cross-sectional, density-weighted images of the left tibia at 4 per cent, 14 per cent, 38 per cent and 66 per cent length

## Bone stress injury: Classifications and pathophysiology

The spectrum of acute bone injury ranges from stress reaction with bone oedema but no loss of bone continuity, to stress fracture sometimes involving discontinuity, to traumatic fracture with obvious discontinuity of bone. Chronic bone injury may include chronic bone stress, such as the common condition of 'Medial Tibial Stress Syndrome' ('shin splints') or periostitis, or stress fractures.

### Traumatic fractures

Fractures are defined as a loss of continuity in bone, a complete or incomplete break in a bone that usually results from excessive force or trauma but may occasionally occur as the end-result of chronic bone overload. Since the diagnosis and management of traumatic fractures is well covered in many orthopaedic texts, it will not be discussed in this chapter.

### Bone stress continuum

Bone stress is a continuum associated with disrupted bone metabolism. There are three stages: bone strain, stress reaction and stress fracture. In athletes, bone is constantly under stress due to repetitive loading, but it is only when bone stress becomes symptomatic that it is considered to be an injury.

### i. Bone strain

With bone strain there is radiological evidence of bone stress but no symptoms. Bone strain can only be detected on either nuclear scintigraphy (bone scan) as increased bone turnover, or magnetic resonance imaging (MRI) as bone oedema.

### ii. Stress reaction

A stress reaction is the symptomatic breakdown of bone structure due to repetitive submaximal loading.[1] The difference between a 'stress reaction' and 'stress fracture' is a matter of degree. Both involve a disruption of bone metabolism. Initially the pain due to a stress reaction is not severe and eases quickly with rest but can progress quickly to fracture if ignored. A stress reaction can only be detected on a bone scan or seen as bone oedema on an MRI scan, but there will be no fracture line visible in the bone.[1]

### iii. Stress fracture

Advanced fatigue in bone can cause it to fail to withstand repeated loading and eventually fracture.[3] This phenomenon can occur in any solid material. For example, if we were to repeatedly bend a paper clip until it snapped, that would be a form of stress fracture. Stress fractures cause pain and tenderness which are well localised. They also cause swelling and increased temperature in the area of fatigued bone. Since a stress fracture is characterised by bone discontinuity, a fracture line will be visible on CT scan, MRI or X-ray.

> Both bone and MRI scans will show heightened bone activity many months after symptoms have completely resolved, so scans do not need to be 'normal' before an athlete can return to training and competition. This should be a clinical decision rather than one based on imaging.

## Pathophysiology of chronic bone stress

Bone stress injury occurs when there is an imbalance between bone damage (induced by mechanical loading) and bone remodelling. Activities that increase the magnitude or the rate of bone loading (or both) may contribute to damage formation with subsequent progression to a stress fracture.[3] Figure 16.3 shows a schematic of the possible mechanisms.

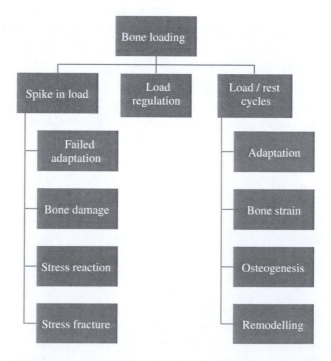

*Figure 16.3* Proposed pathophysiology of bone strain and stress fractures. Adapted from Warden et al. (2006)

## Classification of stress fractures

Stress fractures in athletes may be divided into high-risk and low-risk categories related to both severity and prognosis. High-risk fractures tend to be located on the tension side of a bone, whereas low-risk fractures are located on the compressive side. Fractures with a favourable prognosis that respond well to conservative management, including unassisted weight bearing, are considered low-risk.

Tensile forces and lack of vascularity often lead to a poor healing response in high-risk injuries. They should be managed aggressively, usually with early and prolonged non-weight-bearing and, occasionally, surgery, whereas low-risk fractures tend to respond well to load modification. Risk also relates to severity, so whilst the fibula is normally a low-risk site, a complete stress fracture may progress to non-union and should also be managed aggressively.

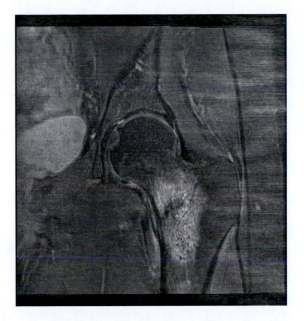

*Figure 16.4* MRI scan of high-risk stress fracture, medial cortex of femoral neck

(Courtesy Andrew Rotstein, Victoria House Medical Imaging)

*Table 16.1* High Risk and Low Risk Stress Fracture Sites

| High Risk Stress Fractures | Low Risk Stress Fractures |
| --- | --- |
| Femoral neck | Femoral shaft |
| Patella | Fibula |
| Anterior cortex of the tibia | Medial tibia |
| Sesamoids | Ribs |
| Tarsal navicular | Calcaneus |
| Neck of the talus | Ulnar shaft |
| Medial malleolus | First to fourth metatarsals |
| Fifth metatarsal | |

## Risk factors for bone injury (intrinsic and extrinsic)

A variety of factors both intrinsic and extrinsic often combine, resulting in the development of a stress fracture.

### Intrinsic risk factors

Intrinsic risk factors are related to an individual's history, morphology or metabolism. Whilst not always easy (and in some cases impossible) to modify these risk factors, an appreciation of them will highlight 'at risk' individuals, marking them as priorities for holistic management. The key intrinsic risk factors are:

### Gender

Females appear to be at greater risk of bone injury than males for a number of reasons. Their more slender bones, gait differences, and unfavourable biomechanical conditions during running caused by a wide pelvis, coxa vara and genu valgum and smaller femoral neck have been offered as possible explanations.[2] Delayed age of menarche and reduced calf girth have been found to be the best independent predictors of stress fractures in women.[6]

Also, an association between stress fractures and the female athlete triad (eating disorder, dysmenorrhea and low bone mineral density), particularly in female distance runners, has been reported.[10] The female athlete triad is discussed in greater detail in chapter 32.

### Vitamin D Deficiency/UV index

Vitamin D plays an important role in bone health via calcium and phosphorous homeostasis, and its deficiency can lead to increased risk of bone injury. Athletes at risk of vitamin D deficiency include those who train indoors or in early morning and late afternoon, have dark skin pigmentation, wear clothing that covers most or all of their body, regularly use sunscreen or consciously avoid the sun, are missing limbs, have gastrointestinal malabsorption (e.g. Coeliac disease or fat malabsorption) or have a family history of bone injury, disorders or vitamin D deficiency.[4]

The principal source of vitamin D comes from exposure to ultraviolet B (UVB) radiation from sunlight.[4] Small amounts of vitamin D can be found in foods but generally will still result in low vitamin D intake. Therefore it is reasonable to advocate dietary supplementation in athletes with low levels found on testing.

### Biomechanics

Higher ground-reaction force and its contributing factors may be associated with the development of lower-limb stress fractures in athletes.[1] Table 16.2 summarises the known biomechanical risk factors in the different sites.

It is important to note that these biomechanical changes can be a sequel to previous injury. For example a previous ankle sprain that has had incomplete rehabilitation may leave the ankle with residual stiffness, leading to poor impulse-dampening strategies and therefore subject to the higher ground-reaction forces that may predispose that foot to stress fractures. Clearly, we need to thoroughly assess athletes' previous injuries to check for residual dysfunction and restore full function to prevent bone stress.

*Table 16.2* Summary of biomechanical risk factors for bone stress injuries

| Site of Bone Stress | Associated Biomechanical Risk/Contributing Factors |
| --- | --- |
| Lower limb | Higher ground-reaction forces, higher rate to peak load, more knee stiffness at impact, rear foot striking |
| Lower limb | Subtalar pronation/rearfoot eversion |
| Pubic bones | Gluteal dysfunction, delayed abdominal activation |
| Ribs | Poor scapular stability under load, thoracic spinal and costovertebral joint dysfunction |
| Navicular | Cavus foot type, metatarsus adductus, short first metatarsal, limited subtalar motion and limited ankle dorsiflexion |
| Pars interarticularis | Poor hip extension, thoracic extension |

## Extrinsic risk factors

Extrinsic factors are those related to the environment or external influences, such as loading magnitudes, direction and frequency, and can influence intrinsic factors or their development.

### Type of sport or activity

Certain sports or activities require a combination of repeated high impact or repeated high rate of mechanical loading. This can occur either through repeated ground impact, as with running, or with repeated high-intensity muscular contraction, as with baseball pitching or rowing.

### Training load

Training load is a potent risk for bone stress injury. In particular, sudden increases in training volume after a period of decreased activity (off-season or injury) and monotonous training (lack of variation) can be associated with fracture risk. However, changes in volume are not always associated with stress fracture development.[3] In fact, variations in training volume are actually required for positive adaptation, but it is the sudden spikes in load, combined with other extrinsic factors or intrinsic factors that are the most likely reason for the onset of a stress fracture. Load monitoring and appropriate management is critical to the identification of and reduction in the risk factors associated with bone injuries.

### Training equipment

In general, equipment can act to absorb or redistribute loads, which can act to alter fracture risk. For example a change from traditional to minimalist running shoes may lead to alterations in bone loading, and we therefore recommend a gradual transition to any new equipment.

### Environmental risk factors

It would seem logical to assume that running on hard surfaces would be a risk factor for bone stress injury. This does not seem to be the case,[3] however, and adaptation to training surface appears be a key factor here; as long as sufficient rest is allowed between loading sessions, the athlete's bones will positively adapt. On the other hand, a *change* in surface, just like a change in training volume, will affect the amount of impact loading rate (increasing when changing to a harder surface) and stabilization musculature required (when changing from hard to soft surface).

## Management of bone stress injuries in athletes

As we can see, the development of bone stress injuries is multidimensional, and so prevention and management responses need to be holistic and consider training load and technique modification, as well as nutritional, medical and, where indicated, psychological intervention.

Bone cells respond to high-magnitude loads, applied rapidly and in different loading distribution from that to which the bone is accustomed. The number of loading cycles required to stimulate osteogenesis is also an important determinant of the adaptive process. The fact that the osteogenic response to loading becomes saturated after relatively few loading cycles has led to the notion that bone cells become desensitised to prolonged mechanical stimulation. However, bone cell mechanosensitivity returns following a period of no loading, and short periods of rest may re-sensitise bone cells to the next bout of loading.[1]

Accordingly, the application of loading to enhance osteogenesis should be done in short bouts separated by rest intervals and may begin with low loads, e.g. low box jumps with 10-second test intervals, progressing to higher loads up to 90 cycles within a bout, but with at least four hours rest between training bouts. In a basketball training camp situation, this may translate to a concept of two shorter sessions of jumping and landing drills separated by rest, rather than one long session followed by a game.

*Low-risk stress fractures* can be successfully treated with activity restriction and a carefully graduated return to sport. A detailed management plan should be mapped out in consultation with the athlete, coaching team and other members of the interdisciplinary support team. Management should seek to address all the modifiable risk factors present and a two-phase protocol should be used to manage most low-risk stress fractures.

*Phase 1* is pain control with relative rest, ice and oral analgesics. Anti-inflammatory medications should be avoided due to potential delayed bone healing.[4] For lower-body stress fractures, weight bearing as tolerated is allowed for daily activities, but participation in sports will be limited (depending on the sport). Walking boots should be used to allow pain-free ambulation. For upper-body stress fractures, the management is along similar lines: no high-impact or heavy-resisted loads through the arms or upper body. Low-impact cardio-vascular exercise, such as pool running, elliptical trainers and cycling, are options for fitness maintenance in this phase.

*Phase 2* can begin when the athlete has been pain-free for 10–14 days. One week after the localised bony tenderness has eased, loading should be resumed at half the usual intensity. For a runner this will be a slow easy run; for a rower this will be an easy session in a single scull or rowing ergometer. Antigravity treadmills are an emerging approach to management of bone stress injuries in athletes.[8] Antigravity treadmills provide adjustable body-weight support and may help to maintain fitness during the recovery form bone stress, as well as providing a controlled loading environment. Initially, athletes with a healing stress fracture should not increase their load every day but allow the healing bone time to recover between these early sessions. Increments of 25 per cent should be used to gradually increase training loads to the pre-injury level over three to six weeks under strict supervision according to the pain response.

A comprehensive conditioning program to normalize strength, endurance and flexibility of all the lower limb muscles and complete reconditioning of the entire kinetic chain, including all joint ranges of motion and motor control, should be included in the return-to-sport plan.

*High-risk stress fractures* require much more complex management, and referral to a sports physician, orthopaedic surgeon and other specialists is often required. Grades 1 and 2 usually resolve with conservative management, including strict restriction of weight-bearing and/or immobilization until healing has occurred on repeat imaging. To prevent progression to full fracture and associated complications, complete healing must be confirmed before the athlete returns to sport. The site of the fracture, higher grade of fracture, stage of healing or non-union/delayed union and the requirements of the sport will determine whether surgery is the treatment of choice. Pulsed ultrasound therapy, extracorporeal shock wave (ECSW) therapy, and capacitive electric fields (also known as bone stimulators) are non-invasive techniques that have been used for stress fractures to promote healing and hasten recovery, particularly with cases of delayed union,[2] but the evidence for these treatments is as yet inconclusive, so routine clinical use cannot be recommended.

## Summary

Despite the inherent characteristics of bone as having strength, stiffness and toughness, it is still susceptible to structural fatigue and a lowered level of natural resilience when a combination of intrinsic and extrinsic factors interact. With appropriate monitoring and identification of risk factors, one can minimize the potential risk of stress fractures in athletes. Therefore, a well-constructed and global approach to athlete management, including bone strength determination, evaluation and modification of intrinsic and extrinsic risk factors, appropriate load application and load monitoring, will all contribute to optimal recovery from bone stress injury.

## Notes

1  Bennell, K. L., Malcolm, S. A., Thomas, S. A., Reid, S. J., Brukner, P. D., Ebeling, P. R., & Wark, J. D. (1996). Risk factors for stress fractures in track and field athletes: A twelve-month prospective study. *The American Journal of Sports Medicine, 24*(6), 810–818.

2  Chen, Y.-T., Tenforde, A. S., & Fredericson, M. (2013). Update on stress fractures in female athletes: Epidemiology, treatment, and prevention. *Current Reviews in Musculoskeletal Medicine, 6*(2), 173–181.

3  Cosman, F., Ruffing, J., Zion, M., Uhorchak, J., Ralston, S., Tendy, S., … Nieves, J. (2013). Determinants of stress fracture risk in United States Military Academy cadets. *Bone, 55*(2), 359–366.

4  Fonseca, H., Moreira-Gonçalves, D., Coriolano, H.-J., & Duarte, J. (2014). Bone quality: The determinants of bone strength and fragility. *Sports Medicine, 44*(1), 37–53.

5  Frost, H. M., & Schonau, E. (2000). The 'muscle-bone unit' in children and adolescents: A 2000 overview. *Journal of Pediatric Endocrinology and Metabolism, 13*(6), 571–590.

6  Heaney, R. P., Abrams, S., Dawson-Hughes, B., Looker, A., Marcus, R., Matkovic, V., & Weaver, C. (2000). Peak bone mass. *Osteoporosis International, 11*(12), 985–1009.

7  Kobayashi, A., Kobayashi, T., Kato, K., Higuchi, H., & Takagishi, K. (2013). Diagnosis of radiographically occult lumbar spondylolysis in young athletes by magnetic resonance imaging. *The American Journal of Sports Medicine, 41*(1), 169–176.

8 Nattiv, A., Loucks, A. B., Manore, M. M., Sanborn, C. F., Sundgot-Borgen, J., & Warren, M. P. (2007). American College of Sports Medicine position stand: The female athlete triad. *Medicine and Science in Sports and Exercise, 39*(10), 1867–82.

9 Rudolph, B. S., & Smith, A. L. (1999). Strength training for the windmill softball pitcher. *Strength & Conditioning Journal, 21*(4), 27–33.

10 Sarkis, K. S., Pinheiro Mde, M., Szejnfeld, V. L., & Martini, L. A. (2012). High bone density and bone health. *Endocrinologia y nutricion: Organo de la Sociedad Espanola de Endocrinologia y Nutricion, 59*(3), 207–14.

11 Schnackenburg, K. E., Macdonald, H. M., Ferber, R., Wiley, J. P., & Boyd, S. K. (2011). Bone quality and muscle strength in female athletes with lower limb stress fractures. *Medicine and Science in Sports and Exercise, 43*(11), 2110–9.

12 Siu, W. S., Qin, L., & Leung, K. S. (2003). pQCT bone strength index may serve as a better predictor than bone mineral density for long bone breaking strength. *Journal of Bone and Mineral Metabolism, 21*(5), 316–322.

13 Tenforde, A. S., Watanabe, L. M., Moreno, T. J., & Fredericson, M. (2012). Use of an antigravity treadmill for rehabilitation of a pelvic stress injury. *PM&R, 4*(8), 629–631.

14 Tommasini, S. M., Nasser, P., Schaffler, M. B., & Jepsen, K. J. (2005). Relationship between bone morphology and bone quality in male tibias: Implications for stress fracture risk. *Journal of Bone and Mineral Research, 20*(8), 1372–80.

15 Turner, C. H., & Robling, A. G. (2003). Designing exercise regimens to increase bone strength. *Exercise and Sport Sciences Reviews, 31*(1), 45–50.

16 Veale, J. P., Pearce, A. J., Buttifant, D., & Carlson, J. S. (2010). Anthropometric profiling of elite junior and senior Australian football players. *International Journal of Sports Physiology and Performance, 5*(4), 509.

17 Warden, S. J., Burr, D. B., & Brukner, P. D. (2006). Stress fractures: pathophysiology, epidemiology, and risk factors. *Current Osteoporosis Reports, 4*(3), 103–9.

18 Zadpoor, A. A., & Nikooyan, A. A. (2011). The relationship between lower-extremity stress fractures and the ground reaction force: A systematic review. *Clinical Biomechanics, 26*(1), 23–28.

19 Ziltener, J.-L., Leal, S., & Fournier, P.-E. (2010). Non-steroidal anti-inflammatory drugs for athletes: An update. *Annals of Physical and Rehabilitation Medicine, 53*(4), 278–288.

# Chapter 17

# Pain and performance

*David Joyce and David Butler*

## Introduction

The eradication or reduction of pain is the outcome that determines the success of many of the interventions of the rehabilitation professional. However, pain is a phenomenon that is largely misunderstood in the sporting arena. Our knowledge of the processes involved in pain production has taken gigantic leaps forward over the last decade, thanks in part to the use of more sophisticated imaging techniques (such as functional magnetic resonance imaging), and an increase in research into the psychology of pain. A growing awareness of the cost of pain – around 600 billion dollars a year in the United States in 2010[1] and a prevalence of chronic pain at around one in four people[2] has increased stakeholder interest in its treatment. We are beginning to appreciate the multi-faceted nature of pain, but the prevailing approach to its management in sport lags well behind other areas of clinical management in acute pain, the prevention of chronic pain and the relationship of pain to performance. We seek to address these issues in this chapter.

## The challenge of pain

Pain is much more than an unpleasant sensation. It can derail the best-laid short- and long-term plans of the athlete, the support staff and, indeed, the hopes of fans. As such, measures designed to accurately deal with pain are of critical importance to the athletic performance team. And yet, sports injury management is still largely the preserve of clinicians intervening at a tissue disorder level. This predominantly biomedical paradigm is no longer tenable, and there needs to be a concerted drive for more of an evidence-based approach to injury rehabilitation. This *necessarily* leads us to consider a biopsychosocial framework to manage pain and performance. By biopsychosocial we mean a dynamic, reciprocal and complex interaction of biological, social and psychological domains.[3,4] Under this framework, we will discuss pain and performance, and broadly discuss methods of addressing the issue pain in the sporting context.

## Pain as an output of the brain

Pain is an adaptive, attention-demanding brain output of highest cortical priority.[5] Its *raison d'être* is to alert, teach, protect and stimulate a change in bodily behaviour to shield from further threat, and allow optimal healing conditions.

A critical conceptual change point for many may be that pain is far better understood as an output of the brain as opposed to an input. Contrary to popular thought, there are no pain pathways or pain endings, and so the body cannot send 'pain messages' to the brain, as was once thought. In essence, the peripheral nerves enable us to sense the environment – the pressure of a punch, the heat of a flame, or the change in pH from lactic acid build-up, for example – and send a barrage of nociceptive ('danger') impulses to the central nervous system (CNS). Second-order neurones in the dorsal horn of the spinal cord then carry this nociceptive information for processing in numerous areas within the central nervous system. In light of all of this, should this information be interpreted as dangerous to the body, a defensive response, very often pain, may be constructed by the brain. This is why we say that pain is an *output*.

### What happens in our brain when we sprain an ankle?

Consider a sprained ankle. Here, a barrage of impulses sent to the brain essentially warns of danger in the ankle region. The brain weighs up this information in light of past experience – its predictions and expectations of the future (what will happen if these messages are ignored, etc.), societal and familial factors (amongst many other variables) – and then, if it concludes that the body is in danger, will coordinate a multimodal output of which pain is a constituent (others may include swelling, limping, alteration in muscle tone, sympathetic, endocrine, emotional and cognitive responses).[6] Of course, there is potential for error as the brain weighs up all the relevant information. Things may not have been as dangerous as, or may be *more* dangerous than, the brain's decision at that particular time and place.

Significant damage does not always result in significant pain. Equally, nor does a lot of pain always indicate that there is significant tissue damage. This is because the amount of pain we construct is a reflection of the amount of *threat* our brain 'believes' we are under, and not necessarily how much tissue damage we have sustained. In fact, pain is very often a poor correlate of tissue damage,[7] yet most people still believe that pain and tissue damage have a linear relationship.

We all have experienced discovering a bruise on our arm but not remembering the incident that caused it. The evidence of tissue damage is there, but clearly the brain has weighed the circumstances at that particular time and concluded that the threat to our body is so low and therefore pain production is unnecessary. In a similar way, many sportspeople have played on with injury and only realised it at the end of a game. The brain has a choice whether something should hurt or not.

### Neuromatrix and neurosignatures

There is no one area of the brain that is responsible for pain processing. Almost all regions of the brain *can* play a role in an individual pain experience. This collective and distributed processing has led to the establishment of a new paradigm to engage pain, known as the *pain neuromatrix*.[8] This refers to all the neuroanatomical regions within the cerebral cortex that are activated when the brain concludes that the body of a *specific individual* is in danger in a *specific context*.[9]

Whilst there is great variation in the exact brain territory involved in initiating a pain experience between (and even within) individuals, brain imaging studies have revealed a reasonably typical pattern of cortical activation in humans undergoing experimentally induced pain.[10,11,12] Areas activated consistently appear to be the insular cortex, bilateral thalamus, anterior cingulate cortex (ACC), sensory cortex and motor areas, although 400 or more areas may be involved. Together, these form the neuroanatomical basis of the pain neurosignature.[5,13] Some of the areas that have been shown to be involved in pain construction can be seen in Figure 17.1.

The brain territory involved in pain neurosignatures does not only comprise neurones. In fact, neurones represent only around 10 per cent of the cells in the CNS. The majority of the rest are cells such as microglia, astrocytes and oligodendrocytes which have immune functions and intimate bidirectional relationships with neurones.[14,15,16]

Accordingly, a shift away from older neurocentric views into more modern neuroimmune considerations supports biopsychosocial approaches, as it not only allows an appreciation of how infection and injury have neuroimmune consequences, but also how psychosocial

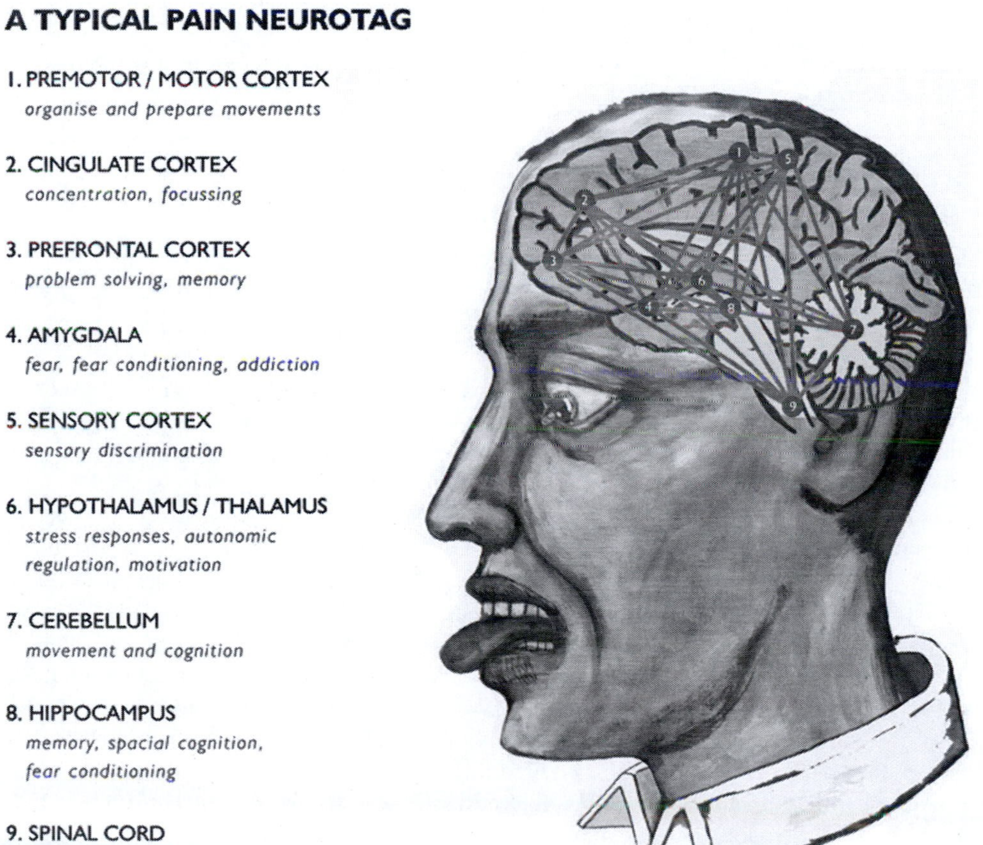

## A TYPICAL PAIN NEUROTAG

1. PREMOTOR / MOTOR CORTEX
*organise and prepare movements*

2. CINGULATE CORTEX
*concentration, focussing*

3. PREFRONTAL CORTEX
*problem solving, memory*

4. AMYGDALA
*fear, fear conditioning, addiction*

5. SENSORY CORTEX
*sensory discrimination*

6. HYPOTHALAMUS / THALAMUS
*stress responses, autonomic regulation, motivation*

7. CEREBELLUM
*movement and cognition*

8. HIPPOCAMPUS
*memory, spacial cognition, fear conditioning*

9. SPINAL CORD
*gating from the periphery*

*Figure 17.1* Likely parts of a pain neurosignature

(From Butler, D. S., & Moseley, G. L. [2013]. *Explain pain* [2nd ed.]. Adelaide, Australia: NOI Group.)

circumstances may influence anti- and pro-inflammatory cytokine balances in the CNS and hence brain outputs.[17] It also informs us that the biomedical model of pain management is clearly limited, and our methods of treating pain must encompass wider domains than just body tissues. It also explains why simply providing an athlete with an aspirin may be completely ineffective.

Microglia and astrocytes are essentially danger surveillance cells as well as players in learning and plasticity; they react temporally and may remain 'experienced' and on alert for many months after injury, even years.[17,18] The athlete overly concerned and vigilant about a body part, enhanced perhaps by unfortunate evocative language (eg 'collapsed arch', 'slipped disc', 'degenerated'), may well have the brain territory representing the body part on alert with enhanced plasticity potential. We often see the athlete who is constantly prodding a troublesome elbow, or wanting adductor 'releases' because their groin is feeling 'tight'. This, if not managed appropriately, can reinforce a chronic alertness, making the neurosignature even harder to shift. We also note in athletes how old pain states can return during time of immunological distress, such as the flu or psychosocial disturbances (breaking up with a partner or exam stress, for example).

> To be truly effective, our management of pain needs to be as sophisticated as the pain construct itself.

## How can we apply the neuromatrix paradigm in sports?

Much of the decision making regarding the status of an injury is currently based upon the athlete's subjective reporting of pain, as though this provides the coach or rehabilitator with an intimate view of how the athlete (including their tissues) are recovering. To a large extent, what the athlete is reporting in terms of pain is influenced by the value that is placed on that sensation. Commonly, we make judgements on fitness to play based on pain levels and talk in terms of injury healing. As we have seen, pain is a complex substrate of many inputs and influences, of which nociception is often (but not necessarily) one, and so it is inappropriately reductive to talk only in terms of tissue damage.

Clearly, factors other than tissue damage that could construct pain neurosignatures need to be taken into account when clinically reasoning. The influence of features, such as past injury profile, adverse experiences with similar injuries, perceptions about pain, current immune health and implications of the injury for employment, are all equally influential in determining whether someone goes on to have a maladaptive pain experience. In short, all the factors that could increase the threat value to the individual need to be considered, as any of these may be collectively adding fuel to the flames. We can categorise these factors as 'the things I hear, the things I say, the things I believe, the things I do, the people I meet, the places I go, and my current biological state'.[19] These factors will differ among people and need to be assessed with as much rigour as the injured tissue is in the structural assessment. This information will then form part of the decision making regarding the relative contribution of tissue-based input factors, the more centrally based factors such as changes in the reactivity of neurones and immune cells in the CNS,[20] and then the influence of other output systems on tissue health. For example changes in outputs other than pain, such as the endocrine, autonomic and motor systems, could influence tissue healing.[6,21,22] This is then used to guide the clinical reasoning process during the management of the injury. This knowledge is what can help guide our judgement about whether or not an athlete is able to play safely in pain while another with no pain should be off the field.

An example of this may be when an athlete exhibits marked stress-type responses when training following an injury. They may not be complaining of pain *per se* but the neuro-endocrine sequelae of stress can impede tissue healing and alter motor patterns – something that can increase re-injury risk. Labelling an athlete 'soft' when they are adversely stressed is common in our sporting culture, but is mostly completely counterproductive. Quite simply, rehabilitation is not complete until the athlete is totally convinced that it is complete.

## All pain experiences are personal

We all have encountered the athlete who tells us that the pain was '10 out of 10' when their little finger was hyperextended. Equally, we all know the person who complains of 'a little bit of a back ache', and when a history is taken, including looking at the scans, you marvel that they are still playing high-level sport. Neither of them is wrong – what they are experiencing is true for them. What it does show us, however, is that pain is a very individual experience and this is because what one person views as a threat, another person is fairly nonchalant about. As a result, just any pain measurement tool cannot necessarily be used as a means for determining the extent of bodily damage. Additionally, it can be seen that it would be inappropriate to compare one person's pain against another's. We can, however, compare different episodes of pain experienced by the same person at different times. For example it would hardly be surprising if a high jumper with a previous history of a significant ankle fracture presented with an exaggerated pain response to a simple ankle sprain sustained a month before the Olympics. This demonstrates the importance of understanding the context of the injury and being aware of the notion of immune surveillance discussed earlier.

---

**Subjective pain reports**

Simply asking the athlete 'How does it feel?' can provide us with an insight into the 'temperature' of their neuromatrix, which in turn, may provide prognostic information, but the response will not necessarily reflect the amount of structural damage.

---

## Pain and sporting performance

Pain has a negative impact on performance, and vice versa. It has the capacity to preferentially demand attention, which distracts conscious attention from other tasks, resulting in poorer performance of these tasks. This impacts upon CNS performance and is known as pain interference.[23] Pain has the capacity to increase reaction times and produce more performance errors during simple tasks.[24,25] This is commonly seen in the athlete who, whilst training, is constantly rubbing a previously injured area. Their attention has been shifted away from the demands of the sport, and onto the demands of a sensitive and anxious nervous system. Undoubtedly, this can sometimes be an appropriate action, but not always and may be something that needs to be dampened. Constant tissue-based 'treatment' can often reinforce the athlete's mindset, and careful consideration needs to be given to whether the athlete needs this intervention.

However, it is not only pain but also that expectation of pain that can affect motor performance. Anxiety levels are high when returning to an important task after injury. It seems reasonable to assert that anxiety levels are higher if the injury occurred during that task, or there was a threat of re-injury upon return to the sport.

To this end, reduction of anxiety when returning to sport needs specific attention. Drills that encourage normal movement and function need to be included as early as is safe and adaptive behaviours encouraged and rewarded. Only when the threat value placed on re-injury by the athlete is removed can the CNS fire at maximum efficiency, a necessary condition for safe return to sport.

Whilst pain is highly demanding of attention, cognitively taxing tasks have been shown to interfere with pain perception and alter activity in the neuromatrix.[11] Some brain areas such as the orbitofrontal cortex and the affective division of the ACC have shown increased activation during cognitively challenging tasks, whilst other areas of the pain matrix dedicated to pain attention and intensity coding showed decreased activity.[11] These findings may support the notion that injury management needs to combine cognitively demanding tasks with physical conditioning. Clearly, we need to help the athlete condition the mind as much as the body.

## Pain and the chronically injured athlete

When we have sustained an injury, our brain places more attention on the harmed area. This can be likened to a process of increasing the numbers of closed circuit television (CCTV) cameras trained on the area of known criminal activity. The brain wants to know *everything* that is going on around there. It's 'looking after us' because it perceives that the threat of further injury (or re-injury) is still high. Unfortunately, these CCTV cameras do not always disappear overnight or even as soon as the physiological process of healing is complete. They are still present for as long as the neuromatrix is concerned about the threat. The process of rehabilitation, therefore, is only complete once:

1 The physiological process of healing is complete;
2 Physical performance is re-instituted; and
3 The brain is satisfied that threat levels have reduced and so has 'turned off its CCTV cameras'.

Often an athlete will tell us that their previously injured part doesn't 'hurt' any more, but it 'feels different' or that they are 'aware of it'. This can be very annoying and is likely to be due to enhanced neuroimmune-inspired brain activity in the neurosignatures of the body part, thus keeping 'tabs' on the previously injured body part. Sensations that would previously have been dealt with unconsciously by the brain (like background music) are now being analysed consciously (like foreground music), even though the healing process is complete. This is their brain looking out for them. It would be irresponsible of the brain *not* to do this. It does become a problem, however, when this process goes on for too long and the CCTV cameras never get turned off. This leads to anxiety and possibly catastrophisation, which not only contribute to slow healing, but also to significant reductions in performance, such as poor skill execution, poor allocation of energy resources and decreased attention to the necessary tasks of the sport.

## What is rehabilitation?

We often think of rehabilitation as a series of steps that physically prepare a person to return to full function by progressively loading and conditioning injured tissues to enable them to withstand stress. While this is undoubtedly true, we believe that this definition is reductive. Rehabilitation is a much more complicated process and it has as much to do with calming down the neuromatrix (progressively reducing the threat levels in order to 'turn off the CCTV cameras') as it does with strengthening local tissues.

## Rehabilitation is for the brain *and* the body!

The key aims in sports injury management are to foster adaptive behaviours in the acute setting and intervene to limit maladaptive behaviours. Reduction of threat by dampening nociceptive mechanisms, education and graduated exposure can help to restore normal movement and function without enhancing the sensitivity of the neuromatrix.[5,26] This is as important an aim in rehabilitation as strengthening a torn muscle or improving lumbar spine mechanics. In essence, we are seeking to rehabilitate the brain's representation of the musculoskeletal system as well as the musculoskeletal system by itself. This would include restoration of a healthy immune balance and brain inhibitory controls.

Given that pain is the brain's response to perceived bodily threat, steps need to be taken to reduce anxiety, fear and misconceptions after injury. It has been shown that laypeople can understand basic neurophysiology of pain[27] and that this understanding reduces the threat value of pain.[5] The corollary here is that evidence-based management of sports injuries must include an explanation of the injury in terms of the neurophysiology. This is powerfully done in the way of analogies and explained in a manner that we have sought to do in this chapter.

The manner in which we present the information on pain to the athlete is critical. We must do so in an assured but reassuring manner that is pragmatic and demonstrates an empathy that is believable and calming. This is critical to minimise the exaggerated cognitive and behavioural responses that can result from a pain experience and is particularly vital when the athlete has a significant pre-conceived idea about the nature of and reason for the pain. One of the most useful therapeutic discussions often focusses on education around 'Hurts do not necessarily equal harm', or similarly, 'You can be sore but safe'. This is particularly relevant to most chronic pain situations but also to some acute pain states. This education often requires some conceptual challenges, but critically, it is not suggesting to an athlete that 'it is all in your head' in a derogatory way. All pain states will include some 'issues in tissues' as well as changes in the representation of tissues and the injury in the brain. In many chronic pain states, tissues may remain unhealthy, unfit and sensitive long past expected healing times, but it is only with the added consideration of the representational changes in the neuromatrix that the best evidence-based assessment and therapy can ensue.

Dividing injuries into 'acute' and 'chronic' is sometimes done arbitrarily and for convenience. Pain signatures are activated in both scenarios, and time elapsed since injury does not necessarily provide an accurate guide to the relative contributions of any specific part of the neuromatrix to the experience. This said, however, chronic pain, where the pain state lasts much longer than tissue healing times would dictate, or where an athlete breaks down at a certain threshold, is likely to have a significant central component, and therapy directed solely at the tissue is likely to be unsuccessful. Attention needs to be shifted to the other areas of the neuromatrix.

Explanation of the rehabilitation process to an injured athlete and providing them with a stepwise recovery process is critical. Focusing on aspects of training that the athlete can achieve (similar to the concept of focusing on what the athlete *can* do as opposed to what they *cannot* to – see chapter 1) provides a calming and restorative environment for the CNS, thus allowing threat levels to be reduced, and, by extension, the multimodal output that is pain.

## Summary

Sports injury rehabilitation is still largely the preserve of professionals intervening at a tissue disorder level. This paradigm is no longer tenable and there needs to be a concerted drive for more of an evidence-based approach to injury rehabilitation. By necessity, this requires a modern biopsychosocial approach to pain and performance. Juxtaposed to the effective management of pain and dysfunction is the improvement in sports performance – the central tenet of sports rehabilitation.

## Notes

1  Institute of Medicine. (2011). *Relieving pain in America: a blueprint for transforming prevention, care, education and research*. Washington D.C.: National Academics Press.
2  Blyth, F. M., et al. (2001). Chronic pain in Australia: A prevalence study. *Pain, 89*(2–3), 127–34.
3  Campbell, C. C., & Edwards, R. R. (2009). Mind-body interactions in pain: The neurophysiology of anxious and catastrophic pain related thoughts. *Translational Research, 153,* 97–101.
4  Gatchel, R. J., et al. (2007). The biopsychosocial approach to chronic pain: Scientific advances and future directions. *Psychological Bulletin, 133,* 581–624.
5  Moseley, G. L. (2003). A pain neuromatrix approach to rehabilitation of chronic pain patients. *Manual Therapy, 8,* 130–140.
6  Butler, D.S ., & Moseley, G. L. (2013). *Explain pain* (2nd ed.). Adelaide, Australia: NOI Group.
7  Melzack, R., & Wall, P. D. (1996). *The Challenge of Pain* (2nd ed.). London: Penguin.
8  Melzack, R. (1999). From the gate to the neuromatrix. *Pain, 82,* S121–S126.
9  Moseley, G. L. (2003). A pain neuromatrix approach to patients with chronic pain. *Manual Therapy, 8*(3), 130–140.
10  Peyron, R., Laurent, B., & Garcia-Larrea, L. (2000). Functional imaging of brain responses to pain: A review and meta-analysis. *Neurophysiologie Clinique, 30*(5), 263–88.
11  Bantick, S., et al. (2002). Imaging how attention modulates pain in humans using functional MRI, *Brain, 125,* 310–319.
12  Apkarian, A. V., et al. (2011). *Pain and the brain: Specificity and plasticity of the brain in clinical chronic pain, Pain, 152,* S49-S64.
13  Melzack, R. (2001). Pain and the neuromatrix in the brain. *Journal of Dental Education, 65,* 1378–1382.
14  Fields, R. D. (2009). *The other brain.* New York: Simon and Schuster.
15  Watkins, L. R., Milligan, E. D., & Maier, S. F. (2003). *Immune and glial involvement in physiological and pathological exaggerated pain states.* In *Progress in pain research and management* (pp. 369–386), J. O. Dostrovsky, D. B. Carr, & M. Kolzenburg (Eds.). Seattle: IASP Press.
16  Yirmiya, R., & Goshen, T. (2011). Immune modulation of learning, memory, neural plasticity and neurogenesis. *Brain, Behaviour and Immunity, 25,* 181–213.
17  Austin, P. J., & Moalem-Taylor, G. (2010). The neuro-immune balance in neuropathic pain: Involvement of inflammatory immune cells, immune like glial cells and cytokines. *Journal of Neuroimmunology, 229,* 23–60.

18  Banati, R. B., et al. (2001). Long-term transynaptic glial responses in the human thalamus after peripheral nerve injury. *Neuroreport, 12*, 3439–3442.
19  Moseley, G. L., & Butler, D. S. (2014). *Explain pain handbook*. Adelaide, Australia: NOI Group.
20  Woolf, C. J. (2011). *Central sensitization: Implications for the diagnosis and treatment of pain*. Pain, *152*(3), S2–15.
21  Gifford, L. S., ed. (1998). *Topical issues in pain*. Falmouth, U.K.: NOI Press.
22  Butler, D. S. (2000). *The sensitive nervous system*. Adelaide, Australia: NOI Group.
23  Crombez, G., et al. (1997). Habituation and interference of pain with task performance. *Pain Forum, 70*, 149–154.
24  Crombez, G., et al. (1999). Fear of pain is more disabling than pain itself. Evidence on the role of pain related fear in chronic back pain disability. *Pain, 80*, 329–340.
25  Moseley, G. L., & Hodges, P. W. (2002). Chronic pain and motor control. In G. Jull & J. Boyling (Eds.), *Grieves modern manual therapy of the vertebral column* (pp. 215–323). Edinburgh, Scotland: Churchill-Livingstone.
26  Gifford, L. S. (1998). Pain, the tissues and the nervous system. *Physiotherapy, 84*, 27–33.
27  Moseley, G. L. (2003). Unravelling the barriers to reconceptualisation of the problem in chronic pain: the actual and perceived ability of patients and health professionals to understand the neurophysiology. *Journal of Pain, 4(4)*, 184–189.

# Chapter 18

# Determining return to play

*Calvin Morriss and Phil Pask*

## Introduction

In an age where sport is a business, and winning and losing impact on much more than just pride, there are normally a number of inputs to the decision making process that determine when an athlete should return to competition. Many of the inputs to an athlete's rehabilitation (rehab) programme are welcomed ones and normally come from the immediate support team. While not exhaustive, the key personnel may often include medical and surgical specialists, sports physicians, physiotherapists, soft tissue therapists, athletic trainers, strength and conditioning (S&C) coaches and the technical coaches. The appropriate synergy of these views and inputs, along with the athlete's own thoughts and feelings, makes a significant contribution to the success of the rehabilitation/reconditioning process.

Including the input of such a wide variety of specialist staff in a fully integrated way makes a lot of sense when one considers what is expected of the athlete when they return to training and competition. These expectations might include:

1    Pain-free and precise movement particular to the sport
2    Strength and power restored to at least pre-injury levels
3    Metabolic and neuromuscular fatigue resistance to high-intensity sporting performance
4    Confidence and competence in the technical performance of sporting skills.

The prioritised balance of these factors will, of course, depend upon the type and severity of the initial injury, as will the associated input of our support team of specialists. A coordinated, truly integrated team effort involves respecting each other's professional abilities. In a poor model, the medical team may perhaps hold onto the athlete too long without involving the S&C coaches (the S&C coaches need to be involved but also to recognise the healing states of the injured tissue). Just as tragic is the model where the technical coaches do not see the player until late in the rehabilitation process, when much low-load technical work could have been completed. Figure 18.1 demonstrates such a poor model for an athlete about to undergo an eight-week rehabilitation programme.

A far better model sees the S&C coaches working hand-in-hand with the physical therapists from very early rehabilitation and the involvement of the technical coaches throughout the process. This would allow the athlete to prepare for 'performance' at the same time as recovering from the initial injury.

What should be clear from the above is that restoring an athlete to competition after injury is actually restoring them to a level of sporting performance and not simply a question of

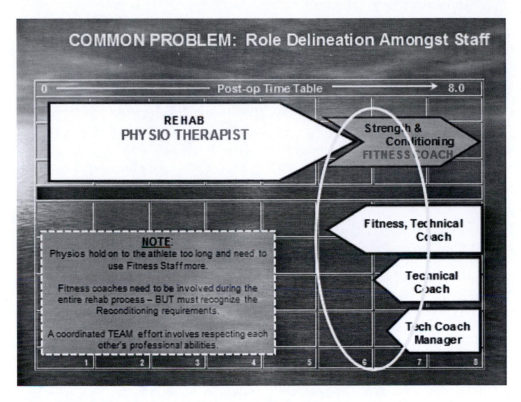

*Figure 18.1* A poor (but common) model of transition from injury to return to competition

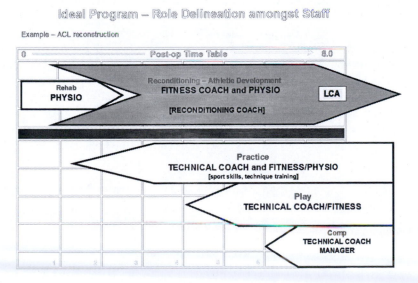

*Figure 18.2* A well-integrated model of the rehabilitation process

(reproduced with permission of Bill Knowles)

the level of healing of the initial injury. Success should not be measured by the speed of the return to play but primarily by the return to a high level of performance and low-level risk of re-injury. The aim of this chapter is to present a robust process for returning a player or athlete to competition following an injury and a subsequent rehabilitation period.

## Return to perform – more than 'medically fit' to play

The decision to return an athlete to a competitive level of performance should be made only when that athlete can 'safely and sensibly' go back to their chosen sport. That athlete must have the physical abilities to perform at levels equal to or above those pre-injury.

So how do we know that an athlete has reached a performance level to compete once more? We need to know the following:

*   Baseline data on the athlete pre-injury. Without this information, it is difficult to know what the 'performance' level really is. Comparing right to left sides can be useful with certain injuries, but if the injury was felt to be due to inadequate strength, flexibility or fatigue resistance, knowing that performance markers have shifted favourably during rehabilitation is critical information.
*   The physiological and biomechanical demands of the sport (and positional demands within team sports). To perform competitively within the sport, the athlete's physical abilities need to adequately match the demands imposed upon the body. The more we understand about the sport's demands, the better we can prepare for those demands.

The physical demands of each sport can be quite different. By including *individualised positional and sport-specific skills* within the rehabilitation programme, the movement patterns that will be required by that athlete can be stressed – and, importantly, stressed under fatigue. It may not be enough for an athlete to have regained strength and flexibility if that cannot be translated into specific skill sets, such as a side-on tackle in rugby, where footwork and a strong body position might also be important performance indicators. The demands in terms of complexity and technique can be progressed as able. The athlete must be able to complete all the physical and technical skills required to perform and perform under fatigue without the fear of re-injury. It would be awful to have all the skill sets to make that vital 'match saving/ winning' tackle, but not have the basic conditioning/fitness to be in a position to make it!

The rehabilitation programme has to contain the right amount of volume and overload to achieve an excellent outcome. Overload that is either too great [damaging] or insufficient [under-adaptive] will be ineffective. Exercise prescription and programme length cannot have a 'cookbook' approach. Athletes will react differently to the same training stimulus.

Programmes should be tailored to the individual and criteria- (not timeline-)driven.

Simple key performance indicators/ key markers along with short-term/long-term objectives with exit criteria written into the programme are essential. These 'performance criteria' are also a great motivational tool for the athlete, as progression can be seen as well as felt.

An example of simply structured, criteria-driven, rehabilitation outline is shown in Table 18.1.

*Table 18.1*  End Stage Rehabilitation Phases: Criteria Driven

| Phase 3 Late/Position Specific | Phase 4 End Stage/Sports Specific | Phase 5 Maintenance |
|---|---|---|
| **Objective:** 1. Functional strength | **Objective:** 1. Return to play | **Objective:** 1. Identify criteria for a screening programme 2. Plan a screening programme 3. Include rehab/prehabilitation into core training programme. 4. Review periodically |
| **Criteria:** • Full range of controlled active movement • No pain • No strain • No substitution | **Criteria:** • Full strength and conditioning programme • Position-specific fitness assessment, including under fatigue conditions • Coach involvement • 10–15% contralateral limb strength | **Criteria** • System homeostasis • Optimal performance |
| **Functional strength** • Hop protocols – single, 3, speed & X over protocols • Isokinetic testing • Closed kinetic chain upper-limb stability test • Single-arm wall push | **Sports-specific** • Positional - coach • Team-specific - coach • Pre-fatigue – physio/S&C • Functional tests based on club screen | **Monitor/Screen** • Weekly • Daily |

The principles apply for any injury. Consider, for example, the process in terms of a simple grade 1 medial collateral ligament (MCL) injury of the knee. The athlete has to progress through the restoration of 'simple' functional control, such as a single-leg squat, before progressing to more 'dynamic' activity, such as hopping. Then comes the 'functional integration' into the more *positional specific* demands, such as twisting and turning, before safely progressing to the more *sport-specific* demands, including force production and force absorption in contact, for example.

The progression through these stages is not a timeline, but criteria-driven – the athlete has to be able to 'perform'.

## End-stage rehabilitation – stressing the athlete fully

The end of a rehabilitation process should involve the athlete being subjected to stresses similar to those experienced in the sport itself. These stresses should be graded and incrementally raised until the athlete and all support staff are satisfied that returning to full sports competition is sensible. In elite sport, both neuromuscular and metabolic fatigue are factors that undeniably affect both performance and injury risk. Knowing this simple fact means that end-stage rehabilitation of an athlete must involve training practices where the player experiences these types of fatigue and successfully adapts to them, restoring fatigue-resistance to pre-injury levels.

## End-stage rehabilitation – high-intensity S&C

Many sports require explosive strength qualities for success, and most injuries will detrimentally affect these qualities if only for a short time period. A thorough rehabilitation programme will incorporate high-intensity S&C work throughout and especially towards the end of the process so that explosive qualities are fully restored and the athlete is ready to train and compete with confidence. There are many devices available, such as GymAware, TendoUnit, MuscleLab and the Ballistic Measurement System that all enable easy quantification of explosive movements conducted within the gym environment. Left/right side comparisons are easy to perform, as are assessments when an athlete performs with a range of loads. These types of assessments provide the opportunity for support staff to explore an athlete's neuromuscular qualities, as well as the symmetry in these qualities, and provide an informed opinion regarding the readiness of the athlete to handle the biomechanical stresses imposed by their sport.

## Quantifying the rehabilitation process: Objective markers and exit criteria to best ensure success

Quantifying an athlete's sporting movements provide extremely valuable information for the rehabilitation process. It enables the biomechanical and physiological stresses placed on the athlete to be better understood and, from this knowledge, athlete-specific training practices to be designed. In many sports, GPS combined with heart rate (HR) tracking systems have enabled support staff to better understand the loadings associated with training sessions, as well as the loadings experienced by players in games.[1] These data are invaluable for creating realistic rehabilitation drills that need to be satisfactorily completed by players in determining fitness to return-to-train or -play criteria.

Table 18.2 (a) shows a selection of variables that were collected from an international rugby match for a player, and Table 18.2 (b) shows the same corresponding variables that were collected during an end-stage rehabilitation fitness assessment. Collection of this data is incredibly useful to place constraints and emphases within the session, whether these be limitations on maximum running speed or match-relevant work:rest ratios, for example.

Table 18.2 Representative GPS and HR data from (a) a rugby match and (b) an end-stage rehabilitation assessment

| Splits | Total Mins | Total km | Km >40% of Max Speed | Km >70% of Max Speed | Metres per Min | Aerobic Training Effect (max=5) | Ave. km/h | Peak km/h | % Max Speed |
|---|---|---|---|---|---|---|---|---|---|
| **Full Match** | 84 | 6.1 | 2.05 | 0.50 | 73 | 4.0 | 4.3 | 26.1 | 89 |

| Splits | Total Mins | Total km | Km >40% of Max Speed | Km >70% of Max Speed | Metres per Min | Aerobic Training Effect (max=5) | Ave. km/h | Peak km/h | % Max Speed |
|---|---|---|---|---|---|---|---|---|---|
| **Rehab** | 40 | 3.1 | 1.52 | 0.83** | 73 | 2.9 | 4.4 | 23.9 | 89 |

**Key**

Total mins – Total minutes played

Total km – Total distance travelled

Km > 40% of max speed – Distance travelled when moving at >40% of individual's previously recorded maximum speed.

Km > 70% of max speed – Distance travelled when moving at >70% of individual's previously recorded maximum speed.

Metres per min – Total distance travelled (m) divided by total minutes played.

Aerobic training effect – Composite figure produced by HR system that corresponds to individual's previously recorded greatest degree of aerobic stress

Ave km/h – average movement speed (km/h)

Peak km/h – peak movement speed (km/h)

% max speed – peak movement speed expressed as a percentage of individual's previously recorded maximum speed.

Simple observation of the data in Table 18.2(b) shows us many things about the rehabilitation session conducted by the athlete. We know that they have run at 89 per cent of maximum pace, which appears similar to their function within a game. They only worked for 40min in the rehabilitation session (half duration of a competitive match) but moved at a work rate equal to that required within a match (73m/min). Notably, the distance covered at a speed above 70 per cent of their maximum pace was 0.83km, 0.33km greater than is normally covered in a game. Fatigue-resistance at relatively high speed was a key factor in this rehabilitation session.

The use of objective data such as GPS/HR enables the support team to be very confident in their return-to-compete judgements regarding athletes.

## Functional performance tests/assessments

Examining the physical qualities of an athlete in a controlled setting, but with stresses and movements performed close to the physical maximum that the athlete can exert, we term functional performance tests/assessments. Let's take the example of a lacrosse player who has injured the medial collateral ligament of their left knee with a prognosis of four to six weeks out of competition. At various stages of the rehabilitation process, functional performance tests might include:

- Dumbbell step-up strength and stability. With this exercise we might be looking for symmetry in strength and control between the right and left sides, as well as a return to the previous strength level of the athlete.
- Single-leg vertical-jump performance. This exercise enables us to look at the symmetry in explosive qualities between the right and left sides. We might choose to look at simply jump height or, if the tests are conducted on a force platform, the similarity in the way that the forces are generated. A similar jump height but lower rate of force development on the injured side provides further direction for the final part of the retraining process.
- Ability to control the landing of a lateral step or hop (performed on a force plate). Again, the force profile provides us with a means of understanding the level of control on

landing between the injured and non-injured sides. If we can see similar rates of force development between the injured and non-injured sides, we can be confident that the athlete has the neuromuscular qualities to absorb and control high-speed landings and so progress to the next stage of the retraining process.

- 3-hop test for distance. When done with maximum exertion, this test asks a lot of the control and explosive qualities of the neuromuscular system. Generally, we would expect the total distance jumped to be less than 10 per cent different between the left and right sides for a healthy athlete. Returning an athlete to these levels of tolerance gives great confidence to staff and the athlete that they are ready to begin much harder training.

These tests are not meant to be exhaustive by any means. They are examples of the types of tests that can provide markers as to the current control and performance level of the athlete. These data can then provide the input to guide the next, more aggressive and stressful aspect of the rehabilitation programme.

## Sport- and position-specific field testing

When an athlete has passed all functional performance tests and is declared 'medically fit', their complete return to sports training should be governed by their performance in a specific field test. This would likely entail movements and movement rates (relative to time) similar to those experienced in a game, be they tackling in football, kicking in taekwondo, landing from a height in mogul skiing or being thrown in judo.

Where appropriate, match-based GPS, accelerometry and HR data would be used to quantify the physiological load of the field test and provide stresses that mirror a section of a game.[2]

Table 18.3 depicts an example of a fitness assessment that compromises high-intensity intervals to pre-fatigue the athlete before entering a rugby-specific circuit designed around a forward's skill set. Ideally a technical coach, physiotherapist and S&C coach would work together during this assessment and have an honest and open discussion with the athlete at the end to determine how well it went.

### Protocol –

- Start on line. On whistle, sprint 10m, touch line, turn and sprint 10m back to start, turn again and sprint 60m
- *Repeat x 6 sprints with 45s rest between runs (drills start at alternate ends)*
- 80s rest
- Rugby-specific circuit below

*Table 18.3* Return to Training/Competition Assessment

| Targets | Total Mins | Total km | Km >40% of Max Speed | Km >70% of Max Speed | Metres per Min | Aerobic Training Effect (max=5) | % Max Speed |
|---------|-----------|----------|----------------------|----------------------|----------------|--------------------------------|-------------|
|         | 40        | 3k       | 1.00                 | 0.2                  | 70             | 5                              | 85+         |

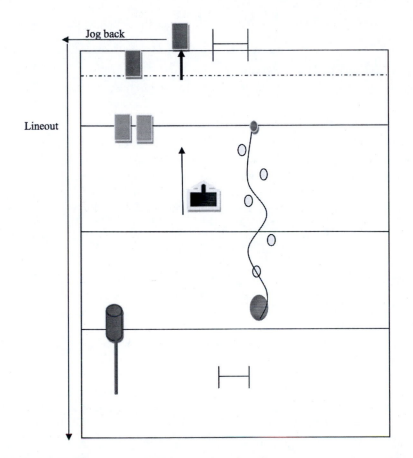

Jog back

Lineout

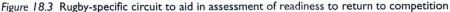

*Figure 18.3* Rugby-specific circuit to aid in assessment of readiness to return to competition

## Training versus 'fitness test'

In many sports, much of the physical load experienced by the athlete occurs in training. Consider, for example, hockey players who typically train for four of the six days between matches. The ability of players to adapt and respond positively to this loading is also a key aspect of a successful rehabilitation process.

As a rule of thumb, many organisations in professional sport will only declare a player fit for selection when they have trained fully for the preceding week. While there are sometimes exceptions, completing a week's training provides a lot of confidence to both athlete and support staff, as the day-to-day loading and subsequent physiological response to training are assessed, rather than the athlete's acute response to an albeit fatiguing and stressful fitness test.

## The role of coach in return to play

While support staff will be able to accurately assess an athlete's physical responses to training and playing, a technical coach is the best judge of the 'effectiveness' of the player's movements from the perspective of performance and technical advice. A coach's experience and technical insight is also very useful in designing appropriate field test criteria that stress the athlete in ways very similar to the game. Involving the coach in the fitness assessment gives the:

• coach confidence in the player's ability to perform
• player confidence and motivation as the coach watches the performance

> The player and coach should collaborate to devise some of the tasks involved in the assessment, identifying and choosing elements that are specific to that player's positional needs or the need of the team. The more the player is involved, the more likely their application and adherence to the programme, as well as their focus on areas or movements with which the player needs to have full confidence for a successful return to playing.

The coach's objective when following the assessment is to be assured that the player has not only the required conditioning and robustness to return to play, but also the skill level that will hold up to the demands of the game. Often a player can be seen through the physical demands of a fitness assessment but the coach has noted a reduction in concentration or skill level, such as passing or position into contact as the player fatigues. The coach then has the necessary information to decide if that player is performing at the level required to be selected.

Injuries notably cause altered movement patterns that need to be retrained to avoid re-injury and also technical proficiency. The coach's role in regaining technical proficiency should not be overlooked, especially as a successful rehabilitation will be measured by a return to performance/competition, not simply that an injury has healed.

## Monitoring the returning athlete

Knowing that the biggest risk factor of injury to an athlete is their previous injury history means that monitoring their exposure to new training and playing loads is very sensible (see Table 18.1 column 5). Indeed, in most high-level sporting organisations, support staff will spend significant time with technical coaches to discuss future training sessions and the grading (if any) needed for training exposure to returning players. GPS and HR data is very useful in determining an athlete's training and playing performance in comparison to peers and historic data. Of equal note are the post-training and playing assessments conducted by the medical staff to evaluate the athlete's response to the training and playing load.

## Summary

A successful rehabilitation programme is one that returns an athlete to pre-injury levels of competition, without fear or increased probability of re-injury and where their sporting performance is no longer compromised. Getting to this point requires the combined and well-planned input of the medical, S&C and coaching teams to ensure that the healing, fitness and sporting requirements of the athlete are all catered to within the reconditioning programme.

The programme should be progressive in terms of loading and movement complexity and should be driven by 'what' the athlete is able to do rather than 'when'. If available, data from competition (for example GPS, accelerometry or heart rate) should be used to design the sports-specific aspects of the programme so that the physical demands placed on the athlete are accurate and reflective of the sport. The final decision to return an athlete to competition should be given when the medical, S&C and coaching teams, as well as the athlete, have the evidence each needs to confirm that the athlete is robust enough, fit enough and performing well enough to compete as often as the sport requires.

## Notes

1 Cahill, N., Lamb, K., Worsfold, P., Headey, R., & Murray, S. (2013). The movement characteristics of English Premiership rugby union players. *Journal of Sport Sciences*, *31*(3), 229–37.
2 Reid, L. C., Cowman, J. R., Green, B. S., & Coughlan, G. F. (2013). Return to play in elite rugby union: application of global positioning system technology in return-to-running programs. *Journal of Sports Rehabilitation*, *22*(2), 122–9.

# Part 4

# Managing the injured athlete

# Chapter 19

# The athletic neck

*Kay Robinson*

## Introduction

The cervical spine is exposed to an immense amount of stress in many sports. Most obvious and dramatic are the high translational, compression and shear forces that are imparted by events such as the collisions in rugby and ice hockey. It is not just the single high-force incident that has the capacity to injure the cervical spine, however – the *accumulation* of lower forces over a period of time can be equally threatening. Common examples of this seen in sport are the high gravitational ('G') forces and vibrations that athletes in motor racing and the ice sliding sports (such as skeleton and bobsled) are exposed to. Whatever the mechanism, these forces can lead to overload and injury in the neck that is not robust enough to tolerate them.

To a large extent, this robustness is contingent upon the capacity of the structure and function of the vertebral architecture, intervertebral discs and complex musculature of the cervical spine to attenuate the forces they are exposed to. Athletes who are unsuccessful in this energy attenuation are exposed to a greater risk of injury or dysfunction. The resulting injuries range from serious vertebral fractures causing spinal instability (and, in severe cases, paralysis), to concussion, through to soft-tissue injuries, where a decrease in range of motion can be barely noticeable.

As professionals in the performance rehabilitation sphere, the greater the understanding we have of neck structure and function, the better placed we are to recognise and intervene in abnormal function. We can then transfer this knowledge into the domain of training and rehabilitation of the neck. This is the purpose of this chapter.

## Prevalence of neck injuries in sport

Sport accounts for almost 10 per cent of all cervical spine injuries (CSI) in the United States,[1] and in the general population, nearly half of us will suffer neck pain at some point in our lives.[2] Sports with some of the highest prevalence of neck injury are:

- American football
- Rugby
- Diving
- Equestrian
- Ski/Snowboarding
- Motor Racing.[3]

Whilst many minor cervical spine injuries will go unreported, nearly a third of high school and freshman American Football players have been reported to show radiological evidence of a previous neck injury, a prevalence that is thought to be rising.[3] Whilst this apparent increase will undoubtedly be attributed in part to better reporting and monitoring of injuries, increases in the physicality of sport, coupled with the fact that neck strength work is often neglected in favour of developing strength everywhere from the 'shoulders down', leaves the cervical spine exposed to ever-increasing loads and therefore vulnerable to injury.

## Causes of neck pain in athletes

Injuries occur when a body part is exposed to an energy or force that exceeds its capacity to absorb or tolerate it. In the neck, as we have discussed, this can be as a result of either an acute incident or chronic loading. Consequently, in order to understand the causes of neck pain, and therefore understand the best ways to both prevent and rehabilitate sporting neck injuries, we need to understand the loading variables that contribute to this equation. These include:

- Magnitude of the forces
- Direction and point of application of these forces
- Velocity of the force application
- Duration of exposure to the forces.

### Injuries as a result of high-force exposure – compression

The principle cause of CSI in sport is axial (compressive) loading.[3] Most commonly, the injury occurs when the axial loading is applied to the cervical spine that is flexed in excess of 30 degrees, a position where there is a loss of the neck's natural lordosis, thus reducing its energy attenuation capability.[3] Compressive forces can also be applied to the posterior elements of the cervical spine when the neck is extended and laterally flexed, with axial compression applied as overpressure. When the natural curves of the neck are eliminated and the normal force attenuation capacities are diminished, loads have to be borne by other structures, increasing the vulnerability to injury of surrounding structures, including the intervertebral discs, vertebral bodies and facet joints.

Situations in which this may occur are in American Football when the ball carrier crashes head first into the defence, or a fall from a height as we might see in a missed landing in gymnastics, or when a rider falls off a horse. This mechanism can be acute or cumulative in its effect, meaning the athlete may be able to recall a singular event, or they might have had multiple exposures to this compression over time.

### Injuries as a result of high-force exposure – acceleration/deceleration

The other common cause of neck injury in sport occurs following sudden acceleration/deceleration movements and is often classified as 'whiplash associated disorders' (WAD).[4] This can be as a result of a direct blow to the head, but also a blow to the trunk. In both cases, the force is transferred to the neck that 'whips' forward and back, which can damage both anterior and posterior vertebral structures.[5] These types of injuries are seen most commonly in high-speed sports such as motor racing and collision sports including martial arts.

### Injuries as a result of high-force exposure – traction/compression

Brachial plexopathies, more commonly known as 'stingers' or 'burners', can either be compressive or distractive in nature and are commonly found in contact sports or following a fall at high velocity onto the shoulder, such as when a mountain biker vaults over the handlebars. Traction stingers occur when a downward force is applied to the shoulder girdle whilst the neck is laterally flexed to the contralateral side. A sudden compressive force that closes down the posterior elements of the ipsilateral side can result in a compressive stinger. Either mechanism can injure or irritate the brachial plexus or nerve roots, most commonly at the seventh cervical level. Symptoms are commonly described as a burning or dead feeling down the arm and a temporary inability to access full muscle power. These effects are often temporary but attention needs to be paid to ensure there are no long-term neurological deficits or altered movement patterns.

### Injuries as a result of chronic force exposure – static postures

It is not just the singular 'big hit' that can lead to pain, injury and dysfunction in the cervical spine. Repeated exposure to lower forces or static postures can accumulate to exceed the tolerance of the cervical spine. Postures adopted in target sports such as archery or shooting that require the athlete to maintain an end-range cervical posture over a long period of time are particularly prone to pain and dysfunction.

### Injuries as a result of chronic force exposure – G forces

Chronic exposure to vibrational or high gravitational forces (Gz) can also lead to neck misery. Sports in which athletes are exposed to high Gz include motor and aircraft racing, high-speed sliding sports and contact sports. Some of the recorded side effects of G-force exposure include dizziness, disorientation, visual disturbances, reduced coordination, delayed reactions, and neck pain.[6] In short, exactly the sort of symptoms that you *do not* want to be experiencing if you are looking to control a high-speed vehicle! These are usually as a result of reduced blood flow to the head, vestibular disturbances and/or the high loads placed on the muscles of the neck.[6]

Along with these acute symptoms, ongoing exposure to high Gz are suggested to leave athletes more at risk of vertebral disc degeneration;[7] therefore, all exposure and loading should be monitored closely, and athletes should be provided with the best possible tools and knowledge as discussed in this chapter to minimise long-term damage.

---

The impact of G forces should also be considered in contact sports where collisions between players may expose the athlete to upwards of 8 Gs.[8] This is the equivalent of a car accident at about 30kph. If this does not sound too impressive, remember that a rugby league player may be involved in upwards of 50 tackles in a match!

---

## Characteristics of a healthy neck

Now that we have discussed the main neck injuries we see in sport, we should take a step back to understand what a healthy neck should look like. We will look at this from the perspective of motion and strength and as a link in a kinetic chain.

## Neck assessment

Movement in the cervical spine is complex, as all intervertebral levels contribute in varying degrees to overall neck motion. For example a vertebral segment may experience its maximal range in flexion or extension prior to the cervical column being in its fully flexed or extended position.[9] Moreover, the change in orientation of the cervical bodies of the mid- to lower cervical spine allows for rotation and flexion but prevents independent lateral flexion, isolating this movement to the upper cervical spine.

Average range of movement of the cervical spine in 20–29-year-olds is 54° flexion, 80° extension, 30–58° lateral flexion and 52–85° rotation to either side.[10] This tends to decrease as we age, and so it is important to take this into account when aiming to determine what is 'normal' in a particular individual.

Radiological examination is thought to be the gold standard for measuring neck ROM; however, this is not possible in most settings due to expense and lack of facilities. Whilst it is common to visually estimate the amount of neck motion an individual has, valid and reliable tools such as the full-circle goniometer (FCG) and cervical range of movement (CROM) instruments are relatively inexpensive and should therefore be employed wherever possible. At the very least, a tape measure should be used and anchor points, which can be seen in Table 19.1.

The primary active stabilisers of the neck, supporting it against gravity in all planes of movement, are collectively known as the deep neck flexors (DNF). These muscles include the *longus capitus, longus colli, rectus capitis anterior* and *rectus capitis laterali*.[2] In practice, it is very difficult to isolate the DNFs from the more superficial neck muscles, but EMG studies suggest that the DNFs are contracted in static neck flexion, as well as working concurrently with the *sternocleidomastoid* and *anterior scalene* through the full range of motion. The DNFs are most active during the commonly prescribed 'chin tuck' (craniocervical flexion), followed by cervical flexion and cervical rotation.[11] This activity is significantly decreased and delayed in subjects with neck pain,[12] reinforcing the need for monitoring neck strength post injury to ensure the neck stability is regained and further injury is prevented.

DNF function can be tested in supine using an inflatable cuff pressure/biofeedback device. With the neck in neutral alignment and the cuff inflated to 20mmHg to fill the cervical lordosis, the athlete is instructed to perform a chin tuck, increasing the pressure within the cuff by 2mmHg increments whilst minimizing the contribution of the more superficial muscles, such as the sternocleidomastoids.[13]

Since the main purpose of the neck is to optimize head position (and in, particular, the sensory structures), we need to consider the mass of the head in all our programming calculations. The head weighs between 3–6kg, and this mass is borne primarily through the upper cervical spine. This highlights the importance of correct posture to ensure equal displacement of the weight and minimise overload to the stabilising muscles.

Table 19.1 Anchor points used to assess cervical range of motion using a tape measure

|  | Flexion | Extension | Lateral Flexion | Rotation |
| --- | --- | --- | --- | --- |
| Anchor point 1 | Tip of chin | Tip of chin | Tragus of ear | Tip of chin |
| Anchor point 2 | Manubrium | Manubrium | Acromion process | Acromion process |

Table 19.2 Prime-mover contribution to cervical motion[14]

| Muscle | Role in Cervical Movement | | |
|---|---|---|---|
| | Agonistic | Antagonistic | Synergistic |
| Sternocleidomastoid | Flexion | Extension | Side Flexion |
| Scalenus medius | Side flexion and extension | Flexion | – |
| Trapezius (mid fibers) | Side flexion and extension | Flexion | – |
| Splenius capitus | Extension | Flexion | Side flexion |
| Semispinalis capitis | Extension | Flexion | Side flexion |

In addition, the other key muscles that we need to consider in any programming are the prime movers of the neck, namely the *sternocleidomastoids, scalenes, trapezius, splenius capitus* and *semispinalis capitis*.[14] The functions of these muscles can be seen in Table 19.2.

Mean flexion and extension forces vary among studies, but consensus in the general population is that flexion force is less than extension force (59 per cent), with extension force having a bias towards an individual's dominant side.[14] Whilst extension is a sagittal plane movement, in the majority of people, there is an element of side flexion coupling that occurs. Therefore, when training, we need to ensure this force difference is evident and focus on specific muscles groups to retrain if it is not. A slight bias to the dominant side is recognised in muscles attributing to lateral flexion and is expected to be more prominent in athletes competing in sports with a performance advantage favouring a particular side, such as tennis and shooting. We should therefore not always see a slight asymmetry as undesirable in these situations.

Although cervical muscle strength testing is not yet commonplace in sport, it is growing in the rugby community, as reflected in a number of recent studies.[15,16,18] It is also widely used in motor sports and in the aviation field, where pilots are exposed to high gravitational and vibrational forces through their necks.

Neck strength and cervical load tolerance capacity can be assessed in a number of ways, including the use of isokinetic and isometric dynamometers. Many of these methods are combined with measuring muscle activity to provide a complete picture of cervical muscle function. All of these methods provide objective data which can be used in monitoring and have a far greater validity than manual muscle testing. Clinicians with access to appropriate facilities should consider use of EMG testing to assess specific muscle activation strength and speed, particularly with athletes returning from neck injury.

To ensure that data is normalised testing data, the following key points should be addressed and replicated across every strength-testing event:

- Torso stabilized to isolate cervical mobilisers
- Feet on wobble cushions on ground to minimise lower extremity involvement

- Measurements made through range (isokinetically or at set ranges isometrically)
- Standardised protocol that includes warm-up through range and non-maximal contractions and familiarisation with apparatus.

### The neck as a part of a kinetic chain

The neck does not function in isolation, and there are strong connections between neck pain and shoulder dysfunction. For example, elite swimmers with a history of shoulder pain demonstrate greater scalene muscle activity during functional and sport-specific tasks, as well as hypertonicity of cervical muscles.[19] Such muscular imbalances alter cervical kinematics, often leading to pain, dysfunction and a heightened risk of further neck injury.

The relationship between the neck and the shoulder girdle is important to consider when planning all conditioning and rehabilitation of athletes to ensure optimal movement patterns and that transmission of forces through the body are maintained. Moreover, we need to consider the maintenance of cervical range of movement throughout any shoulder rehabilitation process.

Along similar lines, since the role of the neck is to position the head, we should also include sporting head injuries in any discussion of the cervical spine. In particular, concussion must be considered. We should have a low index of suspicion for concussion when dealing with an acute neck injury (and vice versa) due to the high forces and impact that is translated between the two areas. Concussion is discussed in more detail in chapter 6.

## Managing neck injuries

Once we understand the mechanisms and force parameters of the loading, as well as the structure and function of the cervical spine, we are better placed to design strategies to ensure that the neck and its surrounding structures are resilient enough to withstand the stress that they will be exposed to.

Since there are a multitude of different injuries that the neck can sustain and it is beyond the scope of this chapter to discuss rehabilitation of each of them, what is presented here is a template that can be adopted for just about every dysfunction. Obviously, the rates of progression between the phases will vary depending on the complexity and chronicity of the injury, but the philosophy of exit criteria–led management as discussed throughout this book should still hold.

### Phase 1 – acute phase

In every case, the athlete should be fully informed about their injury and the plan for their recuperation. This may necessitate imaging studies, nerve conduction studies and external specialist referrals. Once all the information is gathered and the stakeholders agree upon the rehabilitation plan, there is great clarity, something that will provide the athlete with confidence.

The main focus of the first phase of rehabilitation is the reduction of pain and the restoration of range of motion. This should be conducted with the full medical team to ensure the athlete has appropriate analgesia. It is important to note that the longer the dysfunction has been present, the more protracted this pain-reduction process may be. This is discussed in greater detail in chapter 18.

---

Should at any point a serious head or neck injury be suspected, full immobilization, neurological and musculoskeletal assessment should be undertaken by trained personnel and, if necessary, in a hospital setting.

---

If we assume that we have been able to exclude the threat of a serious neck or head injury, our primary focus is to reduce pain and associated muscle spasm.

High-quality evidence to support a specific approach to the management of acute cervical pain is scant,[20] but in practice, a combination of modalities, including massage, electrical stimulation, thermotherapy and analgesics alongside range of movement exercises are often effective.

---

Should the athlete demonstrate marked kinesiophobia (fear of movement), a good strategy to employ in the very early stage is to ask them to keep their neck and head stationary, but to instead rotate their trunk.

---

We should look to commence acute neck pain management in neutral cervical alignment to limit any nerve root, disc or facet joint irritation. This provides us with the ideal opportunity to assess and recruit the DNFs, and cervical-cranial flexion training as discussed previously should commence.

Whilst we want to regain neck ROM, we must remember that the muscles often spasm in the acutely painful neck to provide the body with the stiffness that it feels is necessary for optimal healing. We do know, however, that gentle motion has great analgesic qualities,[21] and so neck mobility work within pain limits should commence as soon as possible. This may initially need to be completed in a gravity-eliminated environment (such as in supine) but should progress to upright as soon as possible.

Aggressive stretching of the muscles in spasm should be avoided in the acute stage, as this can artificially and prematurely reduce the neck's intrinsic stability system, something that can actually lead to even more muscle spasm and stiffness.[22]

As the symptoms subside, it is vital that we regain the motion of all the planes that the neck requires to work in during the sport. This is where understanding the demands of the activity is paramount.

> **To allow progression to phase 2 of rehabilitation, the following exit criteria should be passed:**
>
> 1   Serious injury excluded (fractures, spinal cord or nerve root injury, concussion)
> 2   Pain-free functional active neck ROM
> 3   Absence of any neurological signs and symptoms
> 4   Recruitment of DNFs.

### Phase 2 – early rehabilitation

Once we have established pain-free motion, we can begin the process of neck strengthening. This concept of early strengthening is universally accepted with peripheral joint or muscle injuries (such as shoulder or hamstrings) but seems to be frequently overlooked in the cervical spine. In the early rehabilitation phase we start with isometric contractions in all directions and in a variety of non-provocative positions. Often, a period of time is required to allow for the athlete to learn the technique required, as well as for the neck muscles to adapt to the load.

These contractions can easily be commenced with manual pressure, but use of a handheld dynamometer is very helpful for determining the percentage of maximum voluntary contraction (MVC) that you want your athlete to be working at. Initially, we aim at 30 per cent x MVC and then progress over a number of sessions towards 100 per cent.

It is often helpful to use a pulley/cable system in this phase. The athlete can be seated or standing and a harness attached at one end to the head around the occiput, and at the other to a weight stack. The mass on the pulley system can be easily set to avoid overloading the capacity of the neck and is therefore an effective option to be considered in early stages of strengthening/rehabilitation.

> A good way to assess the competency of the neck as it is challenged by the pulley system mass is to assess the individual's ability to maintain appropriate cervical alignment during the contraction. This also forms the basis for applying duress to the competency of the DNFs.

Initially, isometric training should be carried out at a medium volume and low intensity, until it is ascertained that symptoms are not reproduced. The following isometric exercises should be included:

Cervical flexion – the athlete faces away from the cable machine and performs a chin tuck movement. They then move forward (away from the machine) whilst maintaining the tucked chin posture. Note, many athletes at this stage attempt to perform this motion by extending their neck (poking their chin).

Cervical extension – the athlete faces the pulley system with neck in neutral. They then move away from the machine, resisting the pulley system that will be pulling them into flexion.

Cervical side flexion – face-side onto machine, step or sit away from machine and take weight laterally, repeat to other side. This can also be done in side-lying, resisting manually applied pressure.

These exercises provide an excellent platform, but we also need to consider the functional demands placed upon the athlete in their sport. Specifically, we need to consider orientation of the head when targeting neck strength, taking into account the effects of gravity as well as any other external forces. For example, in skeleton where the athlete lies prone on the sled, we need to move as soon as practical to strengthening in this position. In motor racing, by contrast, we need to be looking to strengthen in-the-cockpit position. Having said that, however, we must also challenge the athlete in other, non-habitual postures, because it is in the positions that the athletes are in less often where many injuries occur, either due to weakness or poor proprioceptive awareness.

Also in this second phase of rehabilitation, submaximal upper limb, scapular and spinal 'core' stability training can be commenced and progressed. This is critical, as the neck is simply part of the entire kinetic chain, and is a clear demonstration of the concept of looking at what the athlete *can* do, as opposed to what they cannot.

---

**To allow progression to phase 3 of rehabilitation, the following exit criteria should be passed:**

1  Pain-free isometric loading
2  Good shoulder girdle stability
3  Good exercise technique
4  No increase in symptoms
5  Increase in post-injury cervical strength.

---

### Phase 3 – mid-stage rehabilitation

Once we are able to progress isometric contraction loading and we have restored asymptomatic ROM, it is then crucial to begin to challenge the neck both concentrically and eccentrically through range. There is a risk of overload using pulley systems at this stage, so manual or dynamometer resistance should be used for higher-volume, medium-intensity work. It is best to commence this in the sagittal plane; then incorporate movement into the coronal plane. Higher-intensity strengthening, including alternating movements between planes, can be completed once the athlete is able to demonstrate control.

Progressive exposure to compressive loadings is important here to increase cervical tolerance. This can commence with manually applied axial compression and then progress to supported headstands, initially in a harness on a soft mat and then eventually to soft flooring. Graduated exposure to tumble turning is also helpful here and serves well to provide the athlete confidence in their neck being subjected to more complex forces.

In keeping with well-established principles of overload, we should not look to suddenly spike training volumes or intensities. Rather a fluctuating programme that seeks to gradually increase demands over a number of weeks is recommended. This is particularly due to the fact that there are many small joints that need stability, as opposed to a single big joint.

> The background of the athlete makes a big difference here. A wrestler that is accustomed to heavy loads applied to his cervical musculature is likely to tolerate loading better than a slender female swimmer. These sessions should be monitored to highlight any postural changes or asymmetries in the shoulder girdle or trunk.

Timescale in this stage of rehabilitation will vary according to initial injury. Range and strength monitoring should continue, and once baseline range, strength and flexion/extension ratios have been achieved, initial integration into sport-specific training can begin.

In collision sports, this may include the use of controlled contact (using tackle bags), and in artistic sports, such as gymnastics and figure skating, we may commence low-difficulty vaulting/pirouetting tasks, so long as the athlete is confident, competent and symptom-free.

It is in this phase where we can introduce low-level vibration and G forces, if this is a demand that the athlete will face in their sport. Regular training involving graduated exposure to Gz and the practice of neck positioning techniques adopted in the sporting environment is helpful in the prevention, as well as the rehabilitation, of neck pain.[23]

> It is critical to understand the impact that exposure to Gz has on the athlete (not just their neck). It has been found to increase heart rate, oxygen consumption and peripheral vascular resistance.[24] Therefore a combination of high-resistance whole-body strength training to withstand the Gz and moderate aerobic training to aid recovery between exposure should be delivered to all athletes with exposure to high Gz.

A challenge in setting strengthening programs for athletes whose sport involves exposure to high G forces and vibrations is replicating this in the training environment. Repetition of the exact activity is likely to have negative health risks due to the peak strain of the G force to which the athlete is exposed commonly being greater than contraction. Overexposure also results in fatigue that can have an adverse impact by reducing power. We therefore need to find alternatives, and trampolining is one such option.

Trampolining has been found to produce a vertical G force of +4Gz[25] and shown to be as beneficial as increasing cervical strength and decreasing recovery times in pilots experiencing high levels of Gz. Trampolining also aides enhancement of balance, positional control and stabilization. The additional benefit of this form is its low intensity and the ability to include high repetition to simulate the onset of fatigue without heavy loading.

Alternative methods of replicating exposure to vibrations include performing exercises on 'power plates', or by the professional providing manual perturbations to a large inflatable exercise ball placed behind the athlete's head whilst they perform sports-relevant drills. An example of this may be the athlete performing wall squats with the ball behind their head. The athlete is challenged to maintain correct cervical posture throughout the movement, despite the coach hitting the ball from different angles and with varying intensity.

As confidence and competence increases, the athlete can progress to the forces seen in their sport. In rugby this may involve tackling, being tackled and scrimmaging. In judo, this may involve progressive grappling, throws and landing. In diving, this will be seen by the increasing complexity of the dives and from increasing heights.

---

**To allow progression to phase 4 of rehabilitation, the following exit criteria should be passed:**

1   Pain-free through range loading
2   No increase in symptoms
3   Ability to participate in controlled exposure to normal training (including body contact, compressive force and vibration exposure, depending on the demands of the sport)
4   No change in shoulder/trunk kinematics
5   Cervical strength in line with baseline measures.

---

## Phase 4 – return to performance

The final phase of rehabilitation sees the emphasis firmly move towards the restoration of both competence and confidence of the athlete as they look to return to competition. All athletes should incorporate this phase of strengthening into their training, along with elements of phase 3 to maintain full strength through available range of motion. Return-to-performance (RTP) protocols will vary depending on the type of injury, sport and position the athlete is returning to. The entire interdisciplinary team should contribute to the process to ensure any strength and skill deficits have been addressed to ensure performance is maintained and the risk of further injury is reduced.

During this phase, further adjuncts to training can be put in place to simulate specific sports and forces. One such adjunct is in the training of resiliency against 'Snap G'. Snap G is the phenomenon of a sudden change in the acceleration of a body in space and can be experienced across a range a sports. It is critical to include an aspect of unanticipated load in neck training to train cervical muscle pre-activation to 'brace' for impacts and sudden direction changes. This is found to have a positive effect on maintaining head kinematics, having the potential to decrease neck and concussion injuries.[26]

Combining training approaches there increases the likelihood of adaptations to a number of neural elements involved in motor skill and muscular control, including increased neuromuscular performance, increased coordination and improved mechanical efficiency, which maintains stability.

---

**To allow progression to return to competition, we suggest the following exit criteria are passed:**

1   No increase in symptoms
2   Ability to load through range, including direction change
3   Full exposure to training environment
4   No change in shoulder/trunk kinematics.

---

## Neck injury prevention

Neck training has the potential to reduce injury risk,[2,16,23,25,26,27] and therefore, muscles must be exposed to overload as part of regular training as well as return from injury. Baseline assessment should be made of any athlete entering a programme where they may be exposed to neck injury risk factors. Where they sit on the competency platform as outlined in the four phases described above can be determined by examining their ROM, cervical strength and endurance and Snap G tolerance. They can then follow the progressions as described above until they reach an acceptable level of strength and robustness to be exposed to high-intensity sport-specific loading.

As with any form of athletic training and rehabilitation programming, it is crucial to monitor load and timing of neck strength work within micro- and macrocycles. Neuromuscular fatigue needs to be accounted for, and any new drilling should be positioned when the athlete is fresh and tissue tolerance is high. Once we are confident in the performance of the drills, we may wish to add duress to the system by getting the athlete to perform them under progressively greater levels of tiredness.

---

Neck flexor and extensor strength training is fatiguing, and, indeed, strength can actually be *reduced* for up to a day post loading.[27] This tells us that we should not look to place our neck work within a day of competition.

---

## Summary

Neck assessment should be a regular process used in our sports to form baselines, aid with return to sport and as a monitoring tool. Range of movement, strength, pain scores and training loads should all be gathered to provide a thorough assessment and should be used by all members of the high-performance team.

By understanding the demands of specific sports and the loads being transferred through the cervical spines, practitioners are in the driving seat to minimise injuries by increasing strength, improving movement patterns and educating athletes. The use of baseline and comparative measures are also keys in aiding return to performance.

Training programs for necks vary but should incorporate the following goals, whether they are part of a progressive rehab program or ongoing strengthening block:

- Maintain/regain ROM
- Stabilise shoulder girdle
- Increase muscle strength
- Sport specificity.

As sport evolves and the popularity of extreme sports continues, there is increased research interest into neck and head injuries, and this should be applied to our training environments to reduce injury, maximise performance and produce robust athletes.

# Notes

1 Jeyamohan, S., Harrop, J., Vaccaro, A., & Sharan A. (2008). Athletes returning to play after cervical spine or neurobrachial injury. *Current Review Musculoskeletal Medicine, 1*(3–4), 175–179.
2 Harris, K., Heer, D., Roy, T., Santos, D., Whitman, M., & Wainner, R. (2005). Reliability of a measurement of neck flexor muscle endurance physical therapy. *Physical Therapy, 85*, 1349–1355.
3 Cooper, M., McGee, K., & Anderson, D. (2003). Epidemiology of athletic head and neck injuries. *Clinical Sports Medicine, 22*, 427–443.
4 Michalef, Z., & Ferreira, M. (2012). Physiotherapy rehabilitation for whiplash associated disorder II: A systematic review and meta-analysis of randomised controlled trials. *British Journal of Sports Medicine, 46*(9), 662–663.
5 Bogduk, N., & Yoganandan, N. (2001). Biomechanics of the cervical spine Part 3: Minor injuries. *Clinical Biomechanics, 16*(4), 267–275.
6 Rickards, C. A., & Newman, D. G. (2005). G-induced visual and cognitive disturbances in a survey of 65 operational fighter pilots. *Aviation, Space, and Environmental Medicine, 76*, 496–500.
7 Lange, B., Nielsen, R., Skejo, P., & Toft, P. (2013). Centrifuge-induced neck and back pain in F-16 pilots: A report of four cases. *Aviation, Space, and Environmental Medicine, 84*, 734–738.
8 Wundersitz, D., Gastin, P., Robertson, S., & Netto, K. (2014). Validity of a truck mounted accelerometer to measure physical collisions in contact sports. *International Journal of Sports Physiology and Performance*, In press.
9 Swartz, E., Floyd, R., & Cendoma, M. (2005). Cervical spine functional anatomy and the biomechanics of injury due to compressive loading. *Journal of Athletic Training, 40*(3), 155–161.
10 Youdas, J., Garrett, T., Suman, V., Bogard, C., Hallman, H., & Carer, J. (1992). Normal range of motion of the cervical spine: An initial goniometric study. *Physical Therapy, 72*, 770–780.
11 Falla, D., Jull, G., O'Leary, S., & Dall'Alba, P. (2006). Further evaluation of an EMG technique for assessment of the deep cervical flexor muscles. *Journal of Electromyography and Kinesiology, 16*, 621–628.
12 Fall, D., Jull, G., & Hodges, P. (2004). Neck pain patients demonstrate reduced activation of the deep neck flexor muscles during performance of the cranio-cervical flexion test. *Spine, 29*(19), 2108–14.
13 Jull, G., O'Leary, S., & Falla, D. (2008). Clinical assessment of the deep cervical flexor muscles: The craniocervical flexion test. *Journal of Manipulative and Physiological Therapeutics, 31*(7), 525–533.
14 Gabriel, D., Matsumoto, J., Davis, D., Currier, B., & Kai-Nan, A. (2004). Multidirectional neck strength and electromyographic activity for normal controls. *Clinical Biomechanics, 19*, 653–658.
15 Hamilton, D., & Gatherer, D. (2014). Cervical isometric strength and range of motion of elite rugby union players: A cohort study. *BMC Sports Science, Medicine and Rehabilitation, 6*, 32.
16 Naish, R., Burnett, A., Burrows, S., Andrews, W., & Appleby, B. (2013). Can a specific neck strengthening program decrease cervical spine injuries in a men's professional rugby union team? A retrospective analysis. *Journal of Sports Science and Medicine, 12*, 542–550.
17 Geary, K., Green, B., & Delahunt, E. (2013). Intrarater reliability of neck strength measurement of rugby union players using a handheld dynamometer. *Journal of Manipulative and Physiological Therapeutics, 36*(7), 444–449.
18 Hamilton, D., Gatherer, D., Robson, J., et al. (2014). Comparative cervical profiles of adult and under-18 front-row rugby players: Implications for playing policy. *BMJ Open* 2014;4:e004975. doi:10.1136/bmjopen-2014-004975
19 Hidalgo-Lozano, A., Fernandez-de-las-Penas, C., Madeleine, P., & Arroyo-Morales, M. (2012). Elite swimmers with unilateral shoulder pain demonstrate altered pattern of cervical muscle activation during a functional upper-limb task. *Journal of Orthopaedic & Sports Physical Therapy, 42*(6), 552–558.
20 Philadelphia Panel. (2001). Evidence-based clinical practice guidelines on selected rehabilitaion interventions for neck pain. *Physical Therapy, 81*(10), 1701–1717.
21 Schomacher, J. (2009). The effect of an analgesic mobilization technique when applied at symptomatic or asymptomatic levels of the cervical spine in subjects with neck pain: A randomized controlled trial. *Journal of Manual and Manipulative Therapy, 17*(2), 101–108.

22 Rihn, J., Anderson, D., Lamb, K., Deluca, P., Bata, A., Marchetto, P., Neves, N., & Vaccaro, A. (2009). Cervical spine injuries in American football. *Sports Medicine, 39*(9), 697–708.

23 Seng, K., Lam, P., & Lee, V. (2003). Acceleration effects on neck muscle strength: Pilots vs. non-pilots. *Aviation, Space, and Environmental Medicine, 74*(2), 164–8.

24 Barker, P. (2011). Reduced G tolerance associated with supplement use. *Aviation Space and Environmental Medicine, 82*, 140–3.

25 Sovelius, R., Oksa, J., Rintala, H., Huhtala, H., Ylinen, J. and Siitonen, S. 2006. Trampoline Exercise vs. Strength Training to Reduce Neck Strain in Fighter Pilots. *Aviation, Space, and Environmental Medicine, 77:1.*

26 Eckner, T., Youkeun, K., Joshi, M., Richardson, J., & Ashton-Miller, A. (2014). Effect of neck muscle strength and anticipatory cervical muscle activation on the kinematic response of the head to impulsive loads. *American Journal of Sports Medicine, 42*, 566.

27 Netto, K., Carstairs, G., Kidgell, D., & Aisbett, B. (2010). Neck strength recovery after a single bout of specific strengthening exercise. *Physical Therapy in Sport, 11*(3), 75–80.

# Chapter 20

# The athletic shoulder

*Ian Horsley and Ben Ashworth*

## Introduction

Athletes need shoulders with the functional mobility and stability necessary to cope with the speeds, loads, ranges and repetitions of their sports. Depending on the sport, shoulders can be subjected to considerable stresses. For example the shoulders of competitive swimmers who cover 10 kilometres per day will accumulate 4,000 revolutions in daily training, whilst the highest recorded angular velocities of any human motion are achieved by the shoulders of a professional baseball pitcher, reaching speeds of more than 7,000°/sec.[1]

Stability within the glenohumeral joint (GHJ) is maintained via anatomical factors such as bony congruity, integrity of the capsuloligamentous structures and neuromuscular feedback loops integrated within the central nervous system.[2] Despite all this, the glenohumeral joint is regarded as one of the least stable joints within the body, and as little as 1–2mm of uncontrolled glenohumeral translation can be the difference between a symptomatic and an asymptomatic shoulder.[3]

As such, the ability to maintain shoulder-joint stability is the key factor in the integrated assessment models and rehabilitation programmes that are the focus of this chapter.

## The functional stability threshold

The goal of efficient shoulder function is to ensure the centring of humeral head within the shallow glenoid, avoiding unwanted glenohumeral translation. The outcome of this task is contingent on interplay between the mechanical and neuromuscular control stability mechanisms. This has been labelled the functional stability threshold (FST)[4] and is shown in Figure 20.1.

When the mechanical components fail, the greater demands placed on the neuromuscular system to reach the FST can result in compensatory movement patterns, rigidity, fatigue and, ultimately, an inability to efficiently control an unstable joint.[4] In the shoulder, this often manifests as reduced performance and recurrent symptoms when activity rises above a certain threshold. Little wonder, then, that it is common to see athletes with structural shoulder problems who can effectively compensate . . . but at a cost.

Muscle fatigue, trauma and hyperlaxity all contribute to stresses placed on shoulder mechanoreceptors, reducing feedback to the central nervous system and resulting in delayed or inappropriate responses. When the neuromuscular systems fail in this way, the glenohumeral (GH) joint's relatively poor passive osseous and capsuloligamentous structures are exposed to excessive shear or compressive forces.[4]

## Dynamic defence of the shoulder

Proprioception is a combination of joint position sense (JPS, the ability to identify the position of a limb in space) and kinaesthesia (the perception of active and passive motion).[5] Whilst it is known that JPS is reduced when fatigued, this only seems to be found at an end-of-range position, with JPS in the mid-range not changing. If, following repeated tackling in rugby, for example (see Figure 20.2), the mechanoreceptors are unable to accurately report shoulder

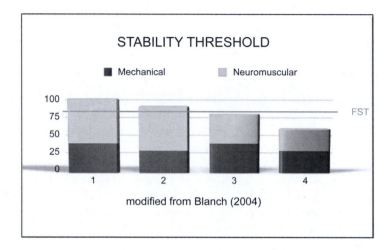

Figure 20.1  Functional stability threshold (FST); Athlete 1 – normal mechanical and neuromuscular stability; Athlete 2 – reduced mechanical stability with compensatory neuromuscular stability; Athlete 3 – normal mechanical stability with reduced neuromuscular stability; Athlete 4 – reduced mechanical and neuromuscular stability

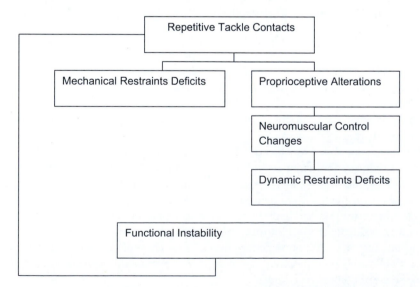

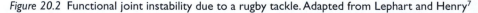

Figure 20.2  Functional joint instability due to a rugby tackle. Adapted from Lephart and Henry[7]

position in the outer range (stretch) position, there is a potential for the anterior structures to become stressed before any protective muscle contraction can take place.[6] These deficits are proposed to contribute to overuse injuries and micro-instability of the glenohumeral joint, which may be related to an increased injury risk.

The sensitivity of the mechanoreceptors can be decreased by muscle fatigue, microtrauma and any disruption to the capsulo-labral mechanism, which potentially exposes the passive structures of the shoulder to increased loading and injury.

## The importance of the scapula

The scapula acts as a link between the lower limb and trunk (e.g. through the fascial connection between gluteus maximus and latissimus dorsi), the glenohumeral joint and upper limb, permitting effective transfer of forces and joint alignment. Establishing a stable scapular platform is essential in minimizing stresses to the shoulder during over-head movements, enabling the rotator cuff muscles to help stabilize the humeral head within the glenoid.

To achieve this stability, active work from the surrounding muscles is critical. If the scapula is not maintained in its optimal position (for example, a 'winging' scapula) the surrounding muscles will be mechanically disadvantaged, resulting in them having to generate higher than desired forces to accomplish their tasks. Over a period of time, this can result in pain and dysfunction. Moreover, since the majority of the muscles that act on the glenohumeral joint originate from the scapula, fatigue of the scapular retractors and/or scapular upward rotators could compromise the subacromial space, fatigue the rotator cuff (especially the external rotators) and cause impingement.

## The importance of the rotator cuff

Anatomically, the moment arms of the rotator cuff muscles suggest a compressive role, acting to maintain humeral head stability against the dominant anterior pull of larger muscles acting on the glenohumeral joint. Isokinetic tests have also confirmed a bias towards internal rotation strength and the anterior shoulder muscles.[8] The presence of such a potential imbalance places the posterior shoulder muscles (rotator cuff and posterior deltoid) at a disadvantage. Therefore, it is suggested that the majority of rehabilitation programmes or pre-session preparation drills will need to address the posterior cuff and posterior deltoid deficits. The mid-back and scapula stabilizer drills outlined below (I's, T's, Y's and W's), have also been shown to activate the posterior cuff, alongside exercises using horizontal extension.[9] In addition, single-arm support work in closed chain positions can be used to bias cuff activity to the posterior shoulder. Rotator cuff exercise prescription for the posterior shoulder can be performed through a variety of different exercises, building fatigue resistance and local muscle capacity through building time under tension at intensities of 30–50 per cent of maximum voluntary contraction (MVC).

## Assessment of integrated shoulder function

Whilst identifying deficits within the sensorimotor system in a clinical setting is not easy, the following assessment tools provide some options when testing proprioception for the upper limb.

## Open chain assessment

Joint angular replication tests thoroughly assess both the static and dynamic shoulder joint stabilisers. An easy way to do this is to passively place the athlete's shoulder into a particular position (generally a combination of abduction and external rotation). The athlete's eyes are closed to negate visual cues and they are then asked to consciously register this position before the arm is returned to a resting position. They are then asked to return the arm to the test position, with errors noted. This is a drill that can be practiced, and over time, the expectation is that the magnitude of the positioning error decreases. Holding a laser pointer is an easy way to provide an external coaching cue as to the accuracy of the repositioning.[10]

*Contralateral arm mirroring* – the athlete's uninvolved shoulder is placed in a position in space (whilst they have their eyes closed) and then asked to mirror that position with the 'involved' limb. The degree of error between the two sides is recorded using goniometry or photography. With the advances in smartphone technology, many reliable bubble inclinometers/goniometers are now available as inexpensive apps that can be used for this.

*Dynamic Rotary Stability Test (DRST) and Dynamic Relocation Test (DRT)* – These functional tests monitor humeral head control and rotator cuff activation through range, assessing directional control deficits as the athlete is required to stabilise their shoulder under progressively more challenging situations.[11] It can be adapted to replicate the point in the range that the athlete experiences their symptoms (pain, weakness, apprehension or instability). The test can be carried out in a sitting or lying position, and the athlete is asked to match the internal or external rotation force provided by the clinician whilst maintaining the humeral and scapular positions. A positive test is indicated by loss of control of the humeral head as detected by the therapist via palpation and/or by the production of pain and loss of rotation force. Retraining of an identified control dysfunction by using dynamic relocation test as a treatment tool can alter the athlete's symptoms and overall presentation on reassessment. Successful retraining through this method is an indication that it is worth persevering with a conservative rehabilitation programme, which is useful in subtle situations where instability is more functional than structural.

## Rehabilitation

Following injury, rehabilitation of the shoulder includes relevant pain management, reduction of inflammation, restoration of optimal muscle strength, and restoration of a functional joint range of motion. Rehabilitation should also progress along a continuum to include functional movements that replicate the demands of the sport. This progression is underpinned by a fundamental requirement for joint control, and as such, there is an inherent need to address proprioceptive awareness, dynamic stabilization, feed-forward mechanisms (through anticipatory muscle responses), and reactive muscle function to athletic demands. Therefore, we need to prioritise proprioceptive training by re-establishing the sensorimotor pathways, as these are fundamental to the success of any rehabilitation programme.

A rehabilitation programme should progress along a continuum of difficulty, which can be seen in Table 20.1, below.

*Table 20.1* Rehabilitation Continuum

|  | *Early Stress* | *End Stage* |
|---|---|---|
| Support | Supported bilateral | Unsupported unilateral |
| Surface | Stable | Unstable |
| Stress | Minimal capsular stress Mid range | Maximal capsular stress Outer range |
| Speed | Slow | Fast |
| Stress application | Predetermined/slow progressive stress | Random/rapid stress |
| Movement pattern | Simple coordination | Complex coordination |

## Restoration of functional range of motion

It is important that a full functional range of motion is restored in the shoulder; restriction in one direction can potentially lead to 'give' (excessive joint play) in another. Posterior shoulder tightness, created by an inability of the shoulder to balance and absorb the stresses created by the high deceleration forces, is often a result of hypertonicity in the posterior cuff.[12] A significant reduction in internal rotation (glenohumeral internal rotation deficit [GIRD]) has been reported as a reliable predictor of shoulder injury and impingement symptoms.[13] Manual therapy and self-stretching techniques (sleeper stretch/cross-body adduction) aimed at restoration of normal tone are vital for improving the length-tension relationships around the glenohumeral joint.[14]

The measure of *total* range of motion in a shoulder is also of importance. A loss of five degrees total range relative to the contralateral arm can be enough to cause symptoms in throwing athletes.[15] Screening an athlete's range of motion and restoring normal range is ideally positioned prior to training. Should the rotator cuff be unable to control anterior humeral head translation, compensation from the larger internal rotator muscle groups (e.g. latissimus dorsi and pectoralis major) to protect the shoulder joint can destabilise the joint further and result in a reduction of functional range. The compensatory muscle actions of larger muscle groups will have an impact on other areas of the kinetic chain (thoracic and lumbar spine and pelvis) and must be addressed both locally and globally.

Accordingly, rather than solely focusing on the glenohumeral joint, we need to consider the shoulder complex as a whole, as well as the entire kinetic chain. For example, the ability to achieve the cocking position in a throw is made up not only of glenohumeral joint rotation, but also scapula and thoracic spine mobility. It is important to incorporate stretching that addresses such restrictions throughout the kinetic chain, as in the combined elevation rollout (Figure 20.3). Tightness in latissimus dorsi in this stretch results in an inability to externally rotate the shoulder required for full elevation and also negatively impacts on optimizing spinal mobility and stability.

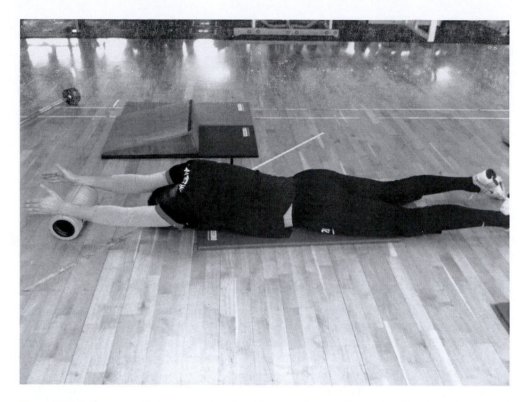

*Figure 20.3* Rollout stretch incorporating thoracic extension, maintenance of lumbo-pelvic neutral arm elevation with scapula upward rotation and glenohumeral external rotation

## Restoration of the sensorimotor system

The goals of neuromuscular rehabilitation are:

- To improve cognitive appreciation of the shoulder relative to position and motion;
- To enhance muscular stabilisation of the joint in the absence of passive restraints;
- Restore synergistic muscular firing and coordinated movement patterns.

Proprioceptive training aims to reconnect and enhance the afferent pathways from the joint to the central nervous system to compensate for changes as a result of injury or fatigue.[5] In order to maximise this, rehabilitation should include movements that replicate the demands of the sport. This will act to enhance JPS and kinaesthetic awareness, dynamic stabilization, and anticipatory as well as reactive muscle responses.

## Closed chain rehabilitation

The use of closed chain (CC) assessments of proprioception and movement patterns around the shoulder highlight deficits that can be addressed through specific CC exercises. CC exercises facilitate the anticipatory rotator cuff function, augmenting joint stability and stimulating muscular co-activation and proprioception. They facilitate the activity of the rotator cuff muscles in safe and congruent positions for the shoulder joint and can be utilised in positions of forward lean standing against a wall, or in four-point kneeling. At the outset, they should be performed with a fixed base of support on a table or wall, encouraging muscular co-activation and scapula stability without increasing shear forces across the shoulder joint. A full range of pain-free motion is the exit criterion for this stage with this series.

These can be progressed to a three-point position (by extending the other arm or either leg) and further progressed to two-point weight bearing which will facilitate the posterior chain to aid with scapular stabilisation, as well as assisting with specific recruitment of scapula stabilisers.

> Although throwing is an open chain (OC) movement, adaptations from CC exercises improve throwing velocity and can be as effective as OC training in promoting maximal strength gains.[17]

CC rehabilitation would then progress from a solid stable surface to a less stable surface (e.g. wobble board, Swiss ball or sling suspension [Figure 20.4]). The quality of the movement and exact local glenohumeral joint and scapula control needs to be monitored, avoiding excessive dominance of scapula-downward rotators and promoting synergistic action of scapula stabilisers (serratus anterior and all components of the trapezius muscle) to produce

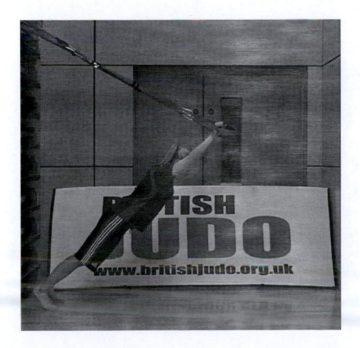

*Figure 20.4* Suspended bodyweight training

an integrated action. Athletes need to be monitored for global rigidity and global muscle dominance around the shoulder, and the lack of ability to dissociate humeral and scapular movement. In addition, it is beneficial to observe the direction of translation of the humeral head.

> It is imperative to notice the resting position of the GHJ prior to movement, to ensure it is not already displaced due to the effects of suboptimal resting tone in neighbouring muscles. Humeral head position can be readily identified with palpation both statically and during dynamic movement.

Another possibility for improving the cognitive awareness of shoulder JPS is to challenge the athlete to find the balance point (Figure 20.5), whereby, in side-lying, they are challenged to place their arm directly perpendicular to the glenoid and, initially, maintain this position against gravity. Asking the patient to maintain this position with a Swiss ball balanced on their hand can further enhance dynamic balance.

To progress this exercise to incorporate the kinetic chain, the patient is asked to stand from this position maintaining balance of the Swiss ball overhead.

The addition of externally applied forces (perturbations) will promote glenohumeral joint co-contraction and rhythmic stabilisation. This is shown in Figure 20.6.

Once we are sure that the patient has good proprioceptive control with active and passive movements, and that there is no pain or global fixation with reactive work to external perturbations, the exercises can be progressed to more functional athletic postures, as body position has a significant influence on an athlete's ability to replicate a target position and to be aware of upper-limb movement.[5] The difficulty of the CC exercise can be progressed for

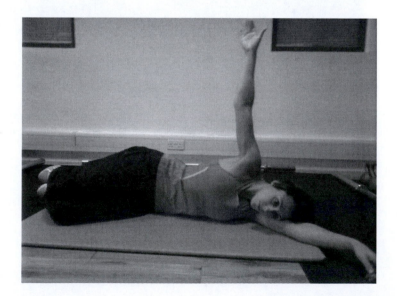

*Figure 20.5* Balance point

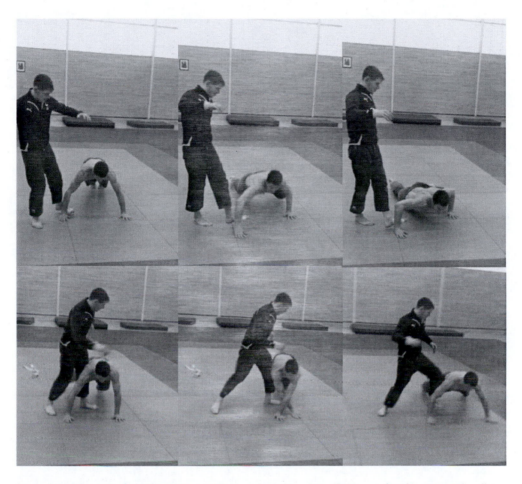

*Figure 20.6* Upper-body walk reaction drills – perturbations into 'Spiderman' and 'crossover' walks

end-stage rehabilitation by incorporating reaction through unexpected perturbations, as in the mat-based judo upper body walk drills seen above.

## Plyometrics

Once an athlete can tolerate the more controlled speeds used with most proprioceptive exercise, it is important that rehabilitation and pre-session preparation progress to include plyometric exercises that attempt to match the speeds and functions required of the shoulder in the athlete's sport. Plyometric drills enhance the reflex joint stabilization (and thus dynamic proprioception) required in a number of overhead sporting tasks such as serving in tennis. They therefore need to be trained specifically. Also, the hand-to-eye coordination required challenges the athlete in a way that improves their performance with repeated and accurate practice of the skill.

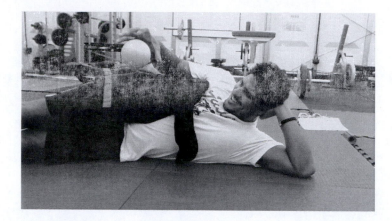

*Figure 20.7* Side-lying external rotation (SLER) ball flips

Common plyometric exercises include: throwing motions, trunk motions, resistive band exercises, ball/wall drills and plyometric push-ups. Rotator cuff force couples appear to play a role in setting 'stiffness' of joint prior to movement.[15, 16] In order to retrain the reactive and protective capacity of the rotator cuff, plyometric exercises can begin with low-level side-lying external rotation (SLER) ball flips (Figure 20.7), which focus on early eccentric work for the infraspinatus and posterior shoulder muscles. Posterior shoulder plyometrics can progress to the more challenging reverse catches, which address deceleration and control through greater range and at higher speeds, and also begin to incorporate more of the kinetic chain in order to train their ability to offload the shoulder by dissipating forces elsewhere in the body (Figure 20.8). It is important to note, however, that as the intensity of the drills increase, the volume should decrease in order to avoid overload.

---

**Plyometric programme design considerations**

**Frequency**: Allow 48–72 hours recovery between sessions.

**Number of contacts**: This will depend on the level of experience and the quality of the tissues, but we generally recommend:

80–100 'contacts' for someone weak or new to upper-limb plyometrics
100–120 for someone averagely strong or with some experience of upper-limb plyometrics
120–140 for someone strong or experienced at upper-limb plyometrics.

**Progression**: Progression to more demanding exercises in terms of frequency, intensity (speed and resistance) and volume is guided by the athlete's ability to demonstrate dynamic control around the shoulder, through full range, with good proprioceptive acuity.

(a)

(b)

(c)

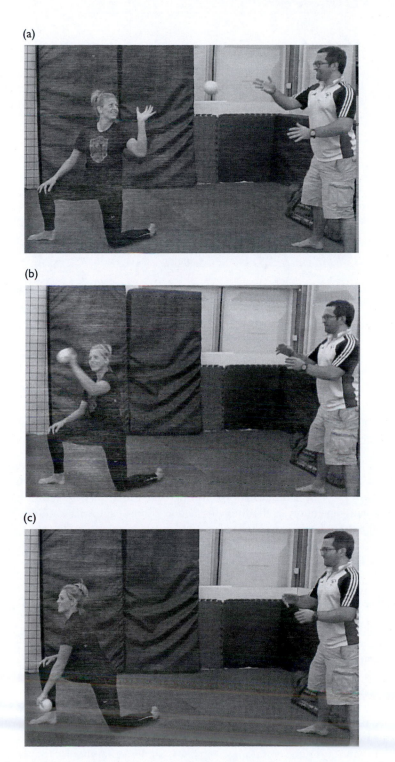

*Figure 20.8* (a, b, c) Reverse catches

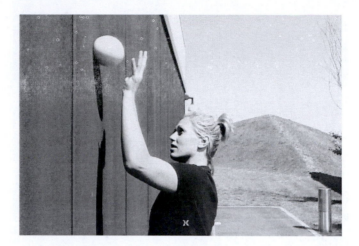

*Figure 20.9* Low-level plyometrics using a jelly med ball in abduction and external rotation

The intensity and volume of the session(s) need to be closely monitored to ensure the quality of the exercise is maintained, the force being produced by the upper limb is consistent and there is good lumbo-pelvic control. Tissue responses may not always be immediate, and so it is important to assess for any adverse reaction 24 hours post training.

> The foundation of good glenohumeral control is a well-sequenced connection from lower limb through the contact surface across the pelvis and trunk and into the scapula and requires efficient transfer of force through each link. Indeed, more than 50 per cent of force generation in the throwing action comes from trunk and lower body.[17] Clearly, the shoulder starts at the feet!

## Rehabilitation of the scapula

Exercising in a scapula plane places the shoulder in a 'safe zone' that minimizes glenohumeral shear, maximizes concavity/compression, and minimizes muscular activation. The scapula is orientated at 30° to 45° anterior to the frontal plane so that the glenoid fossa faces to some extent anteriorly, rather than laterally. In this plane, the inferior glenohumeral capsular ligament is not twisted, and the supraspinatus and deltoid are optimally aligned to elevate the arm. To guide the patient, it would be stressed that, with active movements, they should be able to see their hands throughout the movement without moving their head. The use of similar scapula retraction exercises, often named 'I's, Y's, T's and W's', are an important component of any shoulder rehabilitation or shoulder injury prevention programme.[9]

**Exercise prescription wisdom**

Rather that dictating a pre-determined number of repetitions and sets, only the number of pain-free repetitions that the athlete can execute correctly with consistency should be performed. It is also important to consider the exercises prescribed in terms of degree of challenge and when they are performed. For example, programming complex/challenging drills at end-range towards the end of a rehab session should only be considered in the final stage of rehabilitation. Because fatigue decreases proprioceptive awareness, complex drilling is a risky strategy for the unstable shoulder. Continual assessment of movement patterns and technical execution is imperative prior to progressing the drill's intensity (volume, speed or resistance) or complexity.

## Integrated scapulothoracic rehabilitation

Below is a programme that we advocate to ensure the progression of scapulothoracic retraining over the course of eight weeks. Note that it is a programme encompassing all aspects of the kinetic chain, as well as flexibility, open and closed-kinetic chain drills and finally the progression into plyometrics to add a velocity-based stress to the scapulothoracic articulation.

Table 20.2 Integrated scapulothoracic rehabilitation (adapted from Kibler and McMullen)[18]

| | Weeks (Estimated) | | | | | | | |
|---|---|---|---|---|---|---|---|---|
| | 1 | 2 | 3 | 4 | 5 | 6 | 7 | 8 |
| **Scapular Motion** | | | | | | | | |
| Thoracic Posture Exercises | X | X | X | | | | | |
| Trunk Flexion Extension Rotation | X | X | X | | | | | |
| Lower Abdominal Hip Extension Exercises | X | X | X | X | X | | | |
| **Muscular Flexibility** | | | | | | | | |
| Massage | X | X | | | | | | |
| Electotherapy Modalities | X | X | X | | | | | |
| Stretching | X | X | X | X | X | X | X | X |

(Continued)

*Table 20.2* (Continued)

| | Weeks (Estimated) | | | | | | | |
|---|---|---|---|---|---|---|---|---|
| | 1 | 2 | 3 | 4 | 5 | 6 | 7 | 8 |
| Pectoralis minor stretch | X | X | X | | | | | |
| Sleeper stretch | X | X | X | | | | | |
| **Closed Chain Co-Contraction Exercise** | | | | | | | | |
| Weight transfer | X | X | | | | | | |
| Balance board | X | X | | | | | | |
| Scapular clock exercise | X | X | | | | | | |
| Rhythmic ball stabilization | | X | | | | | | |
| Weight- bearing isometric extension | X | X | | | | | | |
| Wall push-up | | X | | | | | | |
| Table push-up | | | X | X | X | | | |
| Modified to prone push-up | | | | | X | X | X | X |
| **Axially Loaded Active ROM Exercise** | | | | | | | | |
| Scaption | | X | X | X | X | | | |
| Flexion slide | | X | X | X | X | | | |
| Abduction glide | | | X | X | X | | | |
| Diagonal slides | | X | X | X | X | X | | |
| **Integrated Open Kinetic Chain Exercises** | | | | | | | | |
| Scapular motion + arm elevation | | | X | X | X | X | X | X |
| Unilateral/bilateral resistance band pulls + trunk motion | | | | X | X | X | X | X |
| Modified shoulder dump series | | X | X | X | X | X | | |
| Dumbbell punches + progressions | | | | | | X | X | X |
| Lunges with dumbbell reaches | | | | | X | X | X | X |
| **Plyometric Sport-Specific** | | | | | | | | |
| Weighted ball throw and catch | | | | | | X | X | X |
| Resistance tubing plyometics | | | | | | X | X | X |

## Summary

Functional stability of the athlete's shoulder is dependent on co-activation of the muscu-lature, as well as reactive neuromuscular characteristics. Injury to any of the soft tissue structures has been postulated as a cause of disruption of this neuromuscular mecha-nism. Treatment of such a dysfunction needs to consider proprioceptive training and rehabilitation, since the function of the shoulder joint is optimal when proprioception is normalized.

# Notes

1 Allegrucci, M., Whitney, S. L., Lephart, S.M., Irrgang J.J., & Fu, F. H. (1995). Shoulder kinaesthesia in healthy unilateral athletes participating in upper extremity sports. *Journal of Orthopaedic & Sports Physical Therapy, 69,* 220–6.

2 Suprak, D., Osternig, L., van-Donkelaar, P., & Karduna, A. (2006). Shoulder joint position sense improves with elevation angle in a novel, unconstrained task. *Journal of Orthopaedic Research, 24,* 559–568.

3 Cholewinski, J.J., Kusz, D.J., Wojciechowski, P., & Cielinski, L. S. (2008). Ultrasound measurement of rotator cuff thickness and acromio-humeral distance in the diagnosis of subacromial impingement syndrome of the shoulder. *Knee Surgery, Sports Traumatology, Arthroscopy, 16*(4), 408–14.

4 Blanch, P. (2004). Conservative management of shoulder pain in swimming. *Physical Therapy in Sport, 5*(3), 109–124.

5 Janwantanakul, P., Magarey, M., Jones, M., & Danise, B. (2001). Variation in shoulder position sense at mid and extreme range of motion. *Archives of Physical Medicine and Rehabilitation, 82,* 840–844.

6 Herrington, L., Horsley, I., & Rolf, C. (2010). Evaluation of joint position sense in both asymptomatic and rehabilitated professional rugby players and matched controls. *Physical Therapy in Sport, 11*(1), 18–22.

7 Lephart, S., & Henry, T. (1996). The physiological basis for open and closed kinematic chain rehabilitation for the upper extremity. *Journal of Sports Rehabilitation, 5,* 71–87.

8 Moraes, G.F., Faria, C.D., & Teixeira-Salmela, L.F. (2008). Scapular muscle recruitment patterns and isokinetic strength ratios of the shoulder rotator muscles in individuals with and without impingement syndrome. *Journal of Shoulder and Elbow Surgery, 17*(1), S48–S53.

9 Oyama, S., Myers, J.B., Wassinger, C.A., & Lephart, S.M. (2010). Three-dimensional scapular and clavicular kinematics and scapular muscle activity during retraction exercises. *Journal of Orthopaedic & Sports Physical Therapy, 40*(3), 169–179.

10 Lephart, S. M., & Fu, F. H. (2000). *Proprioception and neuromuscular control in joint stability.* Champaign, IL: Human Kinetics Publishers.

11 Magarey, M. E., & Jones, M. A. (2003). Dynamic evaluation and early management of altered motor control around the shoulder complex. *Manual Therapy, 8*(4), 195–206.

12 Myers, J. B., Laudner, K. G., Pasquale, M. R., Bradley, J. P., & Lephart, S. M. (2006). Range of motion deficits and posterior shoulder tightness in throwers with pathologic internal impingement. *The American Journal of Sports Medicine, 34*(3), 385–391.

13 Scher, S., Anderson, K., Weber, N., Bajorek, J., Rand, K., & Bey, M.J. (2010). Associations among hip and shoulder range of motion and shoulder injury in professional baseball players. *Journal of Athletic Training, 45*(2), 191–197.

14 Ellenbecker, T., & Cools, A. (2010). Rehabilitation of shoulder impingement syndrome and rotator cuff injuries: An evidence-based review, *British Journal of Sports Medicine, 44,* 319–327.

15 David, G., Magarey, M. E., Jones, M. A., Dvir, Z., Turker, K. S., & Sharpe, M. (2000). EMG and strength correlates of selected shoulder muscles during rotations of the glenohumeral joint. *Clinical Biomechanics, 15,* 95–102.

16 Hess, S. A., Richardson, C., Darnell, R., Friis, P., Lisle, D., & Myers, P. (2005). Timing of rotator cuff activation during shoulder external rotation in throwers with and without symptoms of pain. *Journal of Orthopaedic & Sports Physical Therapy, 35*(12), 812–20.

17 Prokopy, M.P., Ingersoll, C.D., Nordenschild, E., Katch, F.I., Gaesser, G.A., & Weltman, A. (2008). Closed-kinetic chain upper-body training improves throwing performance of NCAA Division I softball players. *The Journal of Strength & Conditioning Research, 22*(6), 1790–1798.

18 Kibler, W.B., & McMullen, J. (2003). Scapular dyskinesis and its relation to shoulder pain. *Journal of the American Academy of Orthopaedic Surgeons, 11*(2), 142–151.

# Chapter 21

# The athletic elbow

*Adam Olsen and Mike Reinold*

## Introduction

Despite a well-reported susceptibility to injury in many athletic populations, the elbow remains relatively poorly understood in terms of optimal rehabilitation strategies. Athletes who engage in repetitive upper-limb activities are very susceptible to injury at the elbow, either through repetitive microtrauma or acute overload. Whilst collision and contact-related injuries to the elbow are reported in certain sporting groups, the largest impact in keeping athletes on the field can arguably be made by the appropriate evaluation and treatment of overuse injuries.

Rehabilitation of the elbow joint requires a thorough knowledge of the anatomical, biomechanical and pathomechanical factors associated with athletic participation. The purpose of this chapter is to provide an overview of the biomechanics of the sporting elbow followed by an explanation of current techniques in rehabilitation of the elite athlete. The ultimate goal of rehabilitation, as always, is to progressively restore function and return the athlete to competition as quickly and safely as possible.

## Elbow biomechanics in sport

Whilst the following section discusses the biomechanics and pathomechanics of the elbow during three sports that have a high relative incidence of elbow injuries reported in the literature, namely baseball, tennis and golf, we can extrapolate many of the same principles across most other sports, since although the path of the elbow may be different depending upon the sport, similar injury mechanisms can be identified. A large force over a short time or a series of small forces over a lengthened amount of time creates the mechanism for injury. Whether it is the valgus forces during the throwing of a baseball, the rotational activation of the forearm and upper arm during the tennis serve or the co-contraction of the forearm flexors and extensors in golf, knowing the mechanism of injury is vital to understanding how best to rehabilitate the injury.

The baseball pitch can be broken down into six phases: wind-up, stride, arm cocking, arm acceleration, arm deceleration and follow-through (discussed in detail in chapter 11). The majority of force occurs at the transition between cocking and acceleration where the shoulder is in a position of maximal external rotation. As the arm moves into external rotation, a varus torque is produced through the forearm flexors and inertly through the capsule-ligamentous structures to prevent valgus stress.[1] Shortly before maximum external rotation, the elbow is flexed to 95° and a varus torque of approximately 64 Nm is produced.[2] At this critical instant, any excessive valgus strain may cause injury to the medial stabilizing structures of the elbow, particularly the ulna collateral ligament (UCL) and compressive injuries to the lateral compartment of the elbow as the radial head and humeral capitellum are approximated.

In tennis, the overhead serve has been compared to the mechanics of overhead throwing, but with more emphasis on the rotational component of the forearm to produce velocity. The elbow has been reported to extend at 982°/s and pronate at 347°/s during acceleration and deceleration phases of the tennis serve.[3] Morris et al.[4] report high activity of the triceps and pronator teres during the tennis serve in order to produce significant racket velocity, and, as such, the eccentric contraction of the elbow flexors and supinators is critical in the prevention of elbow injuries.

The biomechanics of the golf swing pertaining to elbow and wrist injuries can be broken down into six phases: the address, backswing horizontal, peak of the backswing, downswing horizontal, ball contact (impact) and follow-through horizontal. More than twice as many injuries occur during the downswing compared to the backswing, as the elbow and wrist move approximately three times as fast during this phase.[5] This deceleration of force places a great deal of strain on the forearm musculature as it attempts to maintain control of the club. The majority of elbow injuries take place during impact, as the lateral epicondyle of the lead arm and the medial epicondyle of the back arm are placed under significant strain. The lead elbow extensor mass has been reported to be under even greater stress at impact due to the compressive force from ball impact and divots.[6] At ball contact, the wrist flexor activity significantly increases to approximately 90 per cent of maximal voluntary isometric contraction (MVIC). Additionally, the wrist extensors exhibit EMG activity of almost 60 per cent MVIC.[7]

When comparing the muscular activity patterns of golfers with medial elbow pain (commonly referred to as 'golfer's elbow') and golfers without injuries, those with golfer's elbow exhibit significantly greater wrist flexor muscle activity during the backswing, transition and downswing.[7] It is therefore possible that an imbalance between the wrist flexors and extensors may be implicated in the development in elbow pain, and addressing this in the rehabilitation process will help centralize the joint.

## Elbow rehabilitation

Rehabilitation following elbow injury or elbow surgery follows a sequential and progressive multi-phased approach. The ultimate goal of elbow rehabilitation is to return the athlete to their previous functional level as quickly and safely as possible, while identifying and correcting the kinetic chain faults to mitigate re-injury. Elite performance in all three sports discussed above is characterized by better coordination and utilization of the kinetic chain. In baseball, elite pitchers utilize the lower extremities and trunk more efficiently than amateurs and rely less on the specific muscles of the scapular and rotator cuff muscles to generate the forces for the throw. In the tennis serve, velocity is determined by the effectiveness of the transfer of energy from the lower extremities to the racquet at the end of the chain. In golf, professional players are better able to maintain the shoulder-hip separation from backswing to downswing than high-handicap players because of better control of the trunk muscles.[8] These joint-saving techniques of energy transfer may help to prevent injury in the professional golfer despite higher volumes of playing. These examples point to the importance of properly evaluating the kinetic chain for global weaknesses in the prevention of re-injury.

Initial elbow rehabilitation focuses on minimizing the effects of immobilization and protection of the joint. While completing initial ranging practices for the elbow, wrist and forearm (within specific parameters from the treatment protocol), focus is shifted to total body integration and stabilization. Proper trunk stabilization through the training of the diaphragm, pelvic floor and obliques can create the 'fixation point' for the peripheral joints or 'movable point' to operate off for maximum mobility. This will allow for optimal energy production and dissipation using the entire body.

With global stability training initiated, the movement screen results can be reviewed to focus treatment on possible energy leaks within the kinetic chain. Athletes often exhibit predictable imbalances throughout the muscular system. Janda describes these as Crossed Syndromes, divided into an Upper-Crossed Syndrome and a Lower-Crossed Syndrome.[9] These patterns display clusters of muscles that are weak and lengthened in contrast to others which are over-developed and shortened. When layered upon imbalances inherent to the unilateral athlete, these patterns can become quite profound. Initial stages of rehabilitation for the elbow and wrist are ideal for correcting these muscular imbalances to improve movement dysfunction.

We also need to consider the shoulder complex when assessing elbow function. Proper evaluation of shoulder range of motion, rotator cuff strength and scapular stability can reveal hidden pathology or impairment. Any impairments of the alignment, dynamic movement or ability to stabilize the proximal joints may lead to altered elbow positioning and increased force during functional sport tasks. Integration of total body stabilization[10] with well-established programmes, such as the Thrower's Ten Program, promote proper stabilization patterns through the trunk while strengthening and stabilizing the shoulder (Figure 21.1a–f).

As immobilization and protection guidelines are relaxed, initial focus on the soft tissues through manual scar mobilization and soft tissue mobilization techniques can help promote range-of-motion restoration. In almost every protocol, restoration of elbow extension is paramount. The elbow is predisposed to flexion contractures due to the intimate congruency of the joint articulations, the tightness of the joint capsule and the tendency of the anterior capsule to develop adhesions following injury. In addition to therapist-assisted passive range of motion, low-load long-duration stretching with heat and resistance band loading can assist

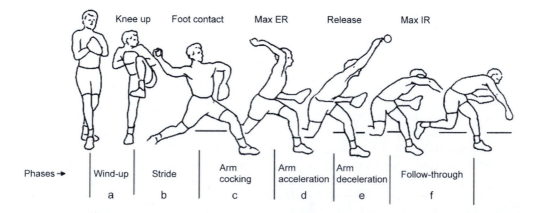

*Figure 21.1* Integration of total body stabilization with well-established programmes, such as the Thrower's Ten Program, promote trunk stability while strengthening and stabilizing the shoulder

with the more stubborn cases. When elbow flexion must be restored, a self-stretch against the wall helps the athlete relax most effectively to regain end range of motion. As range of motion returns, specific nerve flossing helps prevent neurogenic symptoms from becoming the limiting factor, establishing full range of motion.

Isometric strengthening can be supplemented with rhythmic stabilizations in the supine position to begin re-establishing proprioception and neuromuscular control of the upper extremity. This can be seen in Figure 21.2.

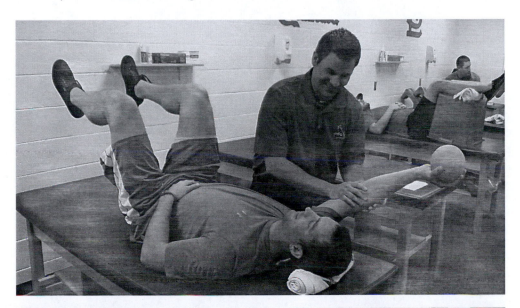

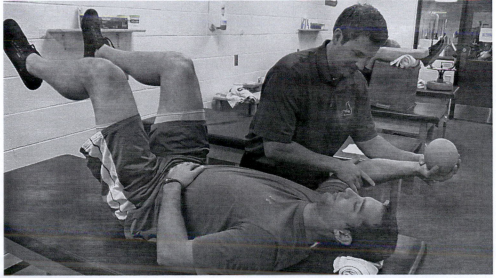

*Figure 21.2 a and b* Rhythmic stabilization in supine. Begin re-establishing proprioception and neuro-muscular control of the upper extremity through rhythmic stabilization at varied arm angles

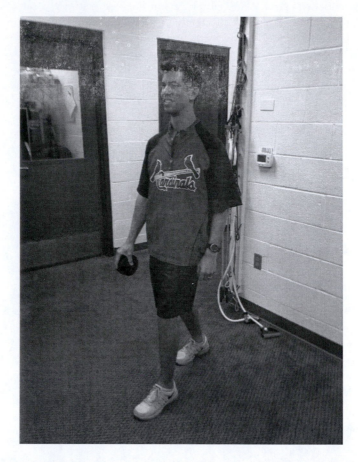

*Figure 21.3* Isometric holds for grip strengthening. Introduce various shapes and weights for isometric grip strengthening

Preference is given to manual strengthening as the athlete progresses to isotonics for consistent resistance through the entire range of motion. Manual biceps combo, which combines elbow flexion, supination and wrist flexion, and manual triceps combo, which combines elbow extension and pronation, promotes multi-joint coordination of movement before re-entry to the weight room for advanced strengthening methods. Progression of this particular exercise includes eccentrics and increase in speed of movement. Manual strengthening of the forearm can be accomplished for all available motions: flexion, extension, supination, pronation, ulnar deviation, radial deviation and phalangeal flexion/extension. Grip strengthening can progress from isometric holds of various weighted objects (Figure 21.3), to rice bucket (Figure 21.4), to plyometrics such as flips and grips (Figure 21.5a–b).

As the athlete approaches return to sport, multi-joint plyometrics (Figure 21.6a–g) bridge the gap to the specific interval sport programmes required to gradually impart the stress that will be encountered upon their return.

In non-surgical cases of chronic elbow pain, such as lateral epicondylalgia (LE), soft tissue mobilization techniques, such as mobilization-with-movement, have been found to have substantial

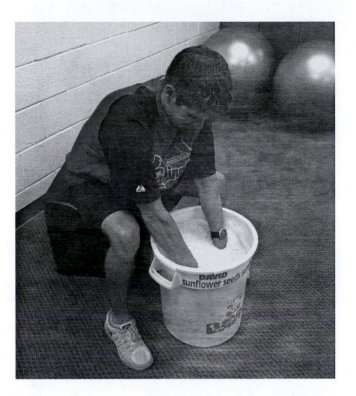

*Figure 21.4* Rice bucket isotonic forearm strengthening. Progress hand and forearm strengthening to include repetitive movements through rice over progressive time intervals

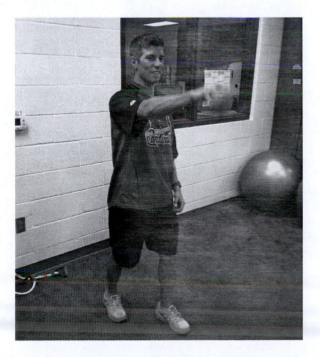

*Figure 21.5a and 21.5b* Plyometric grips and flips. Plyometric strengthening can be performed through the repetitive gripping or flipping of a weighted ball

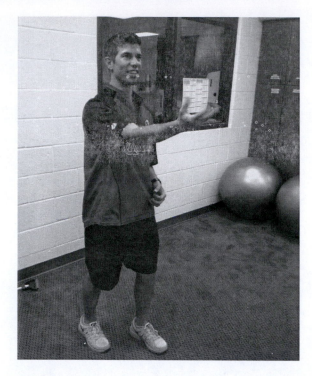

*Figure 21.5a and 21.5b* (Continued)

(a)

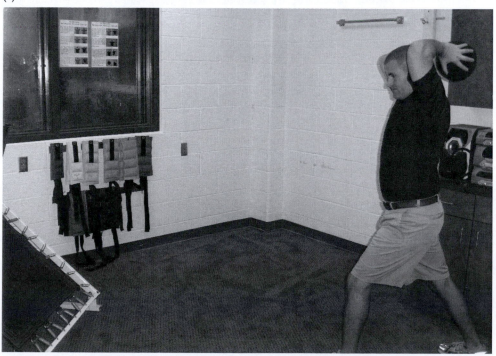

*Figure 21.6 a–g* Upper extremity plyometrics. As the athlete approaches return to sport, multi-joint plyometrics bridge the gap to the specific interval sport programs required to gradually impart the stress that will be encountered upon their return

(b)

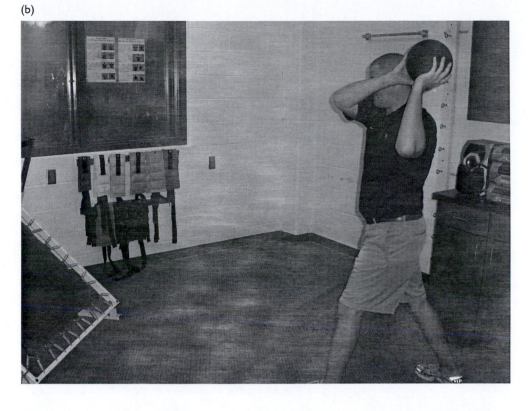

(c)

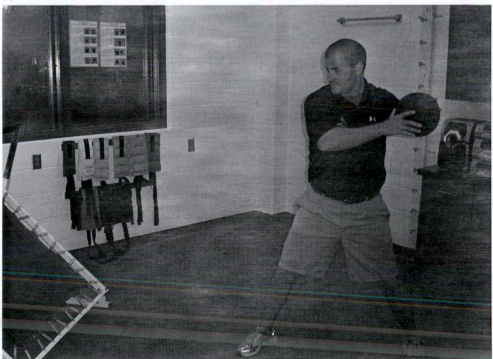

*Figure 21.6* (Continued)

(d)

(e)

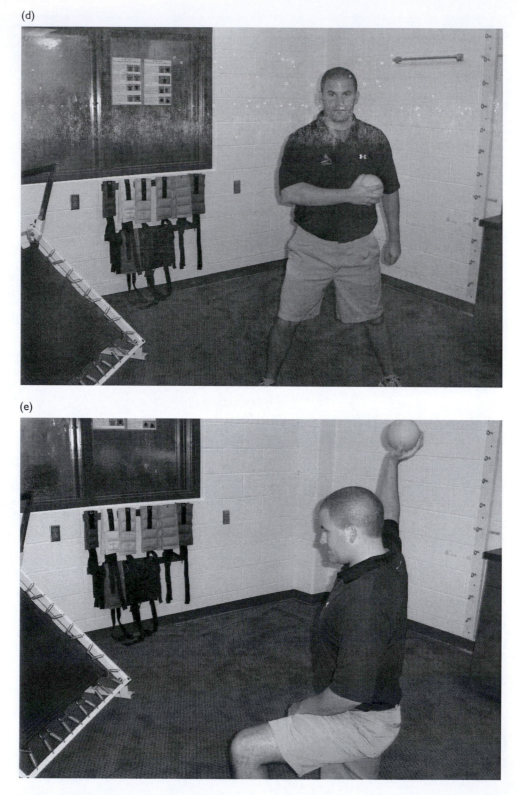

*Figure 21.6* (Continued)

(f)

(g)

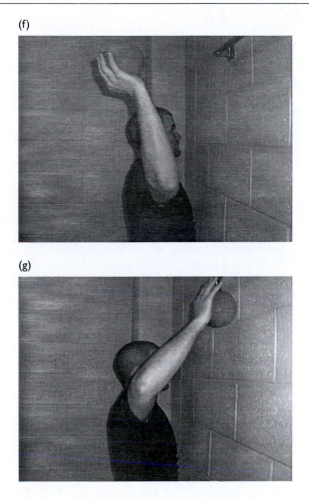

*Figure 21.6* (Continued)

pain-relieving effects,[11] allowing significant increases in grip strength. The proper treatment of medial and lateral epicondylalgia varies depending on the chronicity of the injury and the presence of inflammation process.[12] Acute epicondylitis often resembles a typical tendonitis with tissue inflammation. However, as the tendinopathy becomes more chronic, the presence of an inflammation process is diminished. Treatment for this chronic tendinosis will differ from acute epicondylitis. The emphasis of rehabilitation continues to focus on restoring soft tissue and biomechanical imbalances, as previously mentioned. However, treatment techniques such as deep-tissue friction massage and eccentric exercises are incorporated to promote a healing response to the tissue.[13] For more detail on the principles of tendinopathy management, refer to chapter 15.

Before an athlete is allowed to begin the return-to-activity phase of rehabilitation, the athlete must exhibit full ROM, no pain or tenderness, and a satisfactory clinical examination. The return-to-activity phase involves an interval sport program designed to gradually apply loads to the elbow that are sport-specific.[14]

For the overhead thrower, we initiate a long-toss interval throwing program (Table 21.1). The athlete throws three times per week with a day off from throwing in between each session. Each step is performed at least twice before moving onto the next step, but be aware that throwing is

*Table 21.1* Interval Throwing Program – Phase I – Long Toss

| 45' Phase | 60' Phase | 90' Phase | 120' Phase |
|---|---|---|---|
| Step 1:<br>A) Warm-up Throwing<br>B) 45' (25 Throws)<br>C) Rest 5–10 min.<br>D) Warm-up Throwing<br>E) 45' (25 Throws) | Step 3:<br>A) Warm-up Throwing<br>B) 60'(25 Throws)<br>C) Rest 5–10 min.<br>D) Warm-up Throwing<br>E) 60' (25Throws) | Step 5:<br>A) Warm-up Throwing<br>B) 90' (25 Throws)<br>C) Rest 5–10 min.<br>D) Warm-up Throwing<br>E) 90' (25 Throws) | Step 7:<br>A) Warm-up Throwing<br>B) 120' (25 Throws)<br>C) Rest 5–10 min.<br>D) Warm-up Throwing<br>E) 120' (25 Throws) |
| Step 2:<br>A) Warm-up Throwing<br>B) 45' (25 Throws)<br>C) Rest 5–10 min.<br>D) Warm-up Throwing<br>E) 45' (25 Throws)<br>F) Rest 5–10 min.<br>G) Warm-up Throwing<br>H) 45' (25 Throws) | Step 4:<br>A) Warm-up Throwing<br>B) 60' (25 Throws)<br>C) Rest 5–10 min.<br>D) Warm-up Throwing<br>E) 60' (25 Throws)<br>F) Rest 5–10 min.<br>G) Warm-up Throwing<br>H) 60' (25 Throws) | Step 6:<br>A) Warm-up Throwing<br>B) 90' (25 Throws)<br>C) Rest 5–10 min.<br>D) Warm-up Throwing<br>E) 90' (25 Throws)<br>F) Rest 5–10 min.<br>G) Warm-up Throwing<br>H) 90' (25 Throws) | Step 8:<br>A) Warm-up Throwing<br>B) 120' (25 Throws)<br>C) Rest 5–10 min.<br>D) Warm-up Throwing<br>E) 120' (25 Throws)<br>F) Rest 5–10 min.<br>G) Warm-up throwing<br>H) 120' (25 Throws) |

| 150' Phase | 180' Phase | | |
|---|---|---|---|
| Step 9:<br>A) Warm-up Throwing<br>B) 150' (25 Throws)<br>C) Rest 5–10 min.<br>D) Warm-up Throwing<br>E) 150' (25 Throws) | Step 11:<br>A) Warm-up Throwing<br>B) 180' (25 Throws)<br>C) Rest 5–10 min.<br>D) Warm-up Throwing<br>E) 180' (25 Throws) | Step 13:<br>A) Warm-up Throwing<br>B) 180' (25 Throws)<br>C) Rest 5–10 min.<br>D) Warm-up Throwing<br>E) 180' (25 Throws) | **Throwing Program should be performed every other day.** |
| Step 10:<br>A) Warm-up Throwing<br>B) 150' (25 Throws)<br>C) Rest 5–10 min.<br>D) Warm-up Throwing<br>E) 150' (25 Throws)<br>F) Rest 5–10 min.<br>G) Warm-up Throwing<br>H) 150' (25 Throws) | Step 12:<br>A) Warm-up Throwing<br>B) 180' (25 Throws)<br>C) Rest 5–10 min.<br>D) Warm-up Throwing<br>E) 180' (25 Throws)<br>F) Rest 5–10 min.<br>G) Warm-up Throwing<br>H) 180' (25 Throws) | Step 14:<br>Begin Throwing off the mound or return to respective position. | Perform each step 2 times before progressing to next step. |

**Flat Ground Throwing**
A) Warm-up Throwing
B) Throw 60 ft. (10–15 throws)
C) Throw 90 ft. (10 throws)
D) Throw 120 ft. (10 throws)
E) Throw 60 ft. (flat ground) using pitching mechanics (20–30 throws)

**Flat Throwing**
A) Warm-up Throwing
B) Throw 60 ft. (10–15 throws)
C) Throw 90 ft. (10 throws)
D) Throw 120 ft. (10 throws)
E) Throw 60 ft. (flat ground) using pitching mechanics (20–30 throws)
F) Throw 60–90 ft. (10–15 throws)
G) Throw 60 ft. (flat ground) using pitching mechanics (20 throws)

only to be performed on alternate days. For example Stage One needs to be performed on Monday and Wednesday before moving on to Stage Two on Friday. Throwing should be performed without pain or significant increase in symptoms. If the athlete experiences symptoms at a particular step within the program, they are instructed to regress to the previous stage until symptoms subside. Following the completion of a long-toss program, pitchers will progress to phase II of the throwing program – throwing off a mound (Table 21.2). In phase II, the number of throws, intensity and type of pitch are progressed to gradually increase stress on the elbow joint.

*Table 21.2* Interval Throwing Program – Phase II – Mound Progression

### STAGE ONE: FASTBALLS ONLY

Step 1:   Interval Throwing                          (Use Interval Throwing to 120'
                                                      Phase as warm-up)

          15 Throws off mound 50%
Step 2:   Interval Throwing
          30 Throws off mound 50%
Step 3:   Interval Throwing                          ALL THROWING OFF THE MOUND
                                                     SHOULD BE DONE IN THE PRESENCE
                                                     OF YOUR PITCHING COACH TO
                                                     STRESS PROPER THROWING

          45 Throws off mound 50%
Step 4:   Interval Throwing                          MECHANICS
          60 Throws off mound 50%
Step 5:   Interval Throwing                          (Use speed gun to aid in effort control)
          70 Throws off mound 50%
Step 6:   45 Throws off mound 50%
          30 Throws off mound 75%
Step 7:   30 Throws off mound 50%
          45 Throws off mound 75%
Step 8:   65 Throws off mound 75%
          10 Throws off mound 50%

### STAGE TWO: FASTBALLS ONLY

Step 9:   60 Throws off mound 75%
          15 Throws in Batting Practice
Step 10:  50–60 Throws off mound 75%
          30 Throws in Batting Practice
Step 11:  45–50 Throws off mound 75%
          45 Throws in Batting Practice

### STAGE THREE

Step 12:  30 Throws off mound 75% warm-up
          15 Throws off mound 50% BREAKING BALLS
          45–60 Throws in Batting Practice (fastball only)
Step 13:  30 Throws off mound 75%
          30 Breaking Balls 75%
          30 Throws in Batting Practice
Step 14:  30 throws off mound 75%
          60–90 Throws in Batting Practice (Gradually
          increase breaking balls)
Step 15:  SIMULATED GAME: PROGRESSING BY 15
          THROWS PER WORKOUT (Pitch Count)

*Table 21.3* Interval Tennis Program

| OH – Overhead shots | FH – Forehand shots | | | BH – Backhand shots |
|---|---|---|---|---|
| | MONDAY | WEDNESDAY | FRIDAY | |
| 1st Week | 12 FH | 15 FH | | 15 FH |
| | 8 BH | 8 BH | | 10 BH |
| | 10 min. rest | 10 min. rest | | 10 min. rest |
| | 13 FH | 15 FH | | 15 FH |
| | 7 BH | 7 BH | | 10 BH |
| 2nd Week | 25 FH | 30 FH | 30 FH | |
| | 15 BH | 20 BH | | 25 BH |
| | 10 min. rest | 10 min. rest | | 10 min. rest |
| | 25 FH | 30 FH | | 30 FH |
| | 15 BH | 20 BH | | 15 BH |
| | | | | 10 BH |
| 3rd Week | 30 FH | 30 FH | | 30 FH |
| | 25 BH | 25 BH | | 30 BH |
| | 10 OH | 15 OH | | 15 OH |
| | 10 min. rest | 10 min. rest | | 10 min. rest |
| | 30 FH | 30 FH | | 30 FH |
| | 25 BH | 25 BH | | 15 OH |
| | 10 OH | 15 OH | | 10 min. rest |
| | | | | 30 FH |
| | | | | 30 BH |
| | | | | 15 OH |
| 4th Week | 30 FH | 30 FH | | 30 FH |
| | 30 BH | 30 BH | | 30 BH |
| | 10 OH | 10 OH | | 10 OH |
| | 10 min. rest | 10 min. rest | | 10 min. rest |
| | Play 3 games | Play set | | Play 1½ sets |
| | 10 FH | 10 FH | | 10 FH |
| | 10 BH | 10 BH | | 10 BH |
| | 5 BH | 5 OH | | 3 OH |

*Ice after each day of play

Interval sport programs for tennis and golf follow the same guidelines as the baseball programme. A specific interval programme for tennis is outlined in Table 21.3. As the athlete progresses, the number of forehand and backhand shots are gradually increased. Overhead serving is typically initiated during the third week of the programme, and games are allowed during the fourth week if symptoms have not exacerbated.

Table 21.4 outlines an interval golf programme. The programme begins with simple putting and chipping and progresses to include short-iron swings by the end of week 1, medium

*Table 21.4* Interval Golf Programme

|  | MONDAY | WEDNESDAY | FRIDAY |
|---|---|---|---|
| 1st Week | 10 putts<br>10 chips<br>5' rest<br>15 chips | 15 putts<br>15 chips<br>5' rest<br>25 chipping | 20 putts<br>20 chips<br>5' rest<br>20 putts<br>20 chips<br>5' rest<br>10 chips<br>10 short irons |
| 2nd Week | 20 chips<br>10 short irons<br>5' rest<br>10 short irons<br>15 med. irons (5 iron off tee) | 20 chips<br>15 short irons<br>10' rest<br>15 short irons<br>15 chips Putting 15 med. irons (5 iron/tee) | 15 short irons<br>20 med. irons (5 iron/tee)<br>10' rest<br>20 short irons<br>15 chips |
| 3rd Week | 15 short irons<br>20 medium irons<br>10' rest<br>5 long irons<br>15 short irons<br>15 medium irons<br>10' rest<br>20 chips | 15 short irons<br>15 medium irons<br>10 long irons<br>10' rest<br>10 short irons<br>10 medium irons<br>5 long irons<br>5 wood | 15 short irons<br>15 medium irons<br>10 long irons<br>10' rest<br>10 short irons<br>10 medium irons<br>10 long irons<br>10 wood |
| 4th Week | 15 short irons<br>15 medium irons<br>10 long irons<br>10 drives<br>15' rest<br>Repeat | Play 9 holes | Play 9 holes |
| 5th Week | 9 holes | 9 holes | 18 holes |

Key To Golf Programmes
*Flexibility exercises before hitting   chips – pitching wedge
*Use ice after hitting   short irons – W, 9, 8
(') – abbreviation for minute   medium irons – 7, 6, 5
long irons – 4, 3, 2
woods – 3, 5
drives – driver

irons by week 2, and long irons by week 3. Medium- and long-iron shots are hit using a tee to minimize the forces at the elbow observed while taking a divot. Woods are initiated at the end of week 3 and progressed to include drives by the fourth week. The athlete can play nine holes during the end of the fourth week if asymptomatic.

## Summary

The elbow joint is a common site of injury in the athletic population. Injuries vary widely from repetitive microtraumatic injuries to gross macrotraumatic dislocations. A thorough understanding of the sport-specific anatomy and biomechanics of the joint are necessary for a successful clinical examination, assessment, and rehabilitation prescription. Rehabilitation of the elbow, whether post-injury or postsurgical, must follow a progressive and sequential order to ensure that healing tissues are not overstressed. A rehabilitation programme that limits immobilization, achieves full ROM early, progressively restores strength and neuromuscular control, and gradually incorporates sport-specific activities is essential to successfully return athletes to their previous level of competition as quickly and safely as possible, while correcting the kinetic chain faults to prevent re-injury.

## Notes

1 Werner, S., Fleisig, G. S., Dillman, C. J., et al. (1993). Biomechanics of the elbow during baseball pitching. *Journal of Orthopaedic and Sports Physical Therapy, 17*, 274–278.
2 Fleisig, G. S., & Barrentine, S. W. (1995). Biomechanical aspects of the elbow in sports. *Sports Medicine and Arthroscopy Review, 3*, 149–159.
3 Kibler, W. B. (1994). Clinical biomechanics of the elbow in tennis: implications for evaluation and diagnosis. *Medicine and Science in Sports and Exercise, 26*, 1203–1206.
4 Morris, M., Jobe, F. W., Perry, J., et al. (1989). EMG analysis of elbow function in tennis players. *American Journal of Sports Medicine, 17*, 241–247.
5 McCarroll, J. R. & Gioe, T. J. (1982). Professional golfers and the price they pay. *Physician and Sports Medicine, 10*(7), 64–70.
6 McCarroll, J. R. (1985). Golf. In R. C. Schneider et al. (Eds.). *Sports injuries: Mechanisms, prevention, and treatment* (pp. 290–294). Baltimore: Williams and Wilkins.
7 Glazebrook, M. A., Curwin, S., Islam, M. N., et al. (1994). Medial epicondylitis. an electromyographic analysis and an investigation of intervention strategies. *American Journal of Sports Medicine, 22*, 674–679.
8 Zheng, N., Barrentine, S. W., Fleisig, G. S., & Andrews, J. R. (2008). Kinematic analysis of swing in pro and amateur golfers. *International Journal of Sports Medicine, 29*(6), 487–493.
9 Page, P., Frank, C., & Lardner, R. (2010). *Assessment and treatment of muscle imbalance: The Janda approach.* Champaign, IL: Human Kinetics.
10 Kobesova, A., & Kolar, P. (2013). Developmental kinesiology: three levels of motor control in the assessment and treatment of the motor system. *Journal of Bodywork and Movement Therapy, 18*(10), 23–33.
11 Vicenzino, B., Paungmali, A., Buratowski, S., et al. (2001). Specific manipulative therapy treatment for chronic lateral epicondylalgia produces uniquely characteristic hypoalgesia. *Manual Therapy, 6*(4), 205–212.
12 Ackermann, P. W., & Renstrom, P. (2012). Tendinopathy in sport. *Sports Health, 4*(3), 193–201.
13 Maffulli, N., Longo, U. G., & Denaro, V. (2010). Novel approaches for the management of tendinopathy. *Journal Bone Joint Surgery American, 92*(15), 2604–2613.
14 Reinold, M. M., Wilk, K. E., Reed, J., et al. (2002). Interval sport programs: Guidelines for baseball, tennis, and golf. *Journal of Orthopedic and Sports Physical Therapy, 32*, 293–298.

# Chapter 22

# The athletic spine

*Tim Mitchell, Angus Burnett and Peter O'Sullivan*

## Introduction

Spinal pain can be one of the most debilitating musculoskeletal problems for athletes, often resulting in lost training time, impaired performance and, in severe cases, the premature end of an athlete's career. Low back pain (LBP) accounts for the majority of spinal pain and will be the focus of this chapter.

LBP commonly begins during adolescence. Symptoms often persist beyond 12 months.[24] It does not necessarily begin due to sport, but by the age of 17 years, up to 20 per cent report LBP impacts sports participation.[39] There is conflicting evidence regarding the relationship between sport and spinal pain incidence,[15] as LBP risk is associated with both extremes of exercise (too much and too little).[15, 16] The specific physical demands differ among sports, with injury patterns linked with different spinal demands. Sports commonly associated with high LBP prevalence tend to involve high levels of cyclical spinal loading coupled with side bending and or rotation, such as football (all codes), cricket, gymnastics, rowing, hockey and tennis.

LBP is a complex, multifactorial problem that requires skilled, targeted intervention based on each individual's presentation.[37] Current management of spinal pain in general and sporting populations often do not reflect contemporary knowledge or current best practice guidelines.[14,57] To this end, a framework for athletes with spinal pain has been developed to guide assessment and management of spinal pain within the sporting environment. This chapter will overview elements that the sports medicine and performance team should consider on an individual athlete basis to optimize recovery and prevent recurrence.

## A comprehensive format to assess athletes with spinal pain

When spinal pain is impacting training or competition, the treatment, rehabilitation and return to play processes require a comprehensive approach. It is our experience that athletes 'at risk' of developing a persistent disorder are often overlooked if a comprehensive approach (as outlined in Figure 22.1) is not considered.

The critical things to consider from this framework are:

### 1. Injury mechanism

*Traumatic injuries* to the spine seem to be reduced as a result of preventative measures, including protective equipment and rule modification. However, they still occur in tackling sports as well as high dynamic skill and balance sports, such as snow sports and gymnastics. These injuries usually involve combined movements coupled with load and sudden deceleration and

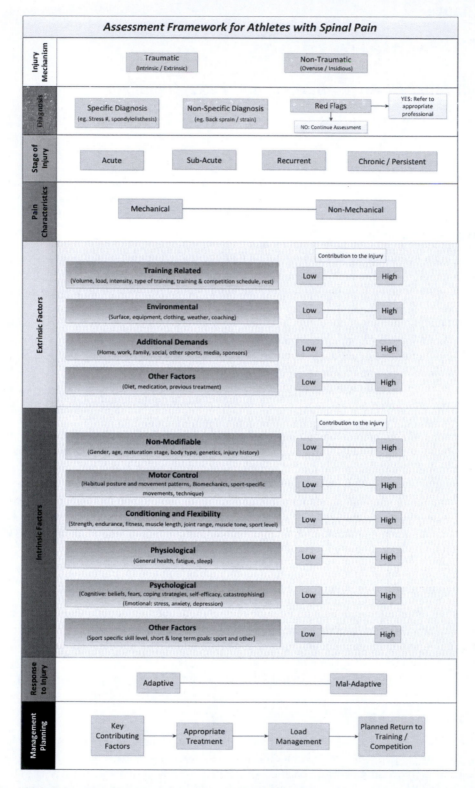

Figure 22.1 Assessment framework for athletes with spinal pain

have the capacity to result in significant injury to both bone and soft-tissue spinal structures. Injury recovery time frames are often predicted by tissue healing rates.

*Non-traumatic injuries* can be linked with either *overuse* or *insidious onset* mechanisms. For the commonly occurring *overuse*-related LBP, there should be a clear link between excess volume- and/or load-related factors which may be coupled with deficits in spine motor control and sensitisation of spinal structures resulting in a gradual onset of symptoms during a specific task/s (e.g. running, jumping, throwing). With this group, the key focus for management involves addressing aspects of training load, motor control factors related to spinal movement and loading, as well as sporting technique.

*Insidious onset* spinal pain occurs when the pain development cannot be linked with trauma or overuse. In this case the athlete may have developed a specific movement pattern or signature (either through training or habitual postures linked to lifestyle-related factors, such as prolonged poor sitting posture), whereby their sport activities further increase tissue strain and sensitisation of spinal structures. This is often coupled with other factors, such as elevated stress, lack of sleep or general malaise, which can further sensitise these structures. When these factors combine, the athlete often reports insidious pain onset. Clear identification of the underlying mechanism/s behind this tissue sensitisation is vital, as this group often fails to return to sport via rest and symptomatic treatment. Directing management towards the underlying lifestyle factors, motor control impairments and targeted conditioning is usually required.

## 2. Diagnosis

In a sporting context, common *specific* LBP disorders are:

- pars stress fracture
- spondyloslisthesis
- disc herniation with radiculopathy.

The proportion of athletes with *specific LBP* is reported to be higher than the general population, due to the high volumes of load placed on the spine during sports.[45] However, a common diagnostic error is to make a patho-anatomical diagnosis based on findings such as degenerative disc and facet joint changes, which are also common in the pain-free pain population.[21] This highlights the need to consider other factors that can contribute to pain sensitisation in LBP.[30]

*Non-specific LBP* occurs when spinal structures become sensitised in the absence of pathology (or the presence of pathology that doesn't correlate with the clinical presentation). This is commonly associated with motor control impairments (often linked to training patterns), resulting in LBP that is mechanically provoked and proportionate to task demands. This is often coupled with other factors related to the sensitisation of spinal structures. In the majority of these cases, management is optimized with consideration of all possible intrinsic and extrinsic contributing factors early in the management process.

## 3. Pain characteristics

Pain with *mechanical* characteristics refers to pain that:

- has a clear and consistent anatomical focus
- has a response that is proportionate to the stimulus
- is clearly provoked and relieved by specific activities and postures.[52]

Pain with *non-mechanical* characteristics refers to pain that is without a clear, consistent anatomical focus, has a response that is disproportionate (absent or exaggerated) to the stimulus and lacks a clear pattern of being provoked or eased by specific activities and postures.[52] Early identification and screening of athletes presenting with LBP with non-mechanical characteristics is important, as it may reflect an underlying inflammatory or neoplastic process or central pain mechanisms, which require very different management from mechanical pain.[27]

## 4. Extrinsic factors

The concept of extrinsic and intrinsic factors contributing to sporting injuries is not new.[58] However, recent research has provided a broader perspective on the range of factors that contribute to injury.[51] Extrinsic factors are external to the individual and are broadly divided into training-related, environmental, additional demands and other potential factors. Individual elements in each category are listed in the framework (Row 5 in Figure 22.1) and are self-explanatory. The influence (or lack) of extrinsic factors on an athlete's presentation should be considered *prior* to physical assessment of the athlete. This information can be gathered from discussion with the athlete, coach and others involved in the athlete's care. A key consideration here is the unique demands of a specific sport (e.g. running, throwing, jumping or lifting).

## 5. Intrinsic factors

Intrinsic factors are factors within the individual that influence the development or maintenance of an injury. These can be divided into non-modifiable factors, motor control (including biomechanics), conditioning and flexibility, physiological, psychological and other factors. Intrinsic factors warranting specific explanation are discussed below. The relevance of these factors for individual athletes can be revealed through questioning the athlete and significant others, combined with physical evaluation.

### Non-modifiable factors

Previous LBP is the strongest predictor of future LBP. Thus, understanding the early course of an athlete's LBP (and injuries to other body regions) can assist management and prevention of recurrence, as the same causative factors are likely still involved. Genetics also strongly influences spinal structure, bone health, the presence of disc degeneration, spondylolisthesis, risk of prolapse and factors such as tissue pain thresholds.[23,33] With this in mind, some athletes may be inherently at greater risk when exposed to high levels of cyclical spinal loading in specific sports.

### Motor control

Individual variations in motor control and spinal biomechanics may place an athlete at greater risk of spinal pain. Some of these postural and movement behaviours are developmental and place individuals at risk for injury,[48] where others reflect maladaptive responses to pain or the threat of pain.[36] Motor control of the spine is highly complex and variable among individuals. This section identifies the key elements considered essential to allow for the analysis of the spine and identify risk for injury. Below are key concepts relating to motor control that are central to the effective diagnosis and management of spinal pain.

Spinal motor control is influenced by a large array of factors, such as:

- genetics and gender
- structural factors, such as connective tissue compliance
- physical factors (task demand, muscle strength, endurance and flexibility)
- lifestyle factors (sleep, activity levels, sedentary behaviours, and diet)
- cognitive and psychological factors.[7,10,32,50]

It involves the integration of a number of body regions moving in multiple planes. Understanding the interaction of the whole kinetic chain (thorax, lumbar spine, pelvis and limb kinematics) assists the ability to analyse likely injury mechanisms for athletes.[5]

There is growing evidence that specific habitual standing (sway, lordotic, laterally shifted and flat back) and sitting postures (slump and hyperlordotic) carry a greater risk for spinal pain.[40,48] These postures are associated with increased LBP risk due to increased end range strain and sub-optimal load transfer strategies linked to altered motor control strategies.[36] Habitual postures provide a platform on which complex movements are built and are predictive of dynamic spinal postures during sporting tasks.[53]

It is critical when analysing static and dynamic lumbar posture that regional differences are considered. The lower and upper lumbar spine have been shown to move independently of each other,[34,53] with the lower lumbar spine being more commonly associated with LBP.[1] The lower lumbar spine is greatly influenced by the pelvis and hips, whereas the upper lumbar spine is influenced by the thorax. Furthermore, the relative movement and control of one region influences that of the other.

Lumbar spine kinematics and patterns of loading are also influenced by combined movements. For example it has been documented that range of axial rotation and side bending in the lumbar spine is reduced when the spine is extended, and the rotation is reduced when it is flexed.[4] This may have implications for tissue loading in sports that involve cyclical loading, where lumbar flexion and/or extension is combined with rotation and side-bending, such as in tennis, cricket and sweep rowing. The combination of poor trunk motor control coupled with high volumes of load may place an athlete at risk of injury. For coaches, clinicians and trainers, a focus on regional spine posture and relative movement of the hips and pelvis during dynamic movement is critical to prevent and manage these LBP disorders.

It is also important to understand how trunk motor control adapts to load and task demand. For example greater levels of trunk muscle co-contraction and intra-abdominal pressure (IAP) occur during high-load and asymmetrical functional loading tasks. This is associated with high levels of spinal stiffness and compressive loading forces on the spine.[31] The motor system must balance the need for spinal control and stability while minimising excessive compression forces known to be risk factors for spinal injury.[41] In sports where there is additional respiratory demand, the motor system needs to adapt to the competing demands of controlling IAP and trunk control while maintaining respiration. Vulnerability to spinal strain may occur where the motor system either fails to control movement effectively (motor control deficit), overestimates the demand resulting in excessive spinal loading (excessive stability) or is unable to coordinate the competing respiratory and stability demands of the sport.

## Conditioning

Conditioning is a key element of optimizing athletic performance and, in some cases, injury prevention. Trunk endurance is influenced by many factors, such as genetics, spinal posture, age, gender, height, psychosocial and lifestyle factors and pain thresholds.[6,28] Deficits in back muscle endurance are associated with increased LBP risk in sports linked to repeated bending such as rowing, and improvements in back muscle endurance reduces this risk.[42] Further, deficits in gluteal muscle strength result in altered patterns of trunk loading and kinematics during single-leg loading, supporting the relationship between lumbo-pelvic conditioning and trunk motor control.[43] Individual aspects, such as strength, endurance, flexibility and available mobility of a region, would need to be considered in context of the athlete's presentation, linking a deficit in these factors with the athlete's pain or altered performance. Also, the concept of relative flexibility can be an important consideration in athletic spinal pain, where regional limitations of flexibility can result in increased spinal loading (see Figure 22.2).

Identification of the athlete's injury mechanism can be achieved through a combination of knowledge of the sport, understanding of the symptoms and assessment of the athlete's function in the specific pain-provocative tasks and postures. See previous work from O'Sullivan[36,37] for more detail about this assessment approach. Examples are provided in Figures 22.3 and 22.4.

Examples of this are sway postures in standing being associated with in increased extension strain in the lower lumbar spine (linked to an impairment of hip or thoracic spine extension) in sports that involve backward bending and rotation, such as ballet, throwing and tennis. Another example is habitual slump sitting, (linked to poor back muscle endurance, limited anterior pelvic rotation and often thoracic extension), predicting greater end-range lumbar flexion strain linked to reduced rotation, such as in cyclists, hockey players and rowers.

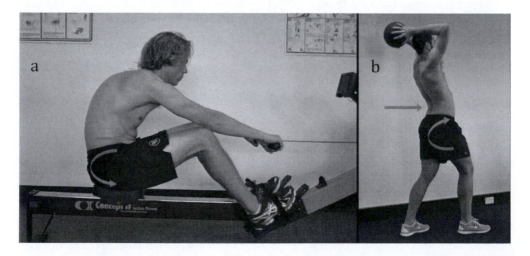

*Figure 22.2* Patterns of movement resulting in increased spinal loading. (a): Posterior pelvic tilt due to sub-optimal movement control patterns ± tight hip extensor muscles can result in increased spinal loading at end range flexion. (b): anterior pelvic tilt due to sub-optimal movement control patterns ± tight flexor muscles can result in increased spinal loading at end-range extension

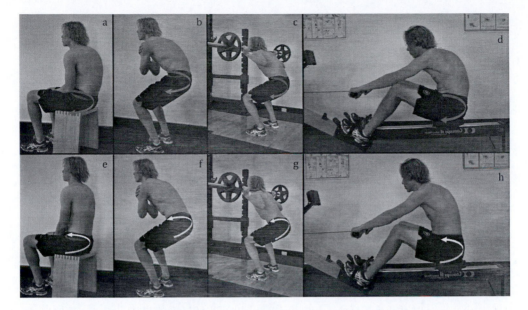

*Figure 22.3* Flexion control impairment resulting in increased thoraco-lumbar flexion in functional tasks and corresponding retraining strategies. (a–d): Habitual thoraco-lumbar flexion with posterior pelvic tilt and flexion of the thorax. (e–h): Functional retaining with emphasis on anterior pelvic tilt and reduction of thoraco-lumbar flexion

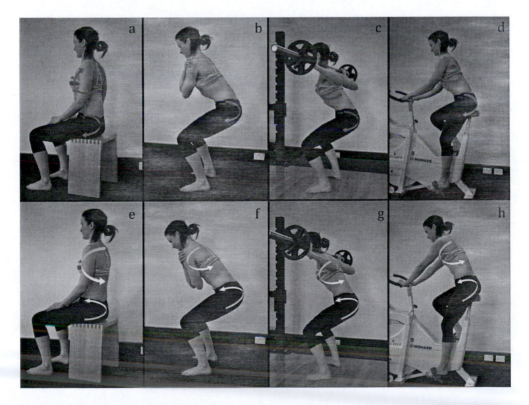

*Figure 22.4* Flexion control impairment with thoracic extension resulting in increased lower lumbar flexion in functional tasks and corresponding retraining strategies. (a–d): Habitual lower lumbar spinal flexion with posterior pelvic tilt and extension of the thorax. (e–h): Functional retaining with emphasis on anterior pelvic tilt and relaxation/flexion through the thorax

In contrast to the lumbar spine, the pelvic girdle is a rigid structure that plays an important role in load bearing and transfer from the lower limbs through the trunk, and vice versa. Motion at the sacroiliac joints is minimal (2–6°) and movement between the pelvic bones is *not* a primary function.[46] Clinical assessment of motion of the sacroiliac joint is neither reliable nor clinically valid,[49] although tests of pain provocation are.[22] Athletes with pelvic girdle pain commonly report inability to tolerate static positions or perform tasks that require load transfer through the pelvis (such as running), whereas pain with movement of the spine and trunk is less common when the sacroiliac joint structures are sensitised.[38] Screening for specific pelvic girdle conditions, such as sacroiliitis and bony stress reactions, is important for athletes presenting with localised pelvic girdle pain.

## Motor responses to pain

While the above section highlights the various motor control strategies that may place athletes without pain at risk of spinal pain, it is also important to understand the motor response to pain and the threat of pain. The nervous system's response to pain, whilst highly variable, is consistently to increase the co-contraction of the muscles of the trunk.[17] In the acute phase, this response may be adaptive as it protects the painful structure from movement and allows for tissue healing, but at the potential cost of increased tissue loading.[17] The greater concern is that these increased patterns of co-contraction persist after the pain has abated and pose a risk for ongoing LBP recurrence.[44]

These patterns are also associated with persistent LBP disorders and represent maladaptive changes that are commonly linked to altered body schema, cognitive and psychological processes (discussed below).[9] In these circumstances, individuals with LBP 'guard' their spine in pain provocative postures (flexed, extended or side-flexed) with increased levels of co-contraction, producing a mechanism for ongoing pain.[9,47] These variable presentations can be broadly sub-grouped based on their direction of pain provocation (extension, flexion, frontal plane or multidirectional), providing targets for effective rehabilitation.[36,42,52] This new knowledge has been slow to be implemented into practice, with the persistence of core stability training that has the potential to, in fact, reinforce these maladaptive patterns.[25,37]

## Physiological factors

This refers primarily to influences on the 'whole system' of the athlete, such as general health, fatigue and poor sleep, often via their influence on immune health and function. This is an area that has gained increased attention in elite sport in recent years, with the introduction of general well-being monitoring as a common component of the management of performance and overuse/overtraining injuries.[20] Further reading on this topic is recommended.[54,55] These factors often influence spinal pain in combination with psychological factors, as outlined below.

## Psychological factors

It is known that psychological factors play a role in the development and persistence of LBP.[36] 'Psychological factors' is an umbrella term that includes cognitive factors (thoughts and beliefs) and affective (emotional) factors.

Cognitive factors relate to how an athlete thinks about and perceives their problem. Beliefs and attitudes can impact positively or negatively on recovery. They are shaped by factors including previous pain experience, culture, familial influences and contextual factors. Consider a minor LBP incident where the amount of perception of threat given to the pain (both by the athlete and health care practitioners) can influence the pain experience. A typical example is how radiological findings are expressed, where a positive message can improve outcome, and a negative impression of scan findings can have the opposite effect.[12] In circumstances of high levels of fear and catastrophising (e.g. believing spinal structure is damaged), the pain response can be magnified beyond the level of tissue damage. This is often associated with exaggerated pain behaviours, such as muscle guarding and antalgic movement patterns. Conversely, some individuals are at risk of further tissue damage and injury due to a lack of attention to noxious stimulus (e.g. an athlete continuing to train with pain associated with lumbar pars stress reaction). Simple observation of an athlete's level of distress relative to the examination findings and history, along with discussion regarding how an athlete perceives their pain, can provide insight into this issue. These issues are discussed in greater detail in chapter 18.

Expectations are another important cognitive factor that have been shown to be a predictor of recovery in back pain.[19] Unrealistic expectations have the potential to adversely affect acceptance and compliance of a management and treatment program. Conversely, positive expectations are associated with more positive outcomes,[35] supporting the idea that appropriate athlete education is an important element of effective management.

Affective factors such as stress, anxiety and depression can magnify pain and disability behaviours.[56] Athletes with elevated psychological distress can be identified through a combination of careful questioning and the use of screening tools (e.g. StartBack questionnaire).[26] The relationship between tissue tolerance and tissue load is highly variable, both within and between individuals.[29] Tissues can become 'pre-sensitized' to normal levels of mechanical loading due to factors including psychological distress, reduced sleep, poor general health, fatigue and genetic factors.[13] Consideration of these factors with individual athletes is important, as they have the potential to reduce tissue tolerance to load and therefore increase the risk of pain and injury associated with higher levels of biomechanical load.

## Management planning

Identification of all contributing intrinsic and extrinsic factors will direct treatment, load management and planning for return to training and competition. From the time the athlete presents with spinal pain, the sports medicine clinician is involved with the athlete's management. However, as the athlete aims to resume performing at pre-injury levels as soon as possible, members of the sports science team need to work side-by-side with the sports medicine clinician(s) for optimal outcomes.

### Managing acute spinal pain

Assuming serious pathology (e.g. spinal fracture) is excluded and after identification of the athlete's injury mechanism, management of acute spinal pain is similar to the management of any acute musculoskeletal injury. The concept of considering acute spinal pain, where there is a clear mechanism of tissue injury, as being equivalent to an acute ankle sprain can be a useful descriptor for the athlete to help remove the common misconception that spinal pain is more dangerous than other injuries.

Key elements of acute management include:

- Reassurance regarding the benign nature of non-specific spinal pain;
- Short period of rest from pain-provocative postures/activities that are associated with adaptive behaviours (3–5 days);
- Medication as appropriate (first choice Paracetamol, second choice NSAIDs);
- Supportive taping in the initial phase to help unload sensitised spinal tissues;
- Clear management plan for athlete's upcoming training and competition;
- Clear communication with relevant groups (e.g. coach , family, etc.)
- Advice to stay active where appropriate, with consideration of alternate exercise options that don't aggravate the athlete's symptoms based on their motor control impairment classification (see section on targeted conditioning below).

## Classification-based cognitive functional therapy

Classification-based cognitive functional therapy is a contemporary approach to managing patients with spinal pain. This approach provides specific targeted intervention directed at the *cognitive* and *functional* factors that have been assessed to be contributing to their condition. Research supports its efficacy for non-specific spinal pain in athletic and non-athletic populations,[42,52] as well as for specific spinal conditions (e.g. spondylolisthesis), where conservative management is indicated.[27]

### Cognitive component

Key cognitive elements include:

- Emphasis on therapeutic alliance
- Education regarding the factors contributing to the ongoing symptoms
- Managing lifestyle, cognitive and affective issues, if present
- Goal setting
- Training motor control through enhanced body awareness with the use of mirrors, videos and movement training
- Teaching the athlete to confront maladaptive behaviours (if present) by providing strategies for optimal spinal loading.

It is essential for athletes to have a clear understanding of their injury to promote active participation in rehabilitation. All staff involved with the athlete should be included at an early stage. Conflicting information is related to poorer outcome from injury, while clear communication and consistent messages are associated with more favourable outcomes.

For athletes identified with strong contributing psychosocial factors (based on screening questionnaires), emphasis must be placed on this aspect of the intervention, with early referral to a sports psychologist as appropriate. This process should be openly discussed with the athlete involved as an active participant. This aspect should be revisited throughout rehabilitation and integrated into the functional aspects of management as the athlete is challenged and exposed to previously provocative tasks.

## Functional component

The aim of functional intervention is to provide the athlete with strategies to normalise their postural and movement behaviours as quickly as possible. This involves three stages: specific movement training, functional integration and targeted conditioning. Specific focus and rate of progression through the stages will be dependent on the individual's presentation.

### Stage 1: Specific movement training

This aspect is directed by the athlete's individual presentation. If the athlete is unable to relax their trunk muscles, they are initially instructed on diaphragm breathing in relaxed postures, such as lying, sitting and standing, prior to movement retraining. Targeted functional postural and movement retraining of painful postures and activities is then based on their movement classification.[36] This approach follows a 'graded exposure' model (see Figure 22.5), where the athlete is trained in a graduated manner using feedback (visual mirrors, video footage, mental imagery and awareness of body responses, such as breath-holding and muscle guarding).

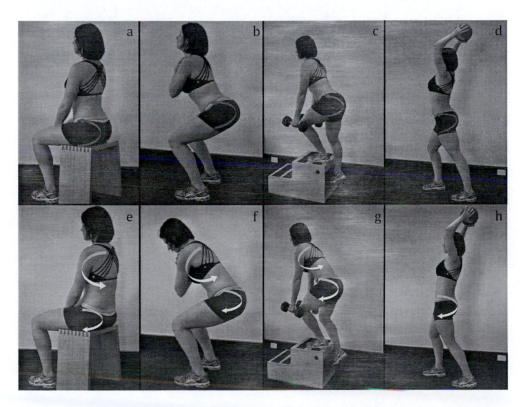

*Figure 22.5* Active extension control impairment resulting in increased lower lumbar extension in functional tasks and corresponding retraining strategies. (a–d): Habitual lower lumbar spinal extension with anterior pelvic tilt and extension of the thorax. (e–h): Functional retaining with emphasis on posterior pelvic tilt and relaxation/flexion through the thorax

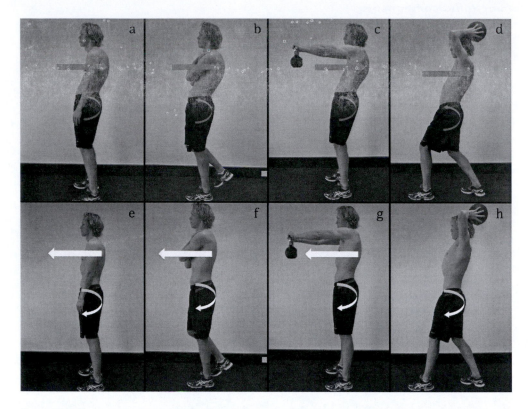

*Figure 22.6* Passive extension control impairment resulting in increased lower lumbar extension in functional tasks and corresponding retraining strategies. (a–d): Habitual lower lumbar spinal extension with anterior pelvic tilt and posterior translation of the thorax with thoracic flexion. (e–h): Functional retaining with emphasis on posterior pelvic tilt and anterior translation and extension of the thorax

Athletes with a major contribution of maladaptive motor control impairment are trained to modify their pain-provocative postures and movement patterns to reduce pain whilst performing the task. For example athletes with a maladaptive flexion 'control impairment' provoked by sitting, bending and lifting are taught to change their pattern of movement to reduce lumbo-sacral flexion during these tasks. They are first taught to dissociate lumbo-pelvic from thoracic movement in sitting to reduce lumbo-pelvic flexion. This is then progressed to bending and lifting with a focus on facilitating hip/pelvic motion to promote neutral lordosis and thoracic flexion in a relaxed manner.[36] See Figure 22.5.

In contrast, an athlete with an active extension control disorder is first taught to relax their spinal muscles and posterior-tilt the pelvis in order to reduce the lumbar lordosis, which is then progressed into functionally specific postures particular to pain provocation linked to the sport. See Figure 22.6. Athletes with a major contribution of maladaptive *movement impairment* require a different management approach, which is described elsewhere.[36]

## Stage 2: Functional integration

Simple low-load exercises are gradually progressed towards higher load and more complex functional-, then sports-specific exercises, as the athlete gains confidence and control in performing the tasks. No more than three or four exercises should be given at any one time. This challenges each athlete to perform previously provocative activities and postures using new functionally enhancing movement behaviours. This is augmented by dynamic practical demonstration of the postures or movement by the clinician, the use of mirrors so they could view their own spines to enhance body schema awareness, written instruction and photographed/videoed exercise routines with correct technique. Typical examples include retraining of base sports-specific postures, such as supine lying, sitting, kneeling and standing, depending on the sport.

## Stage 3: Targeted conditioning

Each athlete's level of conditioning needs to be maintained where possible by considering the movement classification of the athlete's spinal pain. Specifically, the athlete should be exercising in non-provocative spinal postures. For extension overloading (cycling, rowing, arm ergo in relaxed spinal posture), flexion overloading (walking, cross-trainer, swimming, water running) or multidirectional overloading (will depend upon the dominant impairment). Early return to fitness activities can minimise time out of sport for an athlete and is best managed through this individualised exercise modification approach.

A similar approach is taken with return-to-strength and conditioning exercises. While provocative activities are being retrained, other strength and conditioning exercises can be included as long as they involve non-provocative spinal postures or movements.

A good rule of thumb is, if the exercises are pain-free and can be performed with appropriate motor control and biomechanics, then they are probably safe. This process involves liaison with strength and conditioning, rehabilitation and coaching staff to ensure the appropriate rate of exercise progression is consistent.

While general base strengthening exercises are important, when considering athlete rehabilitation or injury prevention, the aim should be to produce a program that develops base, functional and sports-specific elements specific to the athlete's individual skill level, conditioning level, sport and functional deficits. In order to improve performance, the emphasis needs to be on training for the specific tasks involved in combination with general strengthening exercises.[2,3]

High-load exercises, such as squats and deadlifts, are commonly used for high-level athletes requiring optimal strength and power for performance. It is our experience that these exercises can be appropriate for athletes recovering from spinal pain. Importantly, recent unpublished data supports that the optimal posture in terms of maximal leg power and minimal spinal load involves a neutral (not lordotic) lumbar spine. Retraining of such exercises in athletes with spinal pain requires consideration of their individual pain-provocative spinal postures as outlined in Figure 22.6.

## Assessment and monitoring tools

Given that the focus of the athlete with spinal pain is their individual functional impairments, the most adaptable monitoring tool is the patient-specific functional scale.[18] This scale can be used to determine the level of functional disability with tasks relevant to each athlete. For example, if a cyclist has LBP, they may report symptoms with cycling uphill, sitting and, if severe, sleeping. Each of these items can be scored in relation to their ability to perform each task to full capacity. Re-evaluation may then be conducted at appropriate intervals to determine if the athlete's management plan is achieving the key outcome – return to function.

## Return to play considerations

Due to the varying clinical presentation of spinal pain, algorithmic approaches to return to play are lacking in evidence.[11] However, return to sport could follow a general return-to-play model,[8] a process detailed more in chapters 1 and 18. Allowing athletes to return to play or train with on going symptoms will usually result in delayed recovery. As spinal pain significantly impacts motor responses of both the trunk and limbs, there is high risk of developing compensatory motor patterns if the athlete continues to train or compete with pain.

## Prevention of spinal pain

Programmes that follow a recipe-based approach aimed at preventing new or recurrent episodes of spinal pain in athletes are generally unsuccessful. This is likely due to a number of reasons:

- The incorrect assumption that predictors of spinal pain are consistent across individuals;
- Lack of sub-classification of spinal pain based on potential multidimensional mechanisms;
- Difficulty for coaches in striking the balance between setting training volume and intensity to avoid injury, but still maintaining/improving performance.

Arguably, prevention of spinal pain in athletes should target athletes who have had spinal pain before or individuals in high-risk sports. In such individuals, rehabilitation targeted at specific functional deficits may be effective at reducing pain and also improving physical performance. A further key consideration for overuse spinal pain is load management. Tissues are vulnerable to injury when they are overloaded, which can be from excessive levels of load on healthy tissues, or normal levels of loading of vulnerable tissues. From factors outlined earlier, risk of athletes developing spinal pain from repetitive cyclical loading beyond the tissue's capacity to adapt or recover from that loading is high. Therefore, monitoring the athlete's whole well-being along with physical demands is essential.

## The team approach works

In a recent study by Perich,[42] adolescent rowers showed a 61 per cent reduction in LBP during the rowing season, as well as an increase in key performance parameters, following a cognitive functional rehabilitation and prevention programme. Rowers were individually assessed in key aspects of rowing related LBP, including sitting posture, rowing movement patterns, lower-limb muscle flexibility and endurance and cardiovascular fitness. Individual targeted exercise programs were developed along with education of the rowers, parents and coaches regarding key aspects of spinal pain in rowing. In addition, the pre-season training programme and philosophy regarding athlete management for spinal pain were adjusted with cohesive sports medicine and sports science team involvement. This is an example of how multifaceted team approaches can provide the best outcomes for injury prevention and management programmess targeted at specific sports.

## Summary

Spinal pain is a complex multifactorial problem that requires skilled, targeted intervention based on each individual's presentation. In the sporting environment, where the focus of spinal pain management is often on patho-anatomical diagnosis, core stability training and correction of biomechanical faults, a shift towards a broader multifactorial approach, is required. A framework for athletes with spinal pain has been developed to guide assessment and management of spinal pain, based on contemporary evidence. Consideration of all aspects of the framework relevant to the individual athlete's presentation, in the context of a cohesive team environment, will help guide optimal management.

## Notes

1 Adams, M. A., Bogduk, N., Burton, K., et al. (2012). *The Biomechanics of Back Pain* (3rd ed.). Edinburgh: Churchill Livingstone.

2 Alfieri, F. M., Riberto, M., Gatz, L. S., et al. (2010). Functional mobility and balance in community-dwelling elderly submitted to multisensory versus strength exercises. *Journal of Clinical Interventions in Aging, 5*,181–5.

3 Beard, D. J., Dodd, C. A., Trundle, H. R., et al. (1994). Proprioception enhancement for anterior cruciate ligament deficiency: A prospective randomised trial of two physiotherapy regimes. *The Bone & Joint Journal, 76*, 654–9.

4 Burnett, A., O'Sullivan, P., Ankarberg, L., et al. (2008). Lower lumbar spine axial rotation is reduced in end-range sagittal postures when compared to a neutral spine posture. *Manual Therapy 13*, 300–6.

5 Campbell, A., Straker, L., O'Sullivan, P., et al. (2013). Lumbar loading in the elite adolescent tennis serve: A link to low back pain. *Medicine & Science in Sports & Exercise, 45*(8), 1562–1568.

6 Campbell, A. C., Briggs, A. M., O'Sullivan, P. B., et al. (2011). An exploration of the relationship between back muscle endurance and familial, physical, lifestyle, and psychosocial factors in adolescents and young adults. *Journal of Orthopaedic & Sports Physical Therapy, ,41*, 486–95.

7 Chany, A. M., Parakkat, J., Yang, G., et al. (2006). Changes in spine loading patterns throughout the workday as a function of experience, lift frequency, and personality. *The Spine Journal, 6*, 296–305.

8 Creighton, D. W., Shrier, I., Shultz, R., et al. (2010). Return-to-play in sport: A decision-based model. *Clinical Journal of Sport Medicine, 20*, 379–85.

9 Dankaerts, W., O'Sullivan, P., Burnett, A., et al. (2009). Discriminating healthy controls and two clinical subgroups of nonspecific chronic low back pain patients using trunk muscle activation and lumbosacral kinematics of postures and movements: A statistical classification model. *Spine, 34*, 1610–8.

10 Davis, K. G., Marras, W. S., Heaney, C. A., et al. (2002). The impact of mental processing and pacing on spine loading: 2002 Volvo Award in biomechanics. *Spine, 27*, 2645–53.

11 Eddy, D., Congeni, J., & Loud, K. (2005). A review of spine injuries and return to play. *Clinical Journal of Sports Medicine, 15*, 453–8.

12 Flynn, T. W., Smith, B., & Chou, R. (2011). Appropriate use of diagnostic imaging in low back pain: A reminder that unnecessary imaging may do as much harm as good. *Journal of Orthopaedic & Sports Physical Therapy, 41*, 838–46.

13  Gatchel, R. J., Peng, Y. B., Peters, M. L., et al. (2007). The biopsychosocial approach to chronic pain: Scientific advances and future directions. *Psychological Bulletin, 133*, 581–624.

14  Hendrick, P., Mani, R., Bishop, A., et al. (2013). Therapist knowledge, adherence and use of low back pain guidelines to inform clinical decisions – A national survey of manipulative and sports physiotherapists in New Zealand. *Manual Therapy, 18*, 136–42.

15  Heneweer, H., Staes, F., Aufdemkampe, G., et al. (2011). Physical activity and low back pain: a systematic review of recent literature. *European Spine Journal, 20*, 826–45.

16  Heneweer, H., Vanhees, L., & Picavet, H. S. (2009). Physical activity and low back pain: A U-shaped relation? *Pain, 143*, 21–5.

17  Hodges, P. W., Coppieters, M. W., MacDonald, D., et al. (2013). New insight into motor adaptation to pain revealed by a combination of modelling and empirical approaches. *European Journal of Pain, 17*, 1138–46.

18  Horn, K. K., Jennings, S., Richardson, G., et al. (2012). The patient-specific functional scale: Psychometrics, clinimetrics, and application as a clinical outcome measure. *Journal of Orthopaedic & Sports Physical Therapy, 42*, 30–42.

19  Iles, R. A., Davidson, M., & Taylor, N. F. (2008). Psychosocial predictors of failure to return to work in non-chronic non-specific low back pain: A systematic review. *Occupational and Environmental Medicine, 65*, 507–17.

20  Kellmann, M. (2010). Preventing overtraining in athletes in high-intensity sports and stress/recovery monitoring. *Scandinavian Journal of Medicine & Science in Sports, 20*, 95–102.

21  Kjaer, P., Leboeuf-Yde, C., Korsholm, L., et al. (2005). Magnetic resonance imaging and low back pain in adults: A diagnostic imaging study of 40-year-old men and women. *Spine, 30*, 1173–80.

22  Laslett, M., Aprill, C. N., McDonald, B., et al. (2005). Diagnosis of sacroiliac joint pain: Validity of individual provocation tests and composites of tests. *Manual Therapy, 10*, 207–18.

23  Leboeuf-Yde C. (2004). Back pain – individual and genetic factors. *Journal of Electromyography and Kinesiology, 14*, 129–33.

24  Leboeuf-Yde, C., & Kyvik, K. O. (1998). At what age does low back pain become a common problem? A study of 29,424 individuals aged 12–41 years. *Spine, 23*, 228–34.

25  Lederman, E. (2010). The myth of core stability. *J Bodyw Mov Ther, 14*, 84–98.

26  Linton, S. J., Nicholas, M., & MacDonald, S. (2011). Development of a short form of the Orebro Musculoskeletal Pain Screening Questionnaire. *Spine, 36*, 1891–5.

27  Malfait, A. M., & Schnitzer, T. J. (2013). Towards a mechanism-based approach to pain management in osteoarthritis. *Nature Reviews Rheumatology, 9*(11), 654–664.

28  Mannion, A. F., O'Riordan, D., Dvorak, J., et al. (2011). The relationship between psychological factors and performance on the Biering-Sorensen back muscle endurance test. *The Spine Journal, 11*, 849–57.

29  Marras, W. S. (2012). The complex spine: The multidimensional system of causal pathways for low-back disorders. *Human Factors, 54*, 881–9.

30  Maus, T. (2010). Imaging the back pain patient. *Physical Medicine & Rehabilitation Clinics of North America, 21*, 725–66.

31  McGill, S. M., McDermott, A., & Fenwick, C. M. (2009). Comparison of different strongman events: Trunk muscle activation and lumbar spine motion, load, and stiffness. *Journal of Strength and Conditioning Research, 23*, 1148–61.

32  McHardy, A., & Pollard, H. (2005). Muscle activity during the golf swing. *British Journal of Sports Medicine, 39*, 799–804.

33  Miaskowski, C. (2009). Understanding the genetic determinants of pain and pain management. *Seminars in Oncology Nursing, 25*, S1–7.

34  Mitchell, T., O'Sullivan, P. B., Burnett, A. F., et al. (2008). Regional differences in lumbar spinal posture and the influence of low back pain. *BMC Musculoskelet Disorders, 9*, 152.

35  Mondloch, M. V., Cole, D. C., & Frank, J. W. (2001). Does how you do depend on how you think you'll do? A systematic review of the evidence for a relation between patients' recovery expectations and health outcomes. *Canadian Medical Association Journal, 165*, 174–9.

36  O'Sullivan, P. (2005). Diagnosis and classification of chronic low back pain disorders: Maladaptive movement and motor control impairments as underlying mechanism. *Manual Therapy, 10*, 242–55.

37  O'Sullivan, P. (2012). It's time for change with the management of non-specific chronic low back pain. *British Journal of Sports Medicine, 46*, 224–7.

38  O'Sullivan, P. B, & Beales, D. J. (2007). Diagnosis and classification of pelvic girdle pain disorders, Part 2: Illustration of the utility of a classification system via case studies. *Manual Therapy, 12*, e1–e12.

39  O'Sullivan, P. B., Beales, D. J., Smith, A. J., et al. (2012). Low back pain in 17-year-olds has substantial impact and represents an important public health disorder: A cross-sectional study. *BMC Public Health, 12*, 100.

40  O'Sullivan, P. B., Smith, A. J., Beales, D. J., et al. (2011). Association of biopsychosocial factors with degree of slump in sitting posture and self-report of back pain in adolescents: A cross-sectional study. *Physical Therapy, 91*, 470–83.

41  Parkinson, R. J., & Callaghan, J. P. (2009). The role of dynamic flexion in spine injury is altered by increasing dynamic load magnitude. *Clinical Biomechanics, 24*, 148–54.

42  Perich, D., Burnett, A., O'Sullivan, P., et al. (2011). Low back pain in adolescent female rowers: A multi-dimensional intervention study. *Knee Surgery Sports Traumatology and Arthroscopy, 19*, 20–9.

43  Popovich, J. M. Jr., & Kulig, K. (2012). Lumbopelvic landing kinematics and EMG in women with contrasting hip strength. *Medicine & Science in Sports & Exercise, 44*, 146–53.

44  Radebold, A., Cholewicki, J., Panjabi, M. M., et al. (2000). Muscle response pattern to sudden trunk loading in healthy individuals and in patients with chronic low back pain. *Spine, 25*, 947–54.

45  Ranson, C. A., Burnett, A. F., King, M., et al. (2008). The relationship between bowling action classification and three-dimensional lower trunk motion in fast bowlers in cricket. *Journal of Sports Sciences, 26*, 267–76.

46  Ridgeway, K., & Silvernail, J. (2012). Innominate 3D motion modeling: Biomechanically interesting, but clinically irrelevant. *Manual Therapy, 17*, e11–12.

47  Sheeran, L., Sparkes, V., Caterson, B., et al. (2012). Spinal position sense and trunk muscle activity during sitting and standing in nonspecific chronic low back pain: Classification analysis. *Spine, 37*, E486–95.

48  Smith, A., O'Sullivan, P., & Straker, L. (2008). Classification of sagittal thoraco-lumbo-pelvic alignment of the adolescent spine in standing and its relationship to low back pain. *Spine, 33*, 2101–7.

49  Sutton, C., Nono, L., Johnston, R. G., et al. (2013). The effects of experience on the inter-reliability of osteopaths to detect changes in posterior superior iliac spine levels using a hidden heel wedge. *Journal of Bodywork and Movement Therapies, 17*, 143–50.

50  Tijtgat, P., Vanrenterghem, J., Bennett, S. J., et al. (2012). Implicit advance knowledge effects on the interplay between arm movements and postural adjustments in catching. *Neuroscience Letters, 518*, 117–21.

51  van Wilgen, C. P., & Verhagen, E. A. (2012). A qualitative study on overuse injuries: The beliefs of athletes and coaches. *Journal of Science and Medicine in Sport, 15*, 116–21.

52  Vibe Fersum, K., O'Sullivan, P., Skouen, J., et al. (2012). Efficacy of classification-based cognitive functional therapy in patients with non-specific chronic low back pain: A randomized controlled trial. *European Journal of Pain, 17*(6), 916–928.

53  Wade, M., Campbell, A., Smith, A., et al. (2012). Investigation of spinal posture signatures and ground reaction forces during landing in elite female gymnasts. *Journal of Applied Biomechanics, 28*, 677–86.

54  Walsh, N. P., Gleeson, M., Pyne, D. B., et al. (2011). Position statement. Part two: Maintaining immune health. *Exercise Immunology Review, 17*, 64–103.

55  Walsh, N. P., Gleeson, M., Shephard, R. J., et al. (2011). Position statement. Part one: Immune function and exercise. *Exercise Immunology Review, 17*, 6–63.

56  Wiech, K., & Tracey, I. (2009). The influence of negative emotions on pain: Behavioral effects and neural mechanisms. *NeuroImage, 47*, 987–94.

57  Williams, C. M., Maher, C. G., Hancock, M. J., et al. (2010). Low back pain and best practice care: A survey of general practice physicians. *Archives of Internal Medicine, 170*, 271–7.

58  Williams, J.P.G. (1971). Aetiologic classification of sports injuries. *British Journal of Sports Medicine, 4*, 228–30.

# Chapter 23

# The athletic hip and groin

*Enda King*

## Introduction

Hip and groin pain provides a massive challenge for all those involved in the physical preparation and rehabilitation of athletes at all levels. Diagnostically, the region is puzzling due to the complex and overlapping nature of the anatomy, which is further compounded by the fact that there is a poor understanding of the adverse mechanics that predispose the athlete to injury in the first place. On top of this, the nature and significance of what may appear to be 'pathology' when assessed radiologically is still unclear. The end result is that the athlete often suffers from inappropriate diagnosis and poor management. Moreover, there is a lack of definitive rehabilitation guidelines and return to play criteria to guide efficient and successful injury management. This in turn leads to prolonged absence from participation and injury recurrence.

The aim of this chapter is to provide structure and guidelines in a number of areas:

i)   The differential diagnosis of athletic hip and groin pain;
ii)  The pathomechanics that predispose and drive pathology;
iii) The development of robust and comprehensive physical assessments to identify factors driving pain and pathology in the region;
iv)  The development of an athlete back to optimal performance after hip and groin issues.

## The presenting problem

Both the incidence and prevalence of groin and hip injuries in sport have increased over the last decade, with the highest-risk sports being multidirectional field sports such as the various football codes, as well as ice hockey and tennis.[1,2] All these sports share common multidirectional movement demands and have seen large increases in the physical burdens of the game, as well as required training loads.[2,3]

Although acute injury to the hip and/or groin may occur, as a result of slipping or through direct contact, it is much more common for pathology in this region to have an insidious onset associated with a more chronic accumulation of load over time. The most commonly aggravating activities are high load movements, such as acceleration, deceleration, cutting and kicking, that are frequently involved in these sports. Pain may be located in one and often a combination of the following locations:

*   Low abdomen
*   Inner groin

- Pubic region
- Lateral hip.

Typically, symptoms commence gradually and often ease during warm-up, only to become more severe following rest, especially upon rising from bed the following morning. The gradual onset means that athletes often continue to compete even though they are experiencing symptoms, and therefore the true prevalence of the problem may be underreported.

## Differential diagnosis

Making a definitive diagnosis in the hip and groin is complicated for a number of reasons:

i)  The complex and overlapping anatomy with a number of structures that can produce symptoms in the same region, sometimes concurrently;
ii)  The vast array of terms that are used to describe pain to the same structures;
iii)  The level of 'pathology' in the region reported on MRI in asymptomatic athletes.

The key to navigating around all these obstacles, therefore, is to differentiate between the anatomical diagnosis and the biomechanical diagnosis. The *anatomical diagnosis* allows accurate identification of the symptomatic structure(s), and ensures the presentation is suitable for rehabilitation. The *biomechanical diagnosis* identifies movement and control deficits that are driving the athlete's symptoms. It is the biomechanical diagnosis that explains how there can be multiple painful structures in the one area concurrently.

It is important to realize that, for any one anatomical diagnosis, there can be many different biomechanical presentations. For example two athletes may have the same diagnosis (e.g. pubic bone oedema) but present very differently biomechanically. The question is therefore: 'Is the most efficient recovery achieved by prescribing a program for pubic bone oedema, or one that resolves the biomechanical deficits which are causing the pubic overload?'

> Anatomical diagnosis is identifying the victim; biomechanical diagnosis is identifying the culprit.

## Anatomical diagnosis – identifying the victim

It is beyond the scope of this chapter to go into this area in detail, but the anatomy and diagnostic tests are covered in detail in many sports medicine textbooks. Care should be taken when interpreting 'diagnostic tests' in the region given the overlapping anatomy. For example the groin squeeze test will load the adductors but will also load iliopsoas, the pubic bone, the symphysis pubis and the rectus abdominus insertion. The three most commonly used positions are 0° (longest lever), 45° (highest adductor load) and 90° (abdominal stability component as feet off the ground).[4] Similarly, pain presenting during flexion, adduction and internal rotation (FADIR) of the hip has been shown to be diagnostic of labral tear and hip impingement but is also painful with an irritable iliopsoas.[5] In fact, the *absence* rather than the presence of symptoms during these tests may be of greater relevance, as it clears the presence of any hip pathology.[5]

Table 23.1

**Differential and synonymous diagnoses in the hip and groin**

| Hip | Pubic | Adductor | Abdominal |
|---|---|---|---|
| Femoracetabular impingement | Osteitis pubis | Adductor tendinopathy | Gilmore's groin |
| Labral tear | Pubic bone stress | Adductor cleft pain | Sportsman's hernia |
| CAM lesion | Pubic symphysis instability | Anterior plate pain | Posterior inguinal wall insufficiency |
| Chondral lesion | Athletic pubalgia | Adductor enthesopathy | Rectus abdominus tendinopathy |

Equally challenging is navigating through the vast array of labels that have been given to various pathologies and dysfunctions in the hip and groin region, much of which are synonymous and therefore tautological (Table 23.1).

Previous literature has grouped anatomical diagnosis into hip joint, abdominal, adductor, pubic and iliopsoas groups to reduce some of the nomenclature uncertainty,[6] and yet, despite this attempt, there is still confusion. How, for example, do you explain to an athlete that multiple different surgical procedures exist to treat a sportsman's hernia when there is actually no hernia present at all?

Appropriate anatomical diagnosis will identify the painful anatomical structure, the presence of pathology referring symptoms to the anterior pelvis and hip (for example lumbar spine), and indicate whether rehabilitation is appropriate for the presenting problem. For example symptoms emanating from the muscultendionus and osseous structures of the anterior pelvis and groin whose symptoms are modulated by load will be very responsive to rehabilitation.

### The use of MRI in finding the victim

Whilst MRI can be of great use when targeting the 'victim', it does present us with the challenge of determining what are relevant and what are incidental findings in both symptomatic and asymptomatic athletes. Pubic bone stress has been shown to be highly prevalent in asymptomatic multidirectional field athletes;[7] therefore, there is a high chance that should we go looking for a problem we are likely to find one, even if it does not relate to the athlete's symptoms.

> It is essential that MRI is used to confirm the anatomical diagnosis *following* a thorough clinical examination, as opposed to simply using the scan as the main diagnostic tool.

### Using MRI to diagnose impingement

The greatest diagnostic challenge surrounding the relevance of 'pathology' on MRI is at the hip joint, especially in relation to femoroacetabular impingement (FAI). FAI refers to a dynamic abutment of the femoral head in the acetabulum and often involves a subset of morphological changes in hip known as CAM and pincer lesions.[8] CAM lesions refer to changes in the amount of clearance between the femoral head and neck due to an osseous bump on the femoral neck (Ganz lesion). Pincer lesions, on the other hand, refer to an over-coverage of the acetabulum-restricting free passage of the femoral head in the acetabulum. These morphological variants can commence development through adolescence, and their presence means that the athlete has little margin for error in their hip control and high-speed mechanics before impingement occurs.

Care must be taken prior to rushing in to intervene on the basis of these anatomical variants, however, as they have a high prevalence in asymptomatic athletic populations.[9] Indeed, neither CAM nor pincer lesions are diagnoses *per se*, rather descriptions of hip morphology. Whether or not these lesions lead to impingement cannot be diagnosed by a static image, since impingement is dynamic in nature. Bone oedema on the femoral neck, acetabular rim and labral tears are suggestive of the consequences of dynamic impingement, but these are not always present.

### Structural and dynamic impingement

What we should move to, therefore, is an appreciation that there are effectively two forms of impingement: structural and dynamic. *Structural impingement* occurs as a result of the altered hip morphology, especially CAM or pincer lesions. *Dynamic impingement* occurs when there is a failure to maintain control of head of the femur in the acetabulum or avoid end-range articulation during movement. Think of it this way: structural impingement is the truck being too high to pass under the bridge (or the bridge being too low for the truck), whereas dynamic impingement occurs when there is faulty driving leading to the truck clipping the walls of the bridge.

It is important to note that one can lead to the other. Take, for example, the hip joint of an athlete who, through heavy resistance training and poor single-leg control during cutting, running and landing, drives his hip into end-range flexion, adduction and internal rotation repeatedly (dynamic impingement). The body lays down extra bone in response to this load (osteophytes/ CAM lesion), which reduces the clearance of the femoral head, leading to further abutment (structural impingement). Rehabilitation and restoration of dynamic hip control is key to resolving hip symptoms while minimizing the further development of structural impingement.

> Failure to correct dynamic impingement results in increasing hip morphological changes, and as a result, earlier and worsening impingement over time, thus reducing the athlete's 'room for error'. Moreover, surgical intervention to 'correct' this CAM lesion by removing it is unlikely to be successful if the dynamic impingement is not corrected, as the bony stress will reoccur and the CAM lesion will reform.

## Biomechanical assessment of hip and groin – identifying the culprit

Athletic groin pain and hip injury are driven by insufficient control of multi-joint, multiplanar athletic movement. Indeed, for every anatomical diagnosis there can be multiple different biomechanical diagnoses. It is essential to identify all the factors contributing to the athlete's overload and to individualise our management plans based on these specific issues for the most successful and efficient rehabilitation. Optimal performance in the region requires appropriate function of the supporting hip and pelvic musculature to balance load transfer around the hip and pelvis while optimizing multiplanar control throughout the kinetic chain during high-speed multidirectional movement. This keeps the hip and pelvis in relatively neutral positions, especially in the frontal and transverse planes, for optimal loading of the articular and musculoskeletal structures (i.e. avoid excessive pelvic drop, hip abduction/trunk sway).

3D motion capture is the gold standard when analysing high-speed sporting movements. The testing protocol should provide a progressive neuromuscular challenge looking at all aggravating activities, including, jumping, landing, changes of direction (planned and reactive) and kicking. Assessing these sports-specific movements and understanding their link to injury and performance is key to successful outcome. Furthermore, analysing the entire kinetic chain during these tasks will help shed light on the forces, moments and torques placed on the musculotendinous structures and joints around the hip and pelvis.

Take cutting, for example, where athletes often display aberrant movement patterns that increase shearing forces within the hip joint and overload of the musculotendious structures. An increase in trunk sway and rotation away from the direction of intended travel during stance phase has loading implications for the lateral ankle, knee, hip and spine. In particular, it can lead to increased loading toward end-range hip abduction, altered positioning of the resultant hip vector through the acetabulum and a high eccentric load through the adductors and abdominals. These patterns of kinetic linkage when cutting, jumping and landing are outlined in Table 23.2, along with the influence they have on the hip and supporting muscles.

*Table 23.2* Kinetic linkage deficits during jumping, cutting and landing

| | | Hip | Musculotendinous |
|---|---|---|---|
| Trunk-on-pelvis | Increased hip and trunk flexion | Anterior impingement & pubic bone overload | – |
| | Increased trunk sway | Lateral impingement | Adductor longus overload |
| | Increased trunk rotation | – | Rectus abominus and hip flexor overload |
| Pelvis-on-hip | Excess pelvic tilt | Anterior impingement & pubic bone overload | Rectus abdominus & adductor longus overload |
| | Hip internal rotation/ pelvic rotation | Antero-superior impingement & pubic bone overload | Adductor longus overload |
| | Pelvic drop/hip adduction | Anterio-superior impingement & pubic bone overload | Adductor longus overload |
| Knee | Valgus/abduction | Anterio-superior impingement & pubic bone overload | Adductor longus overload |
| | Flexion | Increased hip & pubic loading | – |
| Ankle | Excessive DF | Increased hip & pubic loading | – |
| Foot | External rotation relative to pelvis | Lateral impingement | Increased adductor loading |

Of course, not everyone will have access to a 3D biomechanics laboratory, but that does not mean that these movements should not be assessed with high-definition cameras, which are more readily available. Although accurate measurement, individual joint loads and multiplanar observation will not be possible, moderate to gross deficiencies should be detectable.

## Components of rehabilitation

Once a comprehensive assessment has been carried out, an individualized program can be devised to guide an athlete back to optimal performance. Each program is specific to the athlete's biomechanical deficits, not their anatomical diagnosis and should be phase-based and progressive in design (Figure 23.1).

Whilst it is not imperative that each level of the programme is completed in its entirety before progressing to the next phase, it is important to realize that optimal performance at one level is not possible without competence at a previous level (for example modifying the deleterious influence of poor/uncontrolled lordotic/kyphotic posture on running biomechanics).

A key point during retraining is to ensure all exercises are carried out in the absence of pain. It makes little sense to further stress a joint or musculotendinous structure that is already being overloaded. This does not mean, however, that we should simply provide the athlete with analgesic medications prior to rehabilitation, since pain is often the best guide to the quality of the exercises being carried out. For this reason steroid injection in the region may hinder the process as much as help it, as time is often lost due to post-injection soreness that is better used with rehabilitation and symptom reduction may falsely reflect athlete progress.

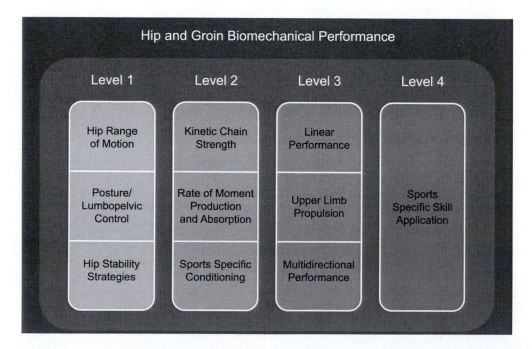

*Figure 23.1* Hip and Groin Biomechanical Performance components

It is also essential to review the key outcome measures (hip range, pain provocation, posture, neuromuscular control) at the end of every session. Appropriate exercise selection and execution will ensure that they have been progressed during every session.

Pain provocation tests provide information regarding the irritability of the athlete's symptoms, efficacy of rehabilitation and readiness to progress to higher load training. The cross-over test is carried out in the Thomas test position. If resisted hip flexion on the lower leg reproduces symptoms on the opposite side, it reflects a high level of irritability. The squeeze test is also useful at assessing load tolerance across the anterior pelvic ring. It can be carried out at 0°, 45° and 90°. Using a pressure cuff can identify the load at the onset of symptoms and the maximum pressure that can be exerted. Effective exercise prescription should see improvements in squeeze test at the end of every rehabilitation session.

## Level I

### Posture/lumbo-pelvic control

Postural control is a key foundation area that is often overlooked during rehabilitation. Restoration of neutral posture is achieved through exercise selection and postural advice. Increased anterior tilt dramatically reduces hip flexion/adduction/internal rotation range of movement, resulting in hip impingement earlier in range.[10]

Compound movements that challenge the athlete's ability to maintain lumbo-pelvic neutral while avoiding aberrant bracing are extremely effective with improving postural control. Deadlifts are useful in this regard, as are 'goblet' squats and split lunges. These are low-load patterning exercises and should be carried out daily, if possible. It is important to improve thoracic extension concurrently and be wary of driving into anterior pelvic tilt during upper body strength training.

### Hip range of motion

Loss of hip range of motion, especially internal hip rotation, is a well-established risk factor for athletic groin pain. Reduction in hip range has also been strongly associated with both athletic groin pain and hip changes.[11,12] This loss of range can be due to:

i)   Hip morphological changes (un-modifiable)
ii)  Hip capsular restriction (modifiable)
iii) Muscular restriction (modifiable).

When assessing hip range it is important to differentiate between the various drivers of loss of range:

i)   Thomas test – hip extension – primarily restricted by *iliopsoas*
ii)  Internal rotation at 90° flexion in supine – primarily restricted by *gluteus maximus*
iii) External Rotation at 90 ° flexion in supine – primarily restricted by joint capsule
iv)  Internal rotation at 0 ° in prone – primarily restricted by joint capsule and the small external rotators
v)   External Rotation at 0 ° in prone – primarily restricted by TFL/*gluteus minimus*.

Capsular restrictions can be improved with mobilisations with band assistance to improve hip glide. Generally speaking, hip flexion and medial rotation restrictions are improved with a posterior glide, and extension and lateral rotation are improved with an anterior glide. Mobilisations should be fluid movements (i.e. without pause) and carried out with high rep ranges (>20) every day. Those athletes who have undergone surgery or have marked hip joint changes should carry out these mobilisations before every session, since the persistent low-grade synovial reaction in the joint, as well as the associated capsular changes, mean they will always have to work to maintain range.

A loss of hip range of motion, especially hip rotation at 90° flexion, is commonly a result of muscle imbalance around the hip joint. Restoration of optimal hip range is an essential component to restoring normal biomechanical loading to the region. While soft tissue massage, foam rolling and dry needling may all temporarily increase range around the joint that has been lost due to muscular tone, this range will not be retained unless the control deficits highlighted above are identified and rectified concurrently.

---

Identifying drivers of hip range-of-motion loss and efficient restoration is key to successful rehabilitation of hip and groin pain.

---

### Hip stability strategies

Dynamic control around the hip and pelvis is a balancing act between torque-producing muscles and stabilizing muscles, as well as between agonists and antagonist muscle groups. This balance is lost when athletes develop patterns of movement that preferentially recruit torque-producing muscles to stabilize, or when previous injury or posture leads to reduced function in stabilizing muscles, with the torque-producing muscles taking up the slack. This leads to two eventual consequences – loss of dynamic stability around the hip and resultant joint impingement OR excessive load through the torque-producing muscles resulting in overload, usually at the musculotendinous junction, tendon or, most commonly, at the attachment site on the pelvis. The high prevalence of concurrent hip and musculotendionous pathology suggests both actions happen simultaneously.[13] There are a number of key muscles around the hip whose function is essential for optimal hip control.

### Iliopsoas

*Iliopsoas* is a vital stabilizer of the anterior hip joint, as well as a flexor of the hip due to its capsular attachment and anatomy.[14] Dysfunction of *iliopsoas* can lead to hip impingement if it is unable to stabilize the anterior hip against a tight posterior capsule or the pull of *tensor fascia lata* (TFL) or *rectus femoris*, as well as the drive of the posterior hip muscles. It also leads to excessive load through the anterior joint towards end-range extension.[14] Concurrently, it may result in *rectus femoris*, as well as TFL overload, as they try to accommodate a poorly functioning agonist.

*Iliopsoas* is best isolated in inner-range hip flexion to avoid over-activity of TFL and *rectus femoris* and is best assessed in supine with the hip in inner range flexion. Isometric holds can be started in supine but quickly progressed to standing with the addition of resistance as tolerated. If carried out appropriately, it is key to feel the hip flexor working through the inguinal crease, as opposed to over-activity in TFL laterally or *rectus femoris* in the upper thigh.

## Gluteus medius/minimus

*Gluteus minimus* and *gluteus medius* are important stabilisers of the lateral hip through their deep and capsular attachments.[15] Poor function leads to an inability to stabilize the hip to counter the superior pull of upper *gluteus maximus* and TFL driving lateral hip impingement (similar to the deltoid and the rotator cuff in the shoulder). They also provide antagonistic stability in single-leg stance to hip adduction and internal rotation which, if absent, leads to overactivity and bias towards the adductors.

*Gluteus medius* and *minimus* work optimally in closed chain positions during inner range abduction, where they have a mechanical advantage over TFL and upper *gluteus maximus*.[16] Hip hitching is a highly effective exercise at achieving this. *Gluteus medius* (posterior) also works as an external rotator and this can be combined with abduction in lateral band marching drills.

## Obliques

*External* and *internal oblique* have both anti-tilt and anti-rotation functions, and therefore optimal performance is carried out isometrically. They are often overpowered by *rectus abdominus*, which is primarily a flexor of the thorax, as it tries to provide stability against pelvic tilt and trunk rotation, which it does not have the mechanical advantage to do. The result is excessive tone and traction at its insertion to pubic symphysis. Exercise strategies should challenge neutral lumbopelvic position while avoiding bracing strategies. Pallof presses, chops and lifts are very useful in this regard.

Groin pain during 'core' exercises is commonly reported and is a reflection of inappropriate exercise selection and execution. Planks are regularly prescribed in supine and side-lying with the athlete collapsing into anterior pelvic tilt, thoracic kyphosis and bracing rectus abdominus, driving ongoing irritation of symptoms and providing no improvement in abdominal control.

## Adductors

The adductors are important stabilisers of the pelvis on the hip joint, especially during single leg stance activities. Adductor strengthening is often prescribed and infrequently required in athletic groin pain athletes. In general, the adductors tend towards hypertonicity, and additional strengthening of overactive/painful muscles is counterproductive. Overload is often driven by poor trunk-on-pelvis and pelvis-on-hip linkage, most commonly during cutting, when there is a high eccentric load through the adductors when swaying into hip abduction.

> Apparent strength deficits are often the result of pain inhibition, rather than actual weakness with adductor strengthening only further aggravating symptoms. However, if there is residual weakness on strength testing once symptoms have been resolved, this should be addressed through closed-chain exercises that replicate their stabilizing role.

Normalising control and tone in the muscles around the hip and pelvis is key for optimizing hip stability and available hip range. There is a high emphasis on the quality of these accessory exercises over quantity but they can be carried out in higher rep ranges (>12 reps; 2–4 sets) 4–5 days per week.

## Level 2

### Kinetic-chain strength

Given the often long-standing nature of symptoms in the region, strength deficits may not be the initial driver of pain in the region but may develop subsequently as a result of pain inhibition and altered movement patterns. Given that the majority of groin presentations are unilateral, this should be reflected in assessment using unilateral leg press or single-leg squat to assess limb strength.

> Whilst there is often a reluctance to prescribe unilateral exercises for athletes with hip, pelvic or groin symptoms, they are, in fact, good to employ from day one. Contrary to popular thought, there is no pubic shear, only excessive musculotendinous traction, when exercises are poorly executed (except in the rarest of post-partum cases).

It is vital to strengthen the entire chain in multiple planes of movement. Despite the fact that these athletes perform in predominantly multidirectional environments, strength training is often limited to the sagittal plane (squats, deadlifts, land lunges).

Lateral sled pulls provide an excellent stimulus in the frontal plane and incorporate all components of the upper limb, trunk and lower limb (Figure 23.2). The dosage prescribed

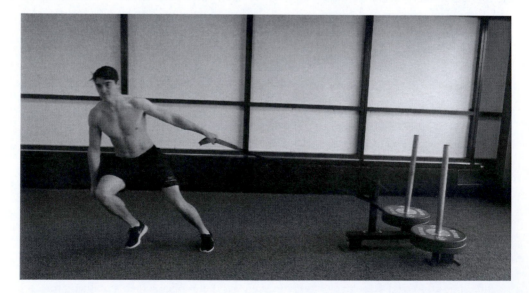

*Figure 23.2* Lateral sled pulls

will depend on the athlete's training history, degree of atrophy and where they are in the season. However most unilateral exercises would fall under accessory exercises, and rep ranges of 6–12 or so three times a week will achieve appropriate stimulus.

### Rate of moment production and absorption

The key characteristic in most field sports is the *rate* at which muscular force is developed. It is critical to be able to identify any side-to-side differences in this quality, as well as deficits compared to baselines. Bilateral assessments are useful, but given the mostly unilateral nature of hip and groin issues, it is also important to examine single-leg force generation qualities. Total force production can be assessed by employing a countermovement jump, while assessing individual joint moments is also useful. Wherever possible, this should be combined with motion analysis to examine for any side-to-side kinematic differences in either force generation or absorption.

Power development should focus on unilateral deficits and begin to resemble the motor patterns they are going to be used for on the field of play. Explosive lunge step-ups re-enforce triple extension patterns utilized in acceleration mechanics, while medball lateral bounds reproduce the explosive frontal plane moments required for multidirectional mechanics. As with all power exercises, they should be carried out with lower rep ranges (< 5), higher recovery times with an emphasis on maximum effort and excellent technique 2–3 times per week.

### The importance of load transfer

Whilst important, a reduction in force production is not the most fundamental factor predisposing an individual to hip and groin problems. We must also examine the athlete's ability to *transfer* this force efficiently. Rate of moment absorption refers to the body's ability to absorb and transfer load as efficiently as possible, improving athletic performance but also minimizing excessive loading of musculotendinous structures. This is often referred to as limb stiffness or reactive strength, and utilises the stretch-shortening cycle (SSC). It can be measured using single-leg drop jumps and calculating the reactive strength index, and is also readily visible qualitatively when looking at running mechanics in the frontal plane. This key attribute is often neglected in rehabilitation and performance programmes in preference for strength and concentric power development.

Low-load SSC exercises can be commenced very early on in rehabilitation and are vital for efficient energy transfer. Many athletes will not have the training history or competency to commence drop jumps during rehabilitation. Single-leg cone hopping can be used in multiple planes to improve 'stiffness' across the lower limb, and introducing overhead arm position can also influence trunk stiffness very effectively. These can be progressed to lateral bounding drills and drop jumps as competency and symptoms allow. The key with these exercises is to minimize the ground contact time by emphasizing good tempo and minimal light ground contact time. Higher repetitions are recommended for the low load plyometric drills, again with an emphasis on excellent technique, 2–3 times per week.

### Sports-specific conditioning

Fatigue has a negative influence on athletic performance and neuromuscular control and also increases injury risk.[17,18] Many athletes with hip and groin issues may have had modified training loads in order to keep going during the season or may have had a long period off trying to resolve the problem and have become deconditioned during this process. Off-feet conditioning can reduce this deconditioning without aggravating symptoms until running is tolerated. Symptom irritability may compromise cross-training choice in the early phases of rehabilitation, but bike work, ropes and swimming are usually well tolerated. Once high-speed running is tolerated, on-feet conditioning can be re-introduced.

## Level 3

Bridging the gap from the gym to the field is often poorly addressed or completely neglected during rehabilitation. Improving on-field mechanics is hugely beneficial for both performance and injury prevention.

### Linear running performance

Linear running is the most common mode of transport on the field of play and therefore plays an essential role in athletic performance and loading of the hip and anterior pelvis. Too often, rehabilitation focuses on static drilling and progressive exposure to running volumes and speed tasks without reviewing and developing linear running performance.

The main deficits that contribute to overload of the hip and groin and reduce performance are:

i) Poor swing-leg recovery – leads to reduced hip flexor recruitment and over-striding;
ii) Prolonged ground contact time – leads to increased joint load and increased musculo-tendinous load through reduced stretch-shortening efficiency;
iii) Over-striding – increased anterior hip load in end-range extension and altered loading of the acetabulum through heel striking in front of the centre of mass;
iv) Pelvic drop/trunk sway – increases hip joint load as well as the demands on hip adductors and abdominals;
v) Excessive trunk rotation – unstable base for leg drive leading to excessive abdominal loading.

Developing drills that challenge neutral lumbopelvic control and optimal swing leg recovery are critical features in optimizing linear running mechanics. The best drills allow the optimal patterns to emerge with minimal coaching. Skipping, barbell running and sled running are highly effective drills and encourage the athlete to improve running posture, leg mechanics and ground contact times. These exercises should be carried out on alternate days during early rehabilitation and as part of every field session warm-up.

### Multidirectional performance

Critical to improving multidirectional mechanics is addressing the neuromuscular control deficits that optimize biomechanical performance in conjunction with reactive or decision making stimuli to replicate sports-specific demands for optimal efficiency upon returning to the field of play. Step drills with bungees and side-to-side shuffle drills with medicine balls both work on optimizing foot placement, body positioning, explosive push off and trunk

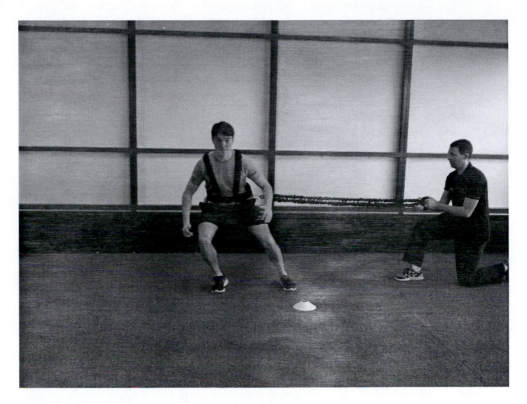

*Figure 23.3* Bungee lateral step drill

stiffness (Figure 23.3). These drills should be progressed to incorporate a reactive component using external stimulus (shadowing) or sports-specific stimulus (passing).

## Upper body propulsion

*Upper body throwing* or swinging patterns should reflect the dominant patterns displayed in the sport. For example a slap shot in hockey, baseball throw and golf swing can all be replicated explosively with medball drills in various positions while adding in external stimulus and perturbations to challenge the pattern of movement.

## Level 4

### Sports-specific skill development

Injury risk and performance decrement can be influenced by technical deficiencies in sports-specific tasks (i.e. tennis serve, throwing technique, kicking mechanics). 3D biomechanics can be used to assess and modify these complex movement patterns, but appropriate intervention requires appropriately qualified and experienced coaches, which is often beyond the scope of practice of an individual physiotherapist or strength and conditioning coaches, and like all interventions, a multi-disciplinary approach works best.

### Return to training/competition

It is important that both the player and the team management understand that a graduated increase in training load from this point is essential to continue the most efficient recovery. Key outcome measures – hip range and pain provocation tests, especially the morning after a session, will indicate how well an athlete is tolerating the training load.

An appropriate guide to progression is:

i)   Commence linear running volume when the athlete demonstrates pain-free crossover test and symmetrical internal hip rotation at 90° of hip flexion;
ii)  Commence multidirectional running volume when the athlete has pain-free squeeze at 45°, symmetrical and appropriate local hip control, pain-free at top sprint speed (low volume);
iii) Commence team training when the athlete demonstrates symmetrical and efficient multidirectional mechanics and pain-free squeeze at 0°, 45° and 90°.

The general rule of thumb is that a player is clear to return to competition once they are able to demonstrate both full confidence and competence with all the demands that the sport places on them. Every movement demand should have been tested during training under fatigued conditions and the athlete should have demonstrated that they have regained full strength, power, speed, stiffness and endurance. Obviously, the longer the athlete has been away from competition the longer they will take to gain full confidence, and so they may require a number of weeks of full training before being considered fully recovered. A more detailed analysis of this decision making process can be found in chapter 18.

## Summary

The pathomechanics, and therefore the rehabilitation, from hip and groin pain in athletes is highly individual. Key to understanding this is differentiating between the anatomical diagnosis and the biomechanical diagnosis, and appreciating that for any one given anatomical diagnosis there are multiple biomechanical presentations. Rehabilitation must therefore address all the factors driving pain and place a high focus on assessing the athlete during high-speed multiplanar movements and optimizing these mechanics. The focus should be on returning the athlete to optimum performance, not only to reduce the risk of re-injury, but also to allow them to hit the ground running on return from injury. Finally, we should be aware of the external factors that contribute to pain and overload in the region and be able to modify them as required to minimize injury risk.

## Notes

1 Falvey, E. C., Franklyn-Miller, A., & McCrory, P. R. (2009). The groin triangle: A patho-anatomical approach to the diagnosis of chronic groin pain in athletes. *British Journal of Sports Medicine, 43*(3), 213–20.

2 Gray, A. J., & Jenkins, D. G. (2010). Match analysis and the physiological demands of Australian football. *Sports Medicine, 40*(4), 347–60.

3 Quarrie, K. L., & Hopkins, W. G. (2007). Changes in player characteristics and match activities in Bledisloe Cup rugby union from 1972 to 2004. *Journal of Sports Sciences, 25*(8), 895–903.

4 Delahunt, E., Kennelly, C., McEntee, B. L., Coughlan, G. F., & Green, B. S. The thigh adductor squeeze test: 45 degrees of hip flexion as the optimal test position for eliciting adductor muscle activity and maximum pressure values. *Manual Therapy, 16*(5), 476–80.

5 Reiman, M. P., Goode, A. P., Hegedus, E. J., Cook, C. E., & Wright, A. A. (2013). Diagnostic accuracy of clinical tests of the hip: A systematic review with meta-analysis. *British Journal of Sports Medicine, 47*(14), 893–902.

6 Holmich, P. (2007). Long-standing groin pain in sportspeople falls into three primary patterns, a 'clinical entity' approach: A prospective study of 207 patients. *British Journal of Sports Medicine, 41*(4), 247–52.

7 Verrall, G. M., Slavotinek, J. P., & Fon, G. T. (2001). Incidence of pubic bone marrow oedema in Australian rules football players: Relation to groin pain. *British Journal of Sports Medicine, 35*(1), 28–33.

8 Pfirrmann, C. W., Mengiardi, B., Dora, C., Kalberer, F., Zanetti, M., & Hodler, J. (2006). Cam and pincer femoroacetabular impingement: Characteristic MR arthrographic findings in 50 patients. *Radiology, 240*(3), 778–85.

9 Kapron, A. L., Anderson, A. E., Aoki, S. K., Phillips, L. G., Petron, D. J., Toth, R., et al. (2011). Radiographic prevalence of femoroacetabular impingement in collegiate football players: AAOS Exhibit Selection. *The Journal of Bone & Joint Surgery, 93*(19), e111(1–10).

10 Ross, J. R., Nepple, J. J., Philippon, M. J., Kelly, B. T., Larson, C. M., & Bedi, A. (2014). Effect of changes in pelvic tilt on range of motion to impingement and radiographic parameters of acetabular morphologic characteristics. *American Journal of Sports Medicine, 42*(10), 2402–9.

11 Verrall, G. M., Slavotinek, J. P., Barnes, P. G., Esterman, A., Oakeshott, R. D., & Spriggins, A. J. (2007). Hip joint range of motion restriction precedes athletic chronic groin injury. *Journal of Science & Medicine in Sport, 10*(6), 463–6.

12 Kubiak-Langer, M., Tannast, M., Murphy, S. B., Siebenrock, K. A., & Langlotz, F. (2007). Range of motion in anterior femoroacetabular impingement. *Clinical Orthopaedics and Related Research, 458*, 117–24.

13 Weir, A., de Vos, R. J., Moen, M., Holmich, P., & Tol, J. L. (2011). Prevalence of radiological signs of femoroacetabular impingement in patients presenting with long-standing adductor-related groin pain. *British Journal of Sports Medicine, 45*(1), 6–9.

14 Lewis, C. L., Sahrmann, S. A., & Moran, D. W. (2007). Anterior hip joint force increases with hip extension, decreased gluteal force, or decreased iliopsoas force. *Journal of Biomechanics, 40*(16), 3725–31.

15 Walters, J., Solomons, M., & Davies, J. (2001). Gluteus minimus: Observations on its insertion. *Journal of Anatomy, 198*, 239–42.

16 Kumagai, M., Shiba, N., Higuchi, F., Nishimura, H., & Inoue, A. (2005). Functional evaluation of hip abductor muscles with use of magnetic resonance imaging. *Journal of Orthopaedic Research, 15*(6), 888–93.

17 Brazen, D. M., Todd, M. K., Ambegaonkar, J. P., Wunderlich, R., & Peterson, C. (2010). The effect of fatigue on landing biomechanics in single-leg drop landings. *Clinical Journal of Sport Medicine, 20*(4), 286–92.

18 Oliver, J., Armstrong, N., & Williams, C. (2008). Changes in jump performance and muscle activity following soccer-specific exercise. *Journal of Sports Sciences, 26*(2), 141–8.

# Chapter 24

# The athletic knee

*Chris Mallac and David Joyce*

## Introduction

Knee injuries are common in the athletic arena. The type of knee injuries sustained by the athlete ranges from the simple bump and bruise, all the way to the more debilitating and rehabilitation-intensive cruciate ligament injuries. In fact, there are in excess of 100 different pathologies that can affect the sporting knee,[1] with many of these requiring surgery and/or lengthy rehabilitation and reconditioning periods.

Returning an athlete with an injured knee to competition requires much more than simply restoring muscle strength and range of movement. An integrated approach encompassing full kinetic-chain function enhancement is required. Additionally, an in-depth knowledge of strength and conditioning principles and how these apply to the systematic rehabilitation process and the long-term reconditioning of the injured knee is essential. Furthermore, ensuring the athlete remains injury-free requires on going management and regular monitoring.

This chapter discusses the relevant anatomy and biomechanics that need to be considered when implementing a holistic knee rehabilitation program. The specific staged 'criteria'-driven rehabilitation process will be explained in detail, with emphasis on specific strength and conditioning principles that need to be considered throughout the reconditioning process. End-stage functional testing forms the integral part of the return-to-competition decision, and the essential aspects of this will also be discussed in this chapter.

## The knee as both a force-absorber and force-generator

For effective performance when running, landing and changing directions, we need efficient lower-limb function. As the 'middle link' in this chain, the knee complex is exposed to a wide variety of stresses, and so it is little wonder that it is commonly injured in sport. To remain injury-free, the knee is reliant on a complex 'symphony orchestra' of joint's structure and its ligamentous and fascio-capsular restraints, as well as the active contractile elements of the surrounding muscles and tendons. All of this is balanced by the delicate sensorimotor (proprioceptive) system.

To understand how to best optimise the function of all these elements, we first need to understand the role of the lower limb in athletic function. As the foot lands on the ground when walking, running and jumping, the joints of the lower limb flex to absorb both the downward force of gravity and the resultant upward ground-reaction force. These forces are worn by the joint structures and the muscle structures that eccentrically work to control this absorbing (dampening) effect. Muscle-tendon-fascial complexes absorb these forces and use the stored elastic energy to recoil (like a spring) into the propulsion or acceleration force of locomotion where the joints are extending. This concept is discussed in more detail in chapter 15, along with its implications in patellar tendon rehabilitation.

Abnormal or excessive stresses, or the inability to absorb these stresses due to inefficient neuromuscular patterns or muscle weakness at one joint, may have an effect on the lower-extremity kinetic chain. Accordingly, hip and ankle kinetics and kinematics during weight-bearing may have a direct impact on knee biomechanics and thus relate to knee injury risk. For example poor ankle dorsiflexion may lead to an increase in the knee flexion moment during landing movements, possibly resulting in injury to the anterior knee components. It is for this reason that any assessment of knee function needs to include the hip and ankle joints.

## Kinetic chain control and alignment: Implications for the knee

Maintaining frontal, sagittal and coronal plane knee alignment during locomotion is important in the prevention of both overuse- and trauma-based injuries. Therefore, maintaining this same alignment during rehabilitation and physical reconditioning is also vital. In the strictest sense, it can be argued that the weight-bearing knee in the sagittal plane (for example when straight-line running or when performing a simple lunge) must stay over the landmarks created by the medial and lateral boundaries of the foot. If the knee falls medial to the foot boundaries, a valgus force will be applied to the knee and the patella that may potentially lead to knee joint injuries, as well as the classic 'tracking' problems associated with the patellofemoral joint.

Let's be practical, though! It is a common feature of many sports that the knee will be forced into a valgus position, for example in slalom skiing or any field/court sport when cutting to change direction is required. In these instances, the forced valgus position is a necessary component of skilled performance and the knee needs to have sufficient structural integrity as well as dynamic control to prevent 'excessive' valgus motion. This is provided by the passive ligamentous constraints around the knee as well as the muscle control of the *quadriceps, hamstrings, popliteus* and *gastrocnemius* around the knee, as well as the hip abductors and external rotators.

In the frontal plane, engaging the limb in stance phase requires a dampening effect in all joints of the lower-limb kinetic chain. Appropriate amounts of subtalar joint pronation, ankle joint dorsiflexion, knee joint flexion and hip joint flexion and eccentric muscle control (see Table 24.1) are required to dampen the impulse ('absorb' the impact) of the resultant ground reaction force as the foot strikes the ground.

Unwanted 'give' in these joints due to a lack of eccentric muscle control in the shock-absorbing muscles will lead to extraneous limb motion, with energy leaked away from the force required for the subsequent propulsion to push off. Conversely, if the joints are too

Table 24.1  Muscles required to function eccentrically to absorb ground reaction forces

| Joint | Muscles |
|---|---|
| Hip | Gluteals and deep hip rotators |
| Knee | Quadriceps, gluteals, popliteus |
| Ankle | Soleus, peroneals |
| Subtalar | Tibialis posterior, long toe flexors |

stiff, insufficient energy will be absorbed by the muscles and instead increased burden will be placed upon the articular surfaces, which may lead to premature degeneration. This kinetic chain analysis is discussed in more detail in chapter 7.

Finally, all lower-limb joints involved in the 'absorption' of downward force are then involved in the 'propulsion' or acceleration phase of locomotion and thus need specific reconditioning to correctly execute the kinetic chain extension movements. We can see, therefore, that we cannot just think of the knee in isolation.

## Phases of rehabilitation

When planning and delivering the stages of our injury prevention and rehabilitation programmes, an understanding of the influence of load exposure, load attenuation and force generation is critical to provide us with a clear understanding of the milestones that need to be achieved and the rate at which they can be pursued. The best way to approach the process, therefore, is to stage the approach to high performance and load resilience using a phased or milestone-based strategy, with each phase feeding into the next. In keeping with the exit-criteria approach (see chapter 1), we do not move between stages according to the passage of time, but the accomplishment of functional goals.

The four primary phases of knee rehabilitation are:

1  Phase One: Protection and healing
2  Phase Two: Restoring muscle strength and range of movement
3  Phase Three: Integrated functional adaptation
4  Phase Four: Sports-specific retraining.

The time frame in each stage will depend primarily on the pathology we are dealing with. For example a postoperative knee reconstruction may require four stages of approximately six weeks duration, returning an athlete back to play in a minimum of 24 weeks, whereas a lateral meniscal repair may require stages that are more compressed, resulting in a 16-week turnaround. Whilst in this chapter we will not discuss individual pathologies *per se*, it is necessary to point out the essential exit criteria for each stage, and these criteria will be reasonably consistent from one pathology to the next. The key objectives for each of the stages are seen in Table 24.2 and are discussed in more detail below.

Table 24.2 The four phases of knee rehabilitation

| Phase | Focus | Key Objectives |
|---|---|---|
| Phase 1 | Protection and healing | Adequate healing |
| | | Restore homeostasis |
| Phase 2 | Motion and strength | Gross muscle mass and strength development |
| | | Range of motion (ROM) restoration |
| | | Propulsive and absorptive force development |
| Phase 3 | Return to function | Functional patterns of movement |
| | | Skill development relevant to the chosen sport |
| | | Multidirectional speed and agility |
| Phase 4 | Return to performance | Technical skill competence |
| | | Competitive confidence |
| | | Resilience |
| | | Training load tolerance |

## Phase 1 – Protection and healing

A critical early intervention following a knee injury is to protect the joint from further damage and to allow a supportive environment in which healing can take place. Dependent on the injury, this may require bracing, taping or even use of crutches. As soon as possible, however, we want to restore normal gait mechanics, as this has positive effects on proprioception and muscle activation. An effective way of graduating this is through an altered weight-bearing environment, such as a pool.

### The importance of removing effusions

A knee joint effusion is an excessive amount of fluid within the synovial capsule of the knee indicating that the knee is inflamed or irritated. The synovial membrane secretes synovial fluid and its secretion will increase in the presence of an intra-articular pathology, as the membrane produces more fluid in attempt to remove the intra-articular debris.

The exact patho-physiological mechanisms for an effusion and the necessary medical interventions are genuine concerns for the rehabilitation practitioner. Even small volumes of fluid (20–30mls) can result in a 50–60 per cent reduction in maximal voluntary muscular activation,[2,3,4,5] a process commonly referred to as 'arthrogenic inhibition'.[6] Moreover, small increases in intra-articular fluid (as modest as 5ml) increases the pressure within the knee joint. This can be a source of discomfort and concern for the athlete.

Furthermore, it has also been found that knee joint effusions will also alter the knee joint mechanics during landing tasks.[7] Those individuals with a knee effusion tend to land with greater ground reaction forces and in greater knee extension, resulting in more force being transferred to the knee joint and its passive restraints.

Effusion will detrimentally affect the function and outcome of the joint in a number of ways:

Increasing intra-articular joint pressure
Altering quadriceps muscle recruitment
Decreasing the stability mechanisms around the knee
Altering limb-loading patterns.

Removing the effusion does make a demonstrable difference to quadriceps function. This can be a frustratingly slow process, however, and so a number of interventions should be prioritised:

1   Regular assessment performed before loading the knee joint and in the subsequent 24 hours, particularly if the load is new and more progressive.
2   Remove the effusion, if present. This can be done with conventional methods, such as elevation, compression with donut felt, effusion massage and reduced weight bearing, or more medically directed interventions, such as non-steroidal anti-inflammatory medication (NSAIDs) or direct needle aspiration, if indicated. Removing the internal fluid will significantly reduce the internal pressure within the knee as well as improving quadriceps strength.
3   Exercise selection. Quadriceps setting exercises that are performed in positions of partial (20°) knee flexion or isometric squats in 20–30° flexion, will allow muscle recruitment without increasing the intra-articular pressure associated with full knee extension.
4   Early pool work provides us with the opportunity to take advantage of hydrostatic pressure to aid with effusion drainage.

### Reactivation of muscles in early phase rehabilitation

Since effective muscle function helps absorb joint loads, a restoration of contractile activity must be seen as a priority, and so in the early stages of knee rehabilitation the focus is on:

*   quadriceps setting exercises
*   quadriceps-hamstring co-contraction exercises
*   isolated hip muscle exercises (particularly gluteals and hip external rotators) in a non-weight-bearing (lying down or sitting) or protected-weight-bearing situation (altered gravity treadmills or pools if available).

The return of quadriceps muscle bulk and thus strength is variable amongst different knee pathologies, and it is not uncommon to see ongoing differences in muscle bulk even after the athlete has returned to full competition. Often these muscle bulk differences will demonstrate equal side-to-side strength comparisons as the athlete returns to full function.

There are many ways to accelerate the return of muscle bulk and gross muscle strength in the early rehabilitation setting. Occlusion training and electrical muscle stimulation can be very helpful in gaining muscle hypertrophy in the early stages of rehabilitation where high mechanical and joint compressive loads are inappropriate.

*Restoring range of motion*

Limitations in range of motion (ROM) are common following a knee injury, particularly in terminal extension. The primary mechanisms that limit the final 5–10° of extension can be broken down into mechanical (intra-articular) and myogenic (muscle tone) reasons. Dependent on the cause, manual therapy aimed at restoring accessory joint motion, effusion aspiration, soft-tissue massage, trigger-point releases and dry needling/acupuncture may help correct ROM restrictions.

---

To allow progression to phase 2 of rehabilitation, we suggest the following exit criteria are passed:

1  Resolution of active inflammatory process
2  Pain-free functional active knee ROM (may lack 5–10° of extension and 20° flexion)
3  Normalised pain-free walking gait
4  Good voluntary muscle action.

---

## Phase 2 – Strength and motion

The second phase of rehabilitation is geared towards the introduction of strength work. This can be broken down simply into knee-dominant and hip-dominant movements. These are essentially exercises done in a sagittal plane and involve the combination movements of ankle dorsiflexion/plantarflexion, knee flexion/extension and hip flexion/extension. In simple terms, examples of the following are:

1  Knee dominant: single-leg squat, single-leg lunge, leg press, Bulgarian (rear-foot-elevated) squat, Nordic hamstring curls
2  Hip dominant: Romanian deadlift, glute-ham raise, hip thruster.

These are initially performed with bodyweight only and with slow controlled tempo and load/speed, and complexity is added as the athlete progresses through the rehabilitation setting. The key feature in this stage is that the joints of the lower limb (knee joint included) are engaging in a coordinated manner that satisfies the kinetic chain requirements of the lower limb.

The joints initially absorb force (slowly in the early stages of rehabilitation) through the eccentric component. They are then required to hold, stabilise and control a loaded position, before finally propelling away from the loaded position whilst maintaining kinetic chain alignment.

Some rules/guidelines to follow when considering the implementation of these traditional clinical/gym-based movements are:

1  Propulsion/acceleration forces. The joints and movements involved in the propulsion phase of locomotion are ankle plantarflexion, knee extension and hip extension (triple-extension phase). This capacity is generally the easiest and safest to develop early, involves concentric muscle force, and requires the least work capacity and the safest joint reaction forces.

2    Absorption/deceleration forces. The joints and movements involved are ankle dorsiflex-
     ion, knee flexion and hip flexion (triple flexion phase). This capacity requires the greatest
     amount of force production as the muscles are working eccentrically and the downward
     effect of gravity and the resultant upward ground reaction force are greatest. This leads
     to the greatest joint stress on the knee and thus is the hardest to develop. However, the
     absorbing/decelerating forces need to be trained to a high level prior to return to compe-
     tition, as knee injuries usually occur in the landing/cutting/deceleration type situations.
3    Temporal constraints. If the athlete is returning from a long absence away from traditional
     strength training and/or sport due to delayed surgery or the pressure to continue to com-
     pete whilst injured, then the focus of strength training is on repetition and volume and not
     load. The emphasis on repetition re-integrates the pathways between the peripheral and
     central nervous systems, and provides a constant proprioceptive-rich training environment
     for the athlete that, by this stage, may have missed many months of training. However if
     an athlete has had a recent surgical procedure – for example two weeks after an acute ACL
     rupture – then the need for high repetition and low load is not as necessary in the early
     postoperative rehabilitation stages. These athletes can push the load variables much faster.
4    Early plyometrics. Introduction of higher-intensity movements with the aim of perfect-
     ing technique for latter stages where load is increased. These can be added early in the
     rehabilitation setting via safe joint-sparing alternatives such as unloaded fast eccentric
     exercises and pool plyometrics.
5    Bilateral transfer. Training the contralateral limb can result in measurable strength and
     performance gains in the affected limb. Early strength work on the unaffected side will
     assist in earlier functional recovery in the affected side.

It is in this phase of the rehabilitation where the athlete needs to spend a lot of time getting
strong under an appropriately qualified performance coach. This strengthening phase needs
to be appropriately periodised, involving fluctuations in volume and intensity, and may last
for a few weeks or as long as four months following an ACL reconstruction.

---

To allow progression to phase 3 of rehabilitation, we suggest the following exit criteria
are passed:

1    Full resolution of any effusion
2    Full range of movement (may lack 10 per cent flexion)
3    Good control of single-leg squat
4    >70 per cent hamstring and quadriceps strength compared to contralateral side.

---

## Phase 3 – Return to function

The third phase is an extension of the second, but the emphasis is now on sport-specific
movements that need to be retrained prior to return to full training and subsequent competition. This is the stage that is characterised by return-to-running protocols and the introduction of agility and cutting movements. A plethora of factors need to be considered and
integrated into a return-to-running programme and many of these are discussed in chapter 9.
From a knee performance perspective, the criteria that need to be satisfied for return to running are shown in Table 24.3.

Table 24.3

| Criterion | Aim | Drills | Coaching cues | Notes |
|---|---|---|---|---|
| Speed and running mechanics | Incorporation of correct lower-limb to upper-limb movement sequencing | Triple flexion of the lower limb joints during swing phase (ankle dorsiflexion/ knee flexion/hip flexion) A drills | 'Heel to butt' | The common tendency for injured athletes is to generate swing phase torque from pure hip flexion and not knee flexion. |
| | Increase force-absorption ability and impulse generation | B drills used to create train impulse generation upon foot strike | 'Light on your feet' | Minimising ground contact time will encourage a more powerful impulse into the stance phase to push off |
| | Reduction of braking forces | Encourage the 'lift' under the buttocks to ensure the foot strikes under the hips and not in front. Running with a skipping rope | 'Foot strike from above (not in front)' | If the athlete consciously thinks about foot strike, then they are more likely to over-stride during stance phase. By foot striking under the hips, braking force is eliminated and ground reaction force is reduced. |
| Acceleration development | To functionally transfer the parallel gains in gross strength/power that is part of the reconditioning process | Short accelerations initially from rolling start and then from a stationary start | 'Quick steps' The focus should be on the first 3–4 steps as being short, fast steps before building into a longer stride length. | Focusing on stride frequency rather than stride length will ensure the athlete can move their inertia into maximum velocity quicker. |
| | Arm drive into flexion/abduction to match the contralateral downward and backward force generated by knee and hip extension in acceleration | Simple wrist taping with a white tape will draw attention to the 'arm drive' being forward in front of the body and in the field of vision. | 'Drive your arm forwards and up' 'Look for the tape in front of your eyes' | The legs push and drive backwards as the arm reaches and drives forward. This will ensure maximum acceleration. |

(Continued)

*Table 24.3* (Continued)

| Criterion | Aim | Drills | Coaching cues | Notes |
|---|---|---|---|---|
| | Symmetrical leg drive | Leaning triple extension drill – hands on a wall. From start position of one leg in triple flexion, aggressively drive leg into triple extension whilst bringing other into triple flexion. | 'Equal force on each leg drive' | A common tendency for a post-knee-injured athlete is to de-power the injured side and to exaggerate the non-injured side. |
| Speed development | To expose the muscle and joint structures to the velocity of contractions and loading forces imposed by high-speed running | Sprint distances will initially need to be kept shorter than 50–60m until the athlete develops a level of speed endurance. | 'Relax and lean' | Encourage the athlete to keep the shoulders slightly forward of the hips at high speed. This will discourage the common over-striding pattern that is evident in post-injured athletes. |
| Deceleration capability development | Often the forgotten element in speed development. Once the athlete has been conditioned to run fast, they also need to be able to decelerate quickly. | Modify deceleration distance with objective marker (cones). Start with easy 20m deceleration distance and reduce to as little as 5m distance. Provide footwork challenges such as ladder drills following an acceleration. | 'Shorten the steps' 'Drop the hips' 'Full foot plant' | The deceleration phase comes with the greatest risk of re-injury, as it causes the greatest joint stress. |

### Developing the capacity to decelerate

Getting the athlete to repeat box landings is helpful in training the ability to arrest body weight. These should be started by jumping onto a box and then progressed to jumping off. Start with double-leg landings and progress to single-leg and then vary the height of the box. The final progression should be jumping and landing for distance, where the athlete is forced to stabilise horizontal propulsion. This progression should take place over the course of a month. Do not try to 'tick all these boxes' in too short a period, as the risk of developing patellar tendinopathy is high if there is a sudden spike in loading (see chapter 15).

We need to be acutely aware of the importance of well-structured running/agility programmes that incorporate the development of the deceleration forces, such as cutting, turning, slowing down, landing and pivoting. Generally speaking, the athlete should be exposed to a number of weeks of increasing volumes of acceleration, deceleration and top-speed drilling before integration into open-skilled training is considered.

To allow progression to phase 4 of rehabilitation, we suggest the following exit criteria are passed:

1   Maintenance of an effusion-free joint
2   Full range of movement (may lack 10 per cent flexion)
3   Good control of single-leg landing from a 40cm box
4   >85 per cent hamstring and quadriceps strength compared to contralateral side
5   Good control of 50° change of direction to either side
6   Return to >85 per cent of pre-injury maximum running speed

## Stage 4 – Return to performance

In the final stage of rehabilitation and reconditioning, the athlete progressively returns to sport-specific skill training. In this stage, high-level rehabilitation exercises that incorporate functional kinetic chain integration (ankle, knee, hip, pelvis, spine and upper limb) need to be implemented in a manner that challenges the athlete's proprioceptive abilities and reactive abilities. The purpose is conditioning the neuro-sensorimotor system to a wide spectrum on unpredictable stimuli so that infinite CNS connections are formed.

The variables that can be manipulated to provide broad spectrum challenges are:

1   Surface. Stable (floor) to unstable (sand, balance boards, trampoline, mats).
2   Body movement. Stable on feet to unstable (rolls to stand, jump variations).
3   External load (cables, dumbbells, vests, asymmetrical weight barbell, kettle bells, suspension trainers, medicine balls).
4   Sensory cues. Variations in responding to sound, vision and touch.
5   Speed. Slow speed to fast movement.
6   Environmental obstacles. Other athletes, cones, hurdles, etc.

There exists a plethora of different training modalities that an athlete may be subjected to in this stage of the rehabilitation/reconditioning process. Two modalities that we have used to great effect are sand-based training and gymnastics-based training.

### Sand-based training

A 5m x 10m sand pit (or, indeed, the beach!) can provide a fantastic and challenging rehabilitation environment for the knee-injured athlete. Simple drills that are also done in stable base training (e.g. grass or gym) can also be used in the sandpit. The benefit of the sandpit is that, due to the shifting surface, it provides a greater proprioceptive challenge, and furthermore, the sand absorbs much of the downward reaction force that is a positive benefit to the load-compromised knee.

1    Running drills. All of the running drills highlighted in stage 3 can be used in a sand-pit. Furthermore, as well as forwards running, the athlete can perform backwards running. Carioca drills, stepping and cutting drills and lateral movement drills in the sand pit.
2    Jump, hop and landing drills. Forward hops, sideways, lateral hops, two legs to one leg, single hops vs. multiple hops are all variations that can be used in the sandpit.
3    Sand displacement drills. Using the planted feet, the athlete can be encouraged to 'move' through the sand by using a twisting motion to displace sand away from the feet. This encourages the development of hip/knee rotation and ankle stability and foot stability. The athlete can move forwards by stepping/lunging into the sand and then twisting the foot prior to the next step. Alternatively they can keep the feet buried and twist side to side to move laterally through the sand.

### Trampoline drills

Full-size trampolines also provide a difficult balance environment for the knee-injured athlete.

1    Run and stop drills. Having the athlete running on the spot and stopping on an auditory or visual cue. This will not only develop reactive abilities to external stimuli, but it will also create greater proprioceptive and balance integration due to the unstable surface the trampoline provides.
2    Hop and landing drills. Single hops, double-leg jumps, forwards, sideways, backwards are all variations that can be used with hop drills.
3    Rolls to balance. Forwards and backwards roll to a squat stance or single-leg stance provides an enormous strength, balance and range-of-movement challenge. Not exactly specific in its application, however, the cross-over effect of this type of balance training can provide immeasurable benefit to the knee-injured athlete.

### Return to contact training

Staging a knee-injured athlete back to a full competitive training situation requires a stepwise progression of drills and skills that resemble the demands of the competition whilst still allowing appropriate protection of the knee at critical stages of recovery. A logical way to prepare the athlete to develop match readiness is to modify the training environment from safe and controlled situations initially to more advanced game-specific events as they progress. For example starting in kneeling positions and then progressing to standing, walking and running positions allows the athlete to confidently practice contact components without fear of further knee injury.

Below is an example of how a knee-injured athlete would progress contact situations for a combative sport such as rugby or American Football. Note that the final stages are of sufficient intensity to be considered as conditioning sessions if repeated, and so this needs to be planned for and taken into account when programming the return-to-performance 'journey' for the athlete.

Table 24.4 Return to contact progressions

| Stage | Intensity | Posture | Aims | Content |
|---|---|---|---|---|
| 1 | Low | Kneel | Simple contact/collision in knee-protected positions | 1. Falling mechanics<br>2. Wrestling mechanics<br>3. Impact absorption<br>4. Forward hits<br>5. Fending |
| 2 | Low | Stand | Simple contact/collision in static stance | As above but at a slightly increased velocity |
| 3 | Low | Walk | Simple contact/collision in safe and controlled walking situations | 1. As above but, again, at a slightly increased velocity<br>2. Hit and spinning |
| 4 | Medium | Walk-jog | Progressions to game simulation in walking | 1. Down + ups<br>2. Specific wrestling<br>3. Being tackled/hit in varying scenarios (high-low)<br>4. Double combined efforts<br>5. Footwork (attack + defence) |
| 5 | Medium | Jog | Increase impact forces | As above but at a slightly increased velocity |
| 6 | Medium | Run | Increase impact forces | As above but at increasing velocities |
| 7 | High | Run | Match situations | Combination of different areas of contact and running |
| 8 | High | Sprint | | Position Specific |
| 9 | High | Maximum | | Position Specific |

## Functional tests

The highest risk for a knee injury is a previous knee injury.[8] In order to do everything we can to reduce this risk to a minimum and be confident that the athlete is not just fit to play but fit to perform, a series of functional, sports-specific tests should be employed. The tests should be objective, measureable and quantifiable tests that include an element of:

- Strength
- Agility
- Power
- Balance
- Neuromuscular status.

The above factors can be incorporated into functional tests, such as hops and agility/movement tests.

The more common hop tests include:

1  Single hop for distance
2  Triple hops

3    Crossover hop
4    6m timed hop.

The ability to maintain isolated single-limb power is important in sports that require significant control in cutting and stepping manoeuvres. This will require the ability to absorb force on a single limb and then to regenerate and redirect the motion. Single-limb testing is critical, as it aids in identifying persistent deficits in lower-limb performance, including deficits in power, force attenuation and postural stability. Moreover, double-limb and modified double-limb tests may not be sensitive enough to demonstrate any asymmetries between sides and the uninvolved limb may mask deficits of the involved limb.[9,10]

Single-leg hopping tests – in particular the crossover hop test (CHT) – are sensitive enough to identify asymmetry. The CHT performed six months after ACL reconstruction is a good predictor of knee function, and the 6m timed test is the most sensitive and indicative of below-normal function at six months postop.[8] Logerstedt et al. (2012) found that, as a predictor of function, patients with below-normal ranges of knee function are five times more likely to have a 6m timed test demonstrating <88 per cent of the contralateral limb, and patients with knee function of above-normal ranges are four times more likely to have a crossover hop test that is >95 per cent of the contralateral limb.[11]

---

To allow progression to full competition, we suggest the following exit criteria are passed:

1    >90 per cent of pre-injury hop distance and cross-over hop test results
2    Return to full sprint speed
3    Return to full acceleration and deceleration velocities
4    Full competence and confidence over the course of a prolonged period of competitive training (as reported by the coaching and support teams, as well as the athlete themselves).
4    >90 per cent hamstring and quadriceps strength compared to contralateral side

---

## The load-compromised athlete

Unfortunately for the athlete suffering from a long-term knee injury, particularly an injury that has involved surgery with a lengthy rehabilitation/reconditioning period, the knee joint pathology needs to be respected for the remainder of the athlete's career. This essentially makes the athlete 'load compromised' against a similar athlete with no history of knee injury, a point emphasised in chapter 1. From a knee perspective, the practical interventions that need to be considered once the athlete is back to competition are:

1    Regular assessment of effusion, particularly after a major change has been implemented, such as a new skill, extra load, plyometric-type training, frequent exposure to competition/training.
2    Regular assessment of functional tests to ensure the athlete stays within acceptable levels.

3   Load monitoring. This can be direct volume and impact monitoring using GPS or, if unavailable, carefully selecting the training sessions the athlete will be involved in. They may need to miss the occasional session to allow knee joint recovery.
4   Regular soft tissue therapy to ensure the myogenic elements are not reacting adversely to load.
5   Education of both athlete and coaches. All interested parties need to be aware that the knee may require periods of de-loading to restore a healthy homeostasis.

## Summary

A knee injury is arguably the highest profile malady of the sportsman or woman. This is on account of the incidence and severity, as well as the performance and financial cost. There is therefore a significant drive to reduce knee injury risks, as well as ensure that the individual who does sustain an injury returns to competition a more resilient and complete athlete. It is vital to stage a rehabilitation process according to performance aims, but the rates of progression between stages is governed by functional competency and tissue tolerance/healing status.

As with any plan, it is critical to start with the end in mind, and so there needs to be functional relevancy to every stage of the rehabilitation process and involvement of the entire interdisciplinary team to ensure all performance goals are met. The rehabilitation and injury prevention professional needs to both understand and coach low- and high-load strength, stability and power and how they integrate into landing and locomotive mechanics. Finally, an appreciation of exit criteria and the importance of manipulating load where required will ensure that the athlete does not just return to training, but returns to high performance.

## Notes

1   Rae, K., & Orchard, J. (2007). The orchard sports injury classification system (OSICS) version 10. *Clinical Journal Sports Medicine*, *17*(3), 201–204.
2   Fahrer, T. G., Rentsch, H. U., Gerber, N. J., Beyeler, C., Hess, C. W., & Grunig, B. (1988). Knee effusion and reflex inhibition of the quadriceps: A bar to effective retraining. *The Journal of Bone and Joint Surgery*, *70-B*(4), 635–638.
3   Hart, J. M., Pietrosimone, B., Hertel, J., & Ingersoll, C.D. (2010). Quadriceps activation following knee injuries: A systematic review. *Journal of Athletic Training*, *45*(1), 87–97.
4   Wood, L., Ferrell, W. R., & Baxendale, R.H. (1988). Pressures in normal and acutely distended human knee joints and effects on quadriceps maximal voluntary contractions. *Quarterly Journal of Experimental Physiology*, *73*, 305–314.
5   Iles, J. F., Stokes, M., & Young, A. (1990). Reflex actions of knee joint afferents during contraction of the human quadriceps. *Clinical Physiology*, *10*(5), 489–500.
6   Young, A. (1993). Current issues in arthrogenous inhibition. *Annals of Rheumatic Diseases*, *52*, 829–834.
7   Palmieri-Smith, R. M., Krienbrick, J., Ashton-Miller, J. A. & Wojtys, E. M. (2007). Quadriceps inhibition induced by an experimental knee joint effusion affects knee joint mechanics during a single legged drop landing. *American Journal of Sports Medicine*, *35*(8), 1269–1275.
8   Walden, M., Hagglund, M., & Ekstrand, J. (2006). High risk of new knee injury in elite footballers with previous anterior cruciate ligament injury. *British Journal of Sports Medicine*, *40*(2), 158–162.
9   Noyes, F. R., Barber, S. D. & Mangine, R. E. (1991). Abnormal lower limb symmetry determined by function hop tests after anterior cruciate ligament rupture. *The American Journal of Sports Medicine*, *19*(5), 513–518.

10 Myer, G. D., Schmitt, L. C., Brent, J. L., Ford, K. R., Barber, K. D., Scherer, . . . Hewett, T. E. (2011). Utilization of modified NFL combine testing to identify functional deficits in athletes following ACL reconstruction. *Journal of Sports Physical Therapy, 41*(6), 377–387.

11 Logerstedt, D., Grindem, H., Lynch, A., Eitzen, I., Engebretsen, L., Risberg, M. A., . . . Snyder-Mackler, L. (2012). Single-legged hop tests as predictors of self-reported knee function after ACL reconstruction: The Delaware-Oslo ACL cohort study. *American Journal of Sports Medicine, 40*(10), 2348–2356.

# Chapter 25

# The athletic shin

*Andy Franklyn-Miller*

## Introduction

Exertional lower-limb pain is very common in running athletes, but the existing literature is confusing, with terms such as overuse lower limb injury (OLLI), exertional lower limb pain (ELLP), medial tibial stress syndrome (MTSS) and chronic exertional compartment syndrome (CECS), along with the colloquial term 'shin splints' widely used to group and differentiate many of the same clinical presentations. The underlying mechanism of these conditions is muscle overload, and accordingly, they should be grouped together as a new diagnosis of *biomechanical overload syndrome* (BOS), rather than viewed as entities on their own.

This chapter will highlight how running kinematics and the timing of muscle recruitment can lead to the development of muscular overload through to bone stress, and how this can be successfully corrected with coaching to alleviate the underlying mechanisms.

## Features of biomechanical overload syndrome

Athletic shin pain can be focal along the medial or lateral tibial border or present more generally across the whole shank (shin) or calf muscle. The pain is always gradual in onset and progressive, described as 'pressure', 'tightening' or 'cramping', and worsens to such a crescendo that continued running is impossible. On occasion, it can additionally present with paraesthesia, 'foot slapping' or colour change, but unless the condition is progressing to fatigue failure and fracture, rest or night pain is uncommon.

Each of the common shin pain conditions is directly related to the muscle groups acting in that muscle compartment and the loading they are subjected to when running, jumping and landing. In *chronic exertional compartment syndrome* (CECS), the underlying pathophysiology was thought to be transient muscle ischemia[1] due to fascial non-compliance or muscle hypertrophy, but, to date, no conclusive proof of tissue necrosis or cell hypoxia has been demonstrated.[2] Moreover, CECS-type symptoms can been described in the anterior, peroneal and deep posterior compartments of the lower leg, making the pathology even less specific.[3] Intra-compartmental pressure measurement peak values show substantial overlap between the pathological and normative values, which, alongside error in variables of measurement technique, throw doubt on the diagnostic process, and as such, the diagnosis in its entirety.[4] Posterior calf pain and lateral calf pain are commonly included in the compartment syndrome bracket – but with much bigger fascial envelopment and no diagnostic pressures ever being confirmed.

*Medial tibial stress syndrome* (MTSS) has been described as a repetitive microtrauma to the tibia resulting from loading of the musculotendinous attachments to the tibial border.[5] The pain arises from the bony attachment of the muscles acting to plantar-flex and invert the foot, and it is the eccentric load on this muscular aponeurosis from the mechanical traction, rather than a torque force alone, which is responsible for the pain.[5]

Runners with a history of tibial stress fracture have been shown to run with greater hip abduction and therefore greater rear foot eversion, which leads to a resultant torque force on the tibia.[6] Greater tibial acceleration forces, and ground reaction forces have been shown to be contributing factors, and it is the lack of proximal muscle control that leads to the overload mechanism.[7]

All of these 'diagnoses' described above have a maladaptation to load that is modifiable by altering running kinematics as their common feature. It is hereby proposed that the label that should be used is *biomechanical overload syndrome*.

## Biomechanical overload syndrome

The common feature of BOS is the initial presentation of pain in various compartments of the lower leg. *Anterior BOS* relates typically to the overuse of the ankle flexors and, in particular, the tibialis anterior, to both lift the foot control it eccentrically in midstance. *Medial BOS* relates to overload of the medial soleus and tibialis posterior, in part due to a lack of forefoot pronation control, whereas *posterior BOS* commonly suggests an exaggerated stretch-contract cycle of the gastrocnemius and soleus. Each of these causative mechanisms will be discussed in turn, but the common features are the smaller muscles of the leg having to work excessively or adapt to a higher workload too quickly, resulting in fatigue failure.

The muscles of the lower limb are designed to absorb the force generated by the impact of landing, jumping and running, and then produce force to enable movement. Failure of the protective action of muscle can be seen as a stress response. Continued loading without the force absorption competency of the fatigued muscles can lead to bony overload and, eventually, to a stress fracture.

These conditions have proved difficult to treat conservatively with limited success of stretching, foam rolling, acupuncture, massage, extracorporeal shockwave therapy and activity modification.[8] Short-term outcomes from surgical decompression or fasciotomy are good in terms of pain relief but not in return to running at the previous level.[9,10]

## Extrinsic risk factors

Commonly, an increase in weekly running mileage is the trigger for BOS. Alternatively, short-term sudden changes in intensity, distance or running surface can be responsible,[11,12,13,14] but these are less frequent than the more gradual change in BOS. Similarly, a sudden change in training content may be able to be identified in the history. For example the new runner who starts to train more formally with a club often has less choice over the content of a training session, and the introduction of hill running or track work can be enough to cause a muscular overload similar to someone starting a new strength program in the gym. This in part can be a desired effect, as in resistance hypertrophy training, where muscle fatigue can be part of training load, but pain that prevents running suggests fatigue failure at the weakest link. As we will explore, this is often due to proximal major muscle groups taking less of the propulsive load than is optimal.

## The effect of shoe selection on shin pain

An extrinsic factor that the runner has control over is that of running shoe selection. The current vogue for minimal drop training shoes can contribute to BOS. These 'minimalistic' shoes offer a much-reduced angle from heel to toe (commonly referred to as 'drop') compared to traditional cushioned running shoes. In a standard running shoe, this can be as much as 14mm fall from heel to toe, but now 3–5mm drop shoes are common alongside zero drop shoes. These shoes are designed to promote a 'lifestyle' style. There is nothing particular about the shoe which alters running kinematics or style; indeed, recent evidence suggests it is perfectly possible to run with a forefoot or rear foot strike in any shoe,[15] and that the shoe does not alter the means of landing and absorbing force.

It is the runner who controls how they run, not the shoe.

Too rapid a transition from traditional to minimalistic shoes results directly in altered muscle loading patterns, in particular of the gastrocnemius and tibialis posterior. Minimalist shoes have also been associated with higher rates of stress fractures, but this is likely to relate to the adaptation, rather than the shoe itself.

Shoe shop running analysis is a burgeoning trend as part of a sales strategy, but any analysis that solely examines the feet gives a very small insight on the overall kinematics, and as such is likely to draw incorrect conclusions about rearfoot and midfoot pronation, which are, of course, normal coping mechanisms. Despite proof that foot pronation is not associated with injury,[16] stability shoes are still prescribed as a means of preventing injury.[17,18]

It seems, therefore, that shoe selection does not matter as much as thought and is purely a personal preference based on feel, fit and comfort and unrelated to injury risk or running gait. Where shoe selection can be useful is as a tool for running re-education; often a thinner sole with a less pronounced drop of 4–8mm can help feedback and, if targeting a midfoot strike, can assist the retraining process, alongside some training sessions barefoot to give enhanced proprioceptive feedback.

## Running technique philosophies

Philosophies regarding running techniques can be another important source of injury risk. Both Chi and Pose running methods purport to have significant weight of injury prevention evidence behind them, but a recent paper suggests there is little evidence that they either reduce injury or are more metabolically efficient.[19] Runners attempting to change their own kinematics can easily overcorrect, and the extremes of technique cues promoted in popular magazines or on weekend courses, if poorly applied, can result in significant muscle loading changes. All technique changes must be graduated to allow time for muscle tolerance to build up and the body to adapt to more proximal control, or the increase in joint moment further up the chain may lead to symptom development.[20]

## Running kinematics and BOS

Understanding the muscle activity and joint angular changes is necessary to understand the kinematics of running, and understanding the kinetics of loading is vital before attempting to alter these variables to manage lower limb pain. To fully understand BOS, we need to appreciate the whole lower limb, and many of the changes need to be made proximally in order to affect a distal change.

The gait cycle is broadly divided into stance and swing phases. Stance phase begins at the initial contact, where the tibialis anterior acts eccentrically to control the foot's force as it strikes the ground. The angle of the tibia at stance phase is important; the potential to overstride here can overload the tibialis anterior.

Stance phase is controlled by the deceleration effect of the gastrocnemius and soleus. This provides us with two potential areas to alter loading. First, reducing ground contact time allows for less pronounced ankle dorsiflexion and reduces the time-under-tension, and thereby mechanical work of the muscles. Second, a stiffer knee allows the posterior chain to take more of the load, reducing anterior knee, shin and calf work. This is in keeping with our philosophy of allowing the 'big muscles to do big jobs'.

Swing phase initiates as the stance limb moves into flight from toe-off. Initially the hip flexors are very active, along with the quadriceps, to return the leg to the correct pre-stance position. Just before foot strike, tensioning of the gluteals, hamstrings and gastrocnemius/soleus is suggested to increase the rate of force development required for propulsion. The gluteals control femoral adduction and internal rotation, so should they be weak or slow to engage and thus unable to adequately resist femoral rotation, patellofemoral and iliotibial band (ITB) symptoms can result. In addition, this loss of control can also lead to issues further down the chain, with tibial rotation giving increased load on tibialis posterior and the plantar flexors, leading to PBOS.

## Kinetics

Changing the range of motion or angle of a joint not only has an immediate effect on the activity of the surrounding musculature, but also changes the direction in which the force is applied and distributed. This force has to go somewhere and can lead to increased anterior knee load unless hamstring stiffness and gluteal speed of action is effectively coached in the gym in addition to the running track.

If we imagine the runner as a single mass on a leg, which is (represented by a spring), it is the stiffness of the spring that controls the explosive force from foot contact. This spring is compressed from foot strike to mid-stance then released to provide forward propulsion. Increasing the rate of force development of the gluteals, hamstrings and lumbar extensors enhances this spring-like stiffness. This results in improved hip extension and propulsion, which provides an opportunity to offload the smaller muscles further down the chain, i.e. the shin.

## Centre of mass

Whilst some popular running schools advocate running with a forward trunk lean to assist the propulsive effect of the hamstrings and gluteals, an excessive anterior pelvic tilt hinders maximal hip extension. Ultimately, this can lead to the ankle being too greatly dorsiflexed in midstance, increasing the demand on the plantar flexors to propel the athlete forward in an attempt to chase their centre of mass (COM). This is the opposite of what we are trying to achieve! As such, a near vertical torso is the most effective position to allow proximal muscle control of the running gait and prevent the overload of the shank muscles.

# Running re-education

## Anterior biomechanical overload

Commonly, the features seen in anterior BOS are:

- over-striding gait with slow cadence
- poor gluteal drive phase
- excessive heel strike with marked dorsiflexion of the ankle in terminal swing phase.

The first set of cues relate to pelvic position and stability of the torso. We focus on an upright body over the centre of mass with a neutral pelvis. The coaching cues can be internal, such as:

- 'Focus on a string pulling your head to the ceiling';
- 'Rest your chin on a shelf.'

or external, such as:

- 'Keep your body still whilst your legs are moving';
- 'Stand tall.'

These can be adapted depending on the response seen in video feedback with the individual.

The second set of cues relate to the thigh position. Asking for an increase in hip flexion by saying 'Close the thigh to the body' (not the body to the thigh) assists the upright body cues

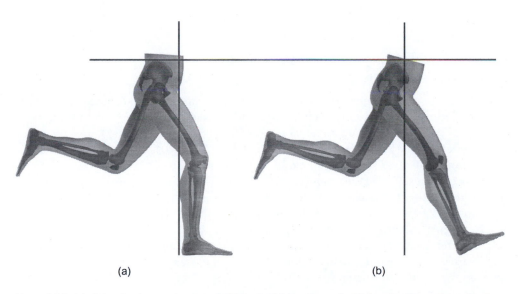

(a)                                                        (b)

Figure 25.1  (a): A level pelvis, with vertical tibia at initial contact and mid-foot landing reduces load on the anterior compartment and is the optimal position for those with anterior shin pain (b): The usual position at foot strike in those with ABOS

and allows the emphasis to be on the downward piston-like action of the leg to increase the propulsion of the hip extensors. In turn, this allows the large proximal muscles to provide the driving force, rather than the smaller muscles of the shank. It is usual to encourage a stamping action and allow it to soften to ensure that the speed of the downward action is emphasized, rather than the speed of the upward action.

> In our experience, 'high knees' is not a good cue here, but the 'piston' cue, like a bicycle pump, is most often successful. 'Slide your heel up a glass window behind your butt' (as opposed to 'kick your butt') can also be effective.

The third set of cues relate to the aim of landing with the mid-foot. Commonly, these athletes are overstriding with a tibial angle approaching 30 degrees from the vertical. Here, we aim to reduce the preload of the dorsiflexors. Barefoot treadmill work can be effective in this group, as are the coaching cues of:

- 'Focus on a downward action of your foot. Start with striking with the front of your foot. Once you've done that, now start to strike on your heel. Gradually oscillate between these two extremes to find the mid-foot balance.'
- 'Imagine an orange under your arch and squash it on every landing.'

The final cue relates to running cadence. Whilst foot position, tibial angle and decreased ground contact time are the most critical issues to try to resolve, by aiming to increase cadence by approximately 2–3 steps per minute above what the athlete presents with (as opposed to prescribing a particular rate), we have found the maintenance of a more vertical tibia that reduces impact loading is facilitated.

### Posterior biomechanical overload and medial tibial stress syndrome

This group of shin pain sufferers often demonstrate prolonged ground contact times, which has the effect of increasing time spent in loaded dorsiflexion, resulting in excessive eccentric loading of the posterior compartmental muscles each stance phase, which, over time, can lead to traction overload on the bone. This, coupled with a rapid rate of pronation and losses of end-range plantar flexor strength, are all are common features.

By coaching a stiffer leg on ground contact and less knee flexion we are seeking to preferentially recruit the large and powerful hip extensors, rather than the ankle plantarflexors. The coaching cues here include a piston-like extension, punching the foot into the ground and externally cueing the upright running style favoured by Michael Johnson. Another way we seek to stiffen a running gait in this group of athletes is by utilizing a 'penguin walk' with stiff legs in order to get the feel of reduced knee flexion in mid-stance. We then look to gradually increase the speed to a penguin run.

As with the anterior symptoms, it is often beneficial here to use the same cues to create a more mid-foot landing and increased hip flexion to both alter the ground reaction force (GRF) and to enhance the spring stiffness.

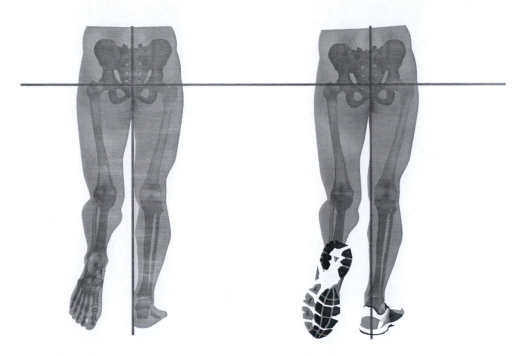

*Figure 25.2* The common decreased gluteal stability results in a crossover gait secondary to femoral rotation, which increases distal loading

A rapid rate of forefoot pronation can increase the eccentric load of the plantar flexors, and it can be useful here to add a stimulus into the shoe. A small rubber disc under the ball of the first metatarsal (MT) can provide a physical cue to encourage the faster rate of force production of tibialis posterior. In this condition, off treadmill work in end-range calf strength is important, along with tibialis posterior strengthening to enhance the control. The focus is to offload these muscles as much as possible, refocusing on the proximal prime movers.

Step width is also important in this population, as any crossover gait reinforces the rate of pronation and lack of eccentric control. It is best viewed from the coronal view and can be corrected by imagining a ball between the calves and running on train tracks, but the best cuing is visual feedback throughout.

## Walk-to-run programming

The philosophy that a deeply ingrained running gait pattern can be easily changed is often met with scepticism. Certainly, making more than one kinematic change at once can be challenging, so we typically utilize a walk-to-run programme, in which athletes are instructed to start a 30-minute session where 4-minute walk and 1-minute running cycles allow for brief focused activity on the coached changes. As this is comfortably completed, it is possible to alter the ratio to 3min:2min, 2min:3 min onwards, until 30 minutes of pain-free running is achieved. Typically these take our patients between four and six weeks, with good retention and follow-up video coaching in between.

## Posterior chain strength

The presence of back pain is a poor indicator in BOS population and commonly attributed to a weak core. It is, however, much more likely to relate to a weak posterior chain (back extensors, gluteals and hamstrings). We have discussed the underlying kinematic changes and the resultant changes to kinetics, but alongside this it is essential that a focus on strength is concurrent. Often the running re-education changes are tiring and require the strengthening of gluteal and lower back muscles to maintain technique and resist fatigue loss of form.

## Rare causes

There are always rare cases which often mimic the BOS presentation, such as:

- popliteal artery entrapment
- tibial nerve root impingement
- lateral popliteal nerve root impingement.

They are, however, far less common than presently described and should be part of a diagnosis of exclusion after running kinematic changes have been attempted.

---

With the feature of rest or night pain, it is prudent to ensure at least a plain X-ray has been carried out to exclude malignancy, which is rare but can present in the long bones.

---

## Summary

Overuse of the shin muscles as a result of incorrect or underuse of the larger, more proximal muscles can lead to overload. Whilst many 'diagnoses' or labels exist for exertional lower limb pain – a condition that ranges from myalgia to periostitis and eventually stress fracture – the terminology used for this continuum should reflect the root cause. Hence, this chapter proposes that the term *biomechanical overload syndrome* (BOS) be adopted to describe all forms of chronic athletic shin pain.

The urgency to make a pathological diagnosis leads many clinicians and coaches to look for a surgical answer when the most important factor is to address running technique. This can be broken down into the pelvis, knee, shin and foot, and many coaching cues are common among the various differential diagnoses.

Different coaching cues will always work better in some individuals than others, and video as well as verbal feedback are essential in making and managing a diagnosis and re-education of the running gait. Changes can be effectively applied over a 4-week period and exciting emerging evidence demonstrates lasting effect change.

## Notes

1 Zhang, Q., & Styf, J. (2004). Abnormally elevated intramuscular pressure impairs muscle blood flow at rest after exercise. *Scandinavian Journal of Medicine & Science in Sports, 14*(4), 215–20.

2  Edmundsson, D., Toolanen, G., Thornell, L. E., & Stal, P. (2010). Evidence for low muscle capillary supply as a pathogenic factor in chronic compartment syndrome. *Scandinavian Journal of Medicine & Science in Sports, 20*(6), 805–13.

3  Thorborg, K., Bandholm, T., Schick, M., Jensen, J., & Holmich, P. (2011) Hip strength assessment using handheld dynamometry is subject to intertester bias when testers are of different sex and strength. *Scandinavian Journal of Medicine & Science in Sports, 23*(4), 487–493.

4  Pedowitz, R. A., Hargens, A. R., Mubarak, S. J., & Gershuni, D. H. (1990). Modified criteria for the objective diagnosis of chronic compartment syndrome of the leg. *The American Journal of Sports Medicine, 18*(1). 35–40.

5  Verrelst, R., De Clercq, D., Vanrenterghem, J., Willems, T., Palmans, T., & Witvrouw, E. (2013). The role of proximal dynamic joint stability in the development of exertional medial tibial pain: a prospective study. *British Journal of Sports Medicine, 48*(5), 388–393.

6  Pohl, M. B., Mullineaux, D. R., Milner, C. E., Hamill, J., & Davis, I. S. (2008). Biomechanical predictors of retrospective tibial stress fractures in runners. *Journal of Biomechanics, 41*(6), 1160–5.

7  Zadpoor, A. A., & Nikooyan, A. A. (2011). The relationship between lower-extremity stress fractures and the ground reaction force: a systematic review. *Clinical Biomechanics, 26*(1), 23–8.

8  Gill, C. S., Halstead, M. E., & Matava, M. J. (2010). Chronic exertional compartment syndrome of the leg in athletes: Evaluation and management. *The Physician and Sportsmedicine, 38*(2), 126–32.

9  Slimmon, D., Bennell, K., Brukner, P., Crossley, K., & Bell, S. N. (2002). Long-term outcome of fasciotomy with partial fasciectomy for chronic exertional compartment syndrome of the lower leg. *The American Journal of Sports Medicine, 30*(4), 581–8.

10  Holmich, P., & Dienst, M. (2006). Differential diagnosis of hip and groin pain: Symptoms and technique for physical examination. *Der Orthopade, 35*(1), 10–5.

11  James, S. L., Bates, B. T., & Osternig, L. R. (1978). Injuries to runners. *The American Journal of Sports Medicine, 6*(2), 40–50.

12  Lysholm, J., & Wiklander, J. (1987). Injuries in runners. *The American Journal of Sports Medicine, 15*(2), 168–71.

13  Marti, B., & Vader, P. (1998). On the epidemiology of running inuries: The 1984 Berlin GrandPrix Study. *American Journal of Sports Medicine, 16*, 285–93.

14  Rochconger, P., Pennes, F., & Carne, W. (1995). Occurrence of running injuries. *Science in Sports, 10*, 15–9.

15  Shih, Y., Lin, K. L., & Shiang, T. Y. (2013). Is the foot striking pattern more important than barefoot or shod conditions in running? *Gait Posture, 38*(3), 490–4.

16  Nielsen, R. O., Buist, I., Parner, E. T., Nohr, E. A, Sorensen, H., Lind, M., et al. (2013). Foot pronation is not associated with increased injury risk in novice runners wearing a neutral shoe: A 1-year prospective cohort study. *British Journal of Sports Medicine, 48*(6), 440–447.

17  Enke, R. C., Laskowski, E. R., & Thomsen, K. M. (2009). Running shoe selection criteria among adolescent cross-country runners. *PM & R, 1*(9), 816–9.

18  Giuliani, J., Masini, B., Alitz, C., & Owens, B. D. (2011). Barefoot-simulating footwear associated with metatarsal stress injury in 2 runners. *Orthopedics, 34*(7), e320–3.

19  Goss, D. L., & Gross, M. T. (2012). A review of mechanics and injury trends among various running styles. *US Army Medical Department Journal,* July–Sept., 62–71.

20  Goss, D. L., & Gross, M. T. (2012). Relationships among self-reported shoe type, footstrike pattern, and injury incidence. *US Army Medical Department Journal,* Oct.–Dec., 25–30.

# Chapter 26

# The athletic foot and ankle

*Dan Lewindon and David Joyce*

## Introduction

Optimal foot and ankle (F+A) function is a vital component of weight-bearing performance. As the only point of contact with the ground, this complex system of bones, joints and muscles must act as both *mobile adaptor* and *spring-like lever* within the same movement, creating a malleable platform for effective balance whilst providing the conduit for explosive force production in dynamic motion.

Success in these tasks is heavily dependent on optimizing the interaction of articular (joint) structure and contractile (muscle) function, a highly specific process orchestrated by a finely tuned sensorimotor system. At the local level, this involves the contribution and interaction of a huge number of articular, capsular and soft tissue receptors in order to pre-determine, evaluate and modify foot/ankle placement and stability, thereby maintaining balance whilst simultaneously ensuring optimal direction and application of force.

During function the athlete's overall economy of motion, speed and evasive ability are all reliant on the efficiency of this local system to use the structural contours of the foot and surrounding tissue to appropriately absorb, store and return ground reaction force (GRF) in the right manner and at the right time. When we consider that all these processes must often occur within a fraction of a second, the importance of a well-tuned, strong and efficient neuromuscular system is clear.

F+A injuries continue to account for a significant proportion of injuries seen at all levels of participation in sports across the world and have high recurrence rates.[1] Moreover, sub-optimal F+A function has been implicated as a significant precursor to injuries higher up the kinetic chain.[2]

This chapter will provide an overview of the relevant anatomy and biomechanics before focusing on the criteria-driven rehabilitation process required to best ensure success following injury to the area.

## Structural overview

Functionally, the ankle is composed of three joints:

1   The talocrual joint (between the talus and the inferior aspect of the tibia)
2   The inferior tibiofibular joint (between the distal ends of the tibia and the fibula)
3   The subtalar joint (between the talus and the calcaneus).

Furthermore, the foot is composed of a proximal row of tarsals (navicular and cuboid), as well as a distal row of tarsal bones (medial, intermediate and lateral cuneiforms). Articulating to the tarsals are the five metatarsals, and then the phalanges and an irregular number of sesamoid bones.

Unlike in large joints such as the hip, the bony architecture of the ankle is only partially responsible for joint stability. The medial and lateral malleoli provide a certain degree of side-to-side stability but in full weight-bearing, all ligaments are in a relaxed state, and so it is the congruency of the talocrual joint that is all-important. The ankle is least stable in plantarflexion (the loose-packed position) and so it comes as no surprise that this is the position most widely implicated in acute ankle injuries. Conversely, the ankle is most stable in dorsiflexion (the close-packed position) and so injuries that occur in this position usually involve significant force and, as such, fractures must often be excluded as part of the diagnostic process. Dynamic stability of the ankle complex is provided by the peroneal muscle group, in particular the peroneus brevis and longus.

## Biomechanics in brief

### Walking

Walking is characterized by three distinct periods of double-limb support within a gait cycle, namely initial contact, mid-stance and toe-off. When performed well, this is a metabolically efficient process, minimising unnecessary muscle action and energy cost through the use of gravity, bony contours, joint articulations and elastic tension.

Efficient gait involves the interaction of three structural contours: the talocrural mortice, calcaneus and first metatarsal head, aptly named the 3-rocker system.[3]

At initial contact, the convex surface of the calcaneus promotes forward motion of the body's centre of mass. This is facilitated by the talocrural mortice, which allows smooth forward translation of the shin. Terminal stance is assisted by the convex surface of the first metatarsal head.

The efficient use of the third 'rocker' and resultant dorsiflexion of the first metatarsophalangeal joint (MTP) also facilitates the tightening of the plantar fascia, which generates stiffness along the longitudinal and transverse arches of the foot and creates an effective platform for motion. This is often termed the Windlass effect.[4]

The coupling of first MTP and talocrural joint dorsiflexion also generates passive tension within the foot and ankle flexors' tensile tissue (including the Acilles tendon), thereby contributing elastic energy at toe-off and reducing the contractile demand of the shank.[5]

Restriction to any aspect of this system may increase the metabolic cost of walking and predispose the individual to aberrant stresses somewhere within the lower-limb chain. Good observational and thorough rehabilitative practice is therefore required when assessing and training gait function to ensure restoration of pre-injury motion.

### The differences between walking and running

In addition to the loss of double-limb support and the introduction of a 'float' phase to the gait cycle, the transition from walking to effective high-speed running involves:

- A progressive reduction in foot contact time
- A progressive increase in vertical and horizontal ground reaction forces
- A change in initial contact position (from heel to mid-foot and from in front of the body to below the body)
- A change in both neuromuscular timing and muscle-tendon demand.

Beyond lowest speed jogging, where athletes may continue to use the first rocker (and therefore heel strike), initial contact will now occur at the mid-foot and/or forefoot with a rapid acceleration through the first MTP into terminal stance.

Clearly this will be a far quicker process, with foot contact times progressively shortening as intensity of running increases, reaching a peak in the elite of below 1/200th second during maximal velocity running. Previous researchers have highlighted the importance of minimising foot contact times in both the acceleration and maximal velocity phases of running,[6] although it should be noted that these studies are restricted to hard, track-like surfaces, rather than a muddy field.

Since foot contact times are shortening and vertical forces are increasing (2–3 times body weight at mid-paced running), the timing and contractile qualities of shank and intrinsic foot musculature are vital for both performance and economy.

Irrespective of the proportion of fast-twitch fibres contained within the shank, it would be inconceivable to generate enough force to provide the optimal platform to counteract vertical forces exceeding 2–3 times bodyweight with such short contact times. Activation of muscles therefore occurs in anticipation of ground contact, to allow time to achieve contraction.[7] Rather than working to a traditional concentric model, the muscle-tendon unit works isometrically to generate an actively 'stiff' F+A complex and brace the limb for impact. On contact with the ground, the contracting muscle then provides the perfect anchor for the free tendon to harness elastic energy through elongation. When performed well this will minimize energy loss by maximising the spring-like potential of series (SE) and parallel elastic tissue (PE) (principally the free tendon).[8]

> High-speed running is heavily reliant on neuromuscular characteristics and timing. When done efficiently the muscles involved act like springs, utilizing the free tendon to maximise both the economy and speed of motion.

## The mobile adaptor

Both the rocker and spring models are fine when dealing with a perfectly flat surface and purely sagittal plane of motion, but in multidirectional activities involving sudden external forces or alterations in the ground underfoot, the F+A must also have the intrinsic strength and malleable qualities to adapt rapidly without loss of movement economy or performance. This process further taxes the sensorimotor system to deliver accurate information at high speeds to moderate muscle tone and output in the appropriate muscle groups. The body uses this information to quickly predict, then adjust tone and foot placement in response to unpredictable demands. Previous studies have highlighted an increase in intrinsic foot muscle activation under perturbing conditions.[9] This is why the F+A complex must function as *both* a spring-like lever and a mobile adaptor. Consequently, both these roles must be taken into account when designing and delivering rehabilitation and injury prevention programmes.

## Consequences of foot and ankle injury

Not only does an injury to the foot and ankle complex require a period of time out of training or competition for recovery (a period that can range from days to months), but there may also be several other less explicit but nonetheless important consequences of the injury that often serve to render the complex more susceptible to further damage. These provide clues to guide the rehabilitation process and highlight the potential mechanical underpinnings of future risk. Common findings following acute and chronic ankle sprains include:

- Reduced joint range of motion
- Reduced rate and peak contractile force development in landing[10]
- Reduced joint position sense and proprioception[11]
- Increased joint landing forces[12]
- Loss of rear-foot and shank coupling in swing phase of gait.[13]

Loss of dorsiflexion (DF) range has the potential to alter gait mechanics and increase peak ground reaction force on landing. Indeed, DF range has consistently been shown to be a marker of future injury risk, both for the ankle and anterior knee.[2]

The remaining effects of injury would appear to be as a result of a loss of neuromuscular function, efficiency and/or timing. The peroneal muscles appear to be particularly affected, with a reduction in both afferent and efferent functioning and coordination of the anticipatory nature of their function reducing the ankle's preparedness to accept body weight at foot strike.[14] This all combines to disrupt the ankle's 'dynamic defence system'.

---

Clearly, the effect of an injury to the foot or ankle can lead to changes that are not confined merely to the injured structure itself, but which overall make this complex less dynamically stable and less efficient. Disruption to either foot and ankle structure or neuromuscular function, therefore, has the potential to increase risk of future injury and will certainly impair athletic performance.

---

## The rehabilitation philosophy

Following any injury, accurate diagnosis must be coupled with a thorough and holistic model of progressive rehabilitation, with the athlete at the centre of the process.

To ensure success, this is not enough, however. There is a vast difference between being judged medically fit to play and being considered ready to perform at the highest level. To achieve this high level of performance following an injury, we must develop a thorough understanding of the athlete, their individual physical and technical capabilities and limitations, and an accurate knowledge of normal training and match-play demands. This will ensure that the benchmarks of match fitness and technical ability are regained or even perhaps superseded before they are given the green light to return to sport.

---

Successful rehabilitation requires the alignment and integration of sports medicine, sports science, strength and conditioning and technical coaching throughout the rehabilitation process, to ensure the best and most timely outcome is achieved.

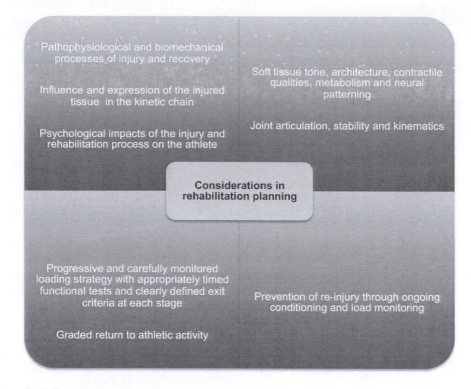

*Figure 26.1* Considerations in rehab

## Foot and ankle rehabilitation

When considering F+A injury rehabilitation and prevention, the primary consideration must be the complex's dual role as *mobile adaptor* and *rigid lever*, as well as our ability to appropriately challenge and develop both dynamic balance and spring stiffness in all three planes of motion and in a sports-specific manner.

### Programme construction

To aid clarity for both the performance team and the athlete, it is preferable to subdivide rehabilitation programmes into clear sections of increasing demand, with each section culminating in a series of exit criteria to allow progression to the next phase. These may include physiological markers of recovery/homeostasis, functional milestones and specific performance targets. Each section should include specific sports medicine/rehabilitation, strength and conditioning (S+C) and coach input, with careful consideration to the restrictions enforced through injury and the overall training volume/load desired.

The construction of this programme begins with athlete-centred planning and goal setting to ensure a good understanding of the process, likely timescales and milestones to be achieved. It also allows the athlete to have an input into their performance goals (both injury related and global).

*Phase I: Acute injury management*

The period immediately following an injury is focused on supporting the healing process of the damaged tissue and preventing excessive inflammation. A detailed account of pathophysiology and tissue healing is beyond the scope of this chapter, but simply put, we must respect the healing tissue's line of stress during this acute phase. Lines of stress are those directions of motion that will place the greatest amount of tensile force on the injured structure. In the case of a lateral ligament sprain, this will be to ensure that excessive inversion and plantarflexion of the foot are avoided, whilst permitting motion in opposing or 'safe' planes. Other examples are listed below:

Table 26.1 Lines of stress

| Injury | Line(s) of Stress |
| --- | --- |
| Deltoid ligament sprain | Eversion |
| Ankle syndesmosis sprain | Dorsiflexion |
| | Axial rotation |
| FHL tendinopathy | First MTP dorsiflexion |
| | Ankle dorsiflexion |

## Acute phase rehabilitation

During this acute phase following an injury, interventions are typically chosen with the aims of:

- Promoting a rapid and successful transition from the inflammatory phase to the early proliferation phase of healing;
- Desensitizing irritated tissue;
- Reducing swelling/effusion; and
- Allowing a timely progression into a functional rehabilitation program.

The presence of localized pain and/or ankle joint swelling in the absence of injury have been shown to result in subsequent weakness to plantar flexion and evertor muscle output, reducing subsequent functional performance and potentially increasing re-injury risk,[15] and so it is vital that pain and inflammation control is established early. Treatment will include some consideration of the P.R.I.C.E. strategy (protect − rest − ice − compress − elevate) and may include the use of strapping, electrotherapy, soft tissue mobilization, manual therapy and weight-bearing adjuncts, depending on the grade of injury and preference of the clinician and athlete.

With specific reference to ankle injuries, previous studies have reported improved outcomes (pain and function) in lateral ankle sprain recovery with an intermittent icing strategy (namely 10 minutes on, 10 minutes off, 10 minutes on every two hours) in comparison to the more typical 20 minutes every two hours application.[16] Although widely used, the physiological benefits of ice are not currently completely defined. At a cellular level, it would appear to reduce metabolism and blood flow and may therefore reduce secondary cell death. Irrespective of healing potential, it certainly blunts local pain response, which in itself will expedite recovery.

The use of low-intensity ultrasound has also been demonstrated to accelerate soft tissue proliferation times and return to pre-injury tensile strength.[17] Typical protocols advocate a daily use of 20 minutes applied to the lesion site.

To fully enhance the 'healing environment' of the injured tissue, the brief use of a pneumatic boot in the initial 48 hours post injury is worthwhile considering, the aim of which is to protect the injured tissue from further damage. Dependent on the severity of the injury, the use of crutches may also be warranted, particularly if the athlete is unable to walk without a pronounced limp.

### Early afferent input is vital

It is generally accepted practice that absolute immobilization of injury must be minimized wherever possible. Following a brief period of protection, early mobilization of soft tissue is essential in order to maintain normal joint, neural and soft tissue afferent input, joint kinematics and motor patterning.[18] With respect to injuries of the foot and ankle, isolated injury within this complex can quickly have a significant and long-lasting effect on neighbouring joints kinematics and overall motion economy. Accordingly, gentle, pain-free motion in 'safe' planes (avoiding lines of stress) should begin within hours of injury in order to:

*   Maintain afferent input to the CNS
*   Maintain pain-free motion within all joints.

> It is not uncommon for the effects of immobilization following injury to the foot and ankle to be the most significant limiting factor in recovery time.

Following the first 24 hours of relative immobilization/unloading, this rehabilitation strategies should include gait re-education/maintenance drills in a weight-supported environment (for example in a shallow pool) to try and maintain the 3-rocker strategy that is so important to gait economy, and encourage normal intrinsic mechanics within the foot – that is challenge its ability to act as mobile adaptor with reduced impact. Tasks such as balance drills, backwards and sideways walking and lunging are all helpful in achieving these aims. The hydrostatic pressure of the pool environment has the added advantage of helping to accelerate the process of effusion reduction.

### S+C: be innovative!

It is important that athletic development is not ignored, even during this initial phase, particularly given the rapid loss of athletic qualities in periods of enforced rest.[18]

Whilst running and heavy/explosive weight-bearing training will not be possible at this point, unloaded and innovative fitness and strength maintenance is both possible and necessary to prevent down-regulation of the athlete's physiology. It is also worth considering that ongoing training may have the potential to directly influence physiological healing and functional restoration through:

- Dynamic crossover of neural patterning[19]
- Positive hormonal stimulation (anabolic pathways).

---

**Examples of appropriate fitness work in phase I of rehabilitation**

**Strength** *(non-affected limb)*

Single leg press + body weight squats
Split stance lunges + calf raises
Hopping/plyometric program
Full upper limb program
Core strength and endurance

**Fitness**

Single-leg row
Seated arm ergometer
Seated boxing

---

## Psychological support

The use of psychology in guiding the athlete through rehabilitation may be extremely important, particularly in high-grade/career-threatening injuries or in athletes with a history of injury.

At a physiological level, strategies to reduce stress (and therefore cortisol levels) may conceivably have an effect on the acute injury recovery process, whilst goal setting, positive thought-processes, performance visualization and emotional support can play a significant role in athlete recovery and bear consideration.

## Exit criteria

Prior to progressing to the next phase of rehabilitation, it is vital that certain milestones are achieved. This helps to eliminate guesswork and ensure that progression to the next level is measured in terms of function and not time. This also helps to ensure that the injured tissue is robust enough to progress to the next phase where, inevitably, the stresses imposed on the injured site will be greater. The advantage of this approach is that the milestones can be communicated to the athlete and coaching staff at the outset, and all are aware of what tasks need to be achieved. It also helps to ensure a consistency of approach to rehabilitation that is focused on function, rather than simply the passage of time. Guidance can be given as to the average time it takes to complete each stage, but neither the performance professional nor the athlete is tied to a discrete time period. Using time as the exit criteria will not be appropriate for every case because of the variables of injury site, injury severity and numerous other individual-specific factors, such as healing rates, previous injury history and compliance with rehabilitation. In contrast, functional exit criteria make the rehabilitation programme applicable to any F+A injury.

---

To allow progression to phase 2 of rehabilitation, we suggest the following exit criteria are passed:

1   Resolution of active inflammatory process
2   Full pain-free active foot and ankle ROM
3   Normalised pain-free walking gait
4   Single-leg weight-bearing control (ability to maintain single leg stance > 30 seconds).

**Considerations in the acute phase**

1   Protect injured tissue's line of stress;
2   Pursue early rehabilitation to maintain afferent and efferent normality;
3   Be innovative in S+C but continue to target athletic development: strength, power, core;
4   Psychological input where necessary;
5   Be guided by exit criteria that confirm that functional progression is possible.

---

## Phase 2: Low-level loading

A heavy emphasis in early F+A rehabilitation is directed towards re-establishing neural pathways and normal motor patterns within the limits of pain and injury irritation. This will involve progressively challenging the foot and ankle's functional control and regulatory systems to adapt to changing surfaces and demands.

## Functional kinematics

This will include restoration of normal gait and balance mechanisms and attention to the 3-rocker system of gait. A common clinical finding following ankle sprain is the loss of talocrural dorsiflexion, which manifests itself in gait with excessive and early pronation and an early heel lift during mid to late stance, with or without an abductory (inward) twist of the hind-foot. A persistent loss of dorsiflexion has been linked to injury risk, both to the lateral ankle ligament complex and more recently at the patella tendon in jumping athletes.[2] It is therefore vital that normal motion is re-trained to minimize the risk of re-injury and new injury alike. This movement can be trained in isolation using gentle weight-bearing techniques, including active knee-to-wall stretches and belt mobilizations.

> Where indicated radiologically, clinically and physiologically, the use of injection therapy may serve as a useful adjunct in resolving a persistent primary effusion or secondary effects of ankle injury such as posterior impingement or synovitis.

From an articular loading perspective, this phase of rehabilitation should begin in a weight-assisted environment (shallow pool or sprung floor), where both gait and balance can be developed without stressing the articular system or risking lateral structures. For most low-grade injuries, a rapid progression from pool gait to land-based drills within 48–72 hours following injury would be targeted, but only once these land-based drills can be performed appropriately.

## Cryokinetics: The role of ice

The use of ice is not only restricted to pain modification and decreasing local cellular demands immediately following injury as it is useful as an adjunct to active rehabilitation. It would appear that icing the affected joint may be effective in improving efferent activation (specifically Hoffman and muscle reflexes) in adjacent muscles, thus blunting the effect of pain/swelling on motor patterning and performance.[20]

Typical protocols will often use 15 minutes of cold-water immersion before rehabilitation drills, with 3–5-minute repeated use every 10 minutes during the session. Whilst this does not have a large and consistent body of affirmative evidence, its underpinning science has merit and this may be an area worth exploring when developing rehabilitation protocols.

## Proprioceptive/balance training

Proprioception can be considered the body's internal awareness or 'GPS', and is broadly comprised of three interactive afferent pathways, namely peripheral mechanoreceptors (articular and peri-articular sensory receptors), vestibular (inner ear) and visual receptors. This system transmits a constant stream of sensory information, which is processed by three distinct hierarchal zones of the central nervous system: the spinal cord, brain stem (cerebellum) and sensory cortex. This multifaceted system allows reflex correction to joint position and muscle force in addition to interpretation by higher centres and therefore permits the potential for conscious learning/skill acquisition and enhancement.

At the F+A, this will involve modulation of shank and intrinsic foot muscles to optimize the position and tone of the mobile adaptor in response to external stress. A significant component of lower-limb rehabilitation should therefore focus on thoroughly re-training balance mechanisms to cope with increasing demands. This should always occur with a view to making the tasks sport relevant.

Typical protocols will progress athletes from tandem or in-line stance onto one limb, with a progressive increase in postural demand through introduction of hand-eye skills, movement out of base of support and unstable surfaces.

## The use of instability training in rehabilitation

Unstable surfaces are often used to stress contractile rate of force development, reactive stability and the foot's ability to act as effective mobile adaptor. These receive mixed reviews amongst many quarters of the S+C world, as they are, in the main, not sports-specific. Their use bears consideration, however, if the desired effect is a greater rate of control than can be achieved on a more stable platform. Additionally, if intrinsic foot strength is to be targeted, this quality can also be specifically enhanced through the use of a soft/pliable surface, so, whilst not 'sports-specific' they can be seen as 'sports-relevant'.

Previous studies have highlighted the use of unstable proprioceptive training protocols in ankle injury prevention with as little as five minutes per day sufficient to produce a significant reduction in non-contact ankle injury risk through a competitive season.[21]

## Positional variation

From a structural perspective, the talocrural joint is least congruent in plantar flexion and therefore more reliant on surrounding musculature and rapid and accurate sensory information to maintain position. Balance drills should therefore start with the foot in a stable position (in dorsiflexion/neutral) but might progress into positions of relative instability (plantar flexion) to greater stress the reactivity of the neuromuscular system as tissue healing and functional ability allow. This has particular relevance for individuals who typically perform in extremes of movement range such as ballet or gymnastics.

---

### Key points

Local reflex balance can be developed through enforced reduction in visual and vestibular contribution or through progressive challenges to the peripheral nervous system/reflex demand, for example:

1   Balance drills with eyes closed
2   Pass/catch/coordination drills
3   Decreasing surface stability such as standing on balance mats or sand.

---

True development of injury saving mechanisms requires repetitive and sports-specific training to develop and ingrain neural pathways. The sole use of a wobble-board will not be enough! This process needs to progress to include dynamic tasks, for example:

1   Footwork and coordination drills
2   Multi-angle and surface hopping
3   Application of external forces (bands, weights, opponents).

## Testing/limb symmetry

Balance performance can be tested using a number of validated tests. One simple quantitative measurement system is the star excursion balance test (SEBT), which measures the ability of the standing leg to maintain balance whilst the free leg reaches as far as possible along eight lines, orientated at 45-degree angles. Previous research has identified this as a sensitive measure of detecting proprioceptive deficits in chronically unstable ankles.[22] This represents a valid test of multi-plane ankle balance, particularly for athletes participating in multidirectional sports. Normally, we would target a limb symmetry of >90 per cent as a reliable indicator of symmetrical balance performance.

## Localized strength

F+A strengthening can begin immediately in cases of isolated ligament or articular injury. In cases of injury involving a muscle, appropriate lines of stress should be considered in the timing and progression of strengthening. Typical rehabilitative practice will involve progressions in loading from gentle isometric midrange contractions to outer-range high-force, high-speed drills as comfort allows.

In the case of an ankle sprain, progressive intrinsic foot strengthening and isometric eversion, inversion and plantarflexion would begin during this phase and would continue as a consideration throughout the entire rehabilitation process.

As previously described in the biomechanical review, economy of motion and performance characteristics in running are partly dependent on optimizing the elastic contribution of the muscle tendon unit through actively stiffening the contractile tissue and therefore allowing the tendon to act as a spring, storing and releasing elastic energy rapidly as required. The use of isometrics should therefore be considered as the first stage in regaining the tensile architecture required for explosive weight-bearing athletic function.

Foot strengthening drills should not be confined purely to rehabilitation. A six-week intrinsic foot-strengthening program has been demonstrated to result in significant increases in jump height,[23] highlighting its significance in developing explosive characteristics.

## S+C: Impact-free

Early rehabilitation should never exclude athletic development. Even in higher grades of peripheral and central injury, as long as practitioners observe the *line(s) of stress*, strength and conditioning can continue/intensify to address agreed areas of deficiency.

There is a growing trend in sports medicine to recognize the 'opportunity' injury affords us to develop athletic function, due to the enforced period of rest from match play and competition. This mind-set has obvious benefits to the athletes' psyche but also highlights the practical possibilities available during an enforced period of rest.

The use of a pneumatic boot or protective taping whilst the athlete completes his upper limb, trunk, unaffected limb S+C will ensure maintenance of the optimal healing environment, whilst allowing potential lower-limb dynamic crossover of neural drive and neuromuscular function as previously described.

To allow progression to phase 3 of rehabilitation, we suggest the following exit criteria are passed:

- Pain-free 90 per cent+ baseline range of motion
- Symmetry/return to baseline static balance
- No reaction to low load functional training.

**Considerations in the low load phase**

1   Surface: progression from pool to sprung surface to land
2   Balance (static): moving from pool to land to soft surface and from dorsiflexion to plantarflexion and from stable to unstable
3   Neuromuscular pathways and optimal movement strategies
4   Contractile tissue qualities and endurance
5   Neural (train unaffected limb) and hormonal benefits of S+C
6   Unloaded fitness maintenance.

## Phase 3: Progressive functional training

The aims of this phase are to:

- Expose the foot/ankle to an increasing program of impact and multi-plane stress; and
- Ensure that the athlete is fully ready to return to maximal intensity, multidirectional training.

Since we are operating on a functional recovery strategy, we must ensure that our exit criteria are robust and valid before the athlete is released to maximal intensity training and a return to unplanned situations and/or collision training.

## Rehabilitation: Control, absorption, deceleration and reactivity

Now that static balance has been restored, the next phase is to add dynamism and ground reaction force to the lower limb to develop the reactive stabilizing and elastic energy mechanisms previously described, and optimize the 'rigid' lever portion of F+A function. These drills will prepare the joints and surrounding surfaces for the impacts faced in weight bearing.

As previously described, plyometric performance in hopping (and therefore, by extension, jogging and sprinting) is dependent in part on the optimization of leg spring stiffness, which serves to harness elastic energy potential from impact whilst simultaneously protecting articular tissues from excessive impact forces. When considering the role of the F+A in propulsion, previous research has demonstrated the significance of the plantar foot afferent receptors in modulating whole-leg spring stiffness and therefore hopping and, again, by extension, sprint performance.[24] Developing these qualities would involve the manipulation of training surface and ankle position to progressively increase the loading demand and elastic contribution:

- Pool counter-movement jumps
- Trampette force absorption and reactivity
- Progressive landing drills
- Progression to force absorption and reactivity/return
- Short shuttles to develop deceleration
- Mini functional plyometric drills (stiff-foot short-step bounds and skipping drills).

From a qualitative point of view, whatever drills are selected, hind-foot and mid-foot control and patterning should be exposed and appropriately trained to ensure that optimal movement patterns are fostered during these drills as previously described in the biomechanics section. Specifically we would look to prevent excessive or asymmetrical frontal plane motion at the subtalar or midtarsal joints, and that quality of force absorption, propulsion and use of the 3-rocker was achieved in all drills. We would seek to limit any limping, early lift-off or asymmetrical loading patterns.

As the athlete progresses through low-level, firm-surface drills, it is not unreasonable for them to resume light treadmill-based jogging drills – although care should be taken to monitor volume-load, particularly in injuries involving an articular component.

### Sand

A surface that bears consideration in lower-limb rehabilitation is sand. This has the dual advantage of reducing impact forces in joint-compromised athletes, whilst also increasing the contractile demand of shank and intrinsic foot muscles. In injuries to contractile tissue around the foot and ankle, this may prove an excellent adjunct to traditional strength programmes. Typical drills would include:

- Rapid deceleration quality training
- Linear and multidirectional footwork
- Early return to hopping and dynamic balance.

When considering the use of sand, be aware of the increased concentric energy demands to the whole lower limb as fatigue will occur more quickly.

### Lateral and torsional stress

The 'lines of stress' previously considered throughout the earlier stages of rehabilitation must at this stage be progressively exposed through lateral and multidirectional static and dynamic balance components in readiness for multidirectional running.

The drills chosen would entirely depend on the specific injury suffered. For example a high-ankle injury (injury to the ligamentous tissues stabilizing the tibia and fibula) would necessitate axial torsion stress in talocrural dorsiflexion, whilst injury to the first metatarsophalangeal joint would require loading of the forefoot in plantarflexion.

In the lateral ankle injury example, this would commonly include:

- One-quarter turn hop
- Lateral step and hold (against external load)
- Maximal lateral hop + stick drills
- Sports-specific movement patterns.

### Central fatigue and motor control

Injury audit data across all sports consistently identifies that a significant proportion of injuries occur in the latter stages of match play/competition, highlighting the potential effects of central and peripheral fatigue on exposure and injury risk.[25] It would therefore be prudent to manipulate rehabilitation progression with a pre-fatigue process before motor control/ balance training to further expose the proprioceptive systems to challenge and contractile tissue to fatigue.

### S+C: Weight-bearing training

With range and static-unloaded balance restored, external loading can safely be resumed through the affected limb. With proprioception (and, in this example, sports-specificity) in mind, the use of single-leg training should form part of this program. To ensure intrinsic foot afferent input, strength and control is simultaneously trained. There is also a strong argument for barefoot strength training (provided this is safe).

Typical drills might include:

- Barbell/dumbbell/kettle bell:
  - Lunge
  - Step up
  - Split-stance dead-lift
  - Aleckna
- Weighted vest endurance circuits
  - Squat, lunge, step up, box switch
- Sled pulls (forward + reverse towing).

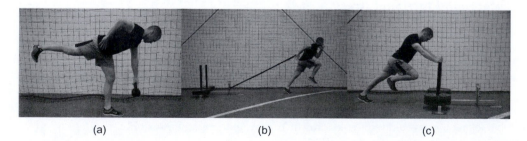

(a)        (b)        (c)

*Figure 26.2* (a) Aleckna, (b) sled pulls, (c) prowler push

## Occlusion training

The use of vascular occlusion training has gained in popularity over recent years as an effective method of developing muscle tissue strength and size without exposure to significant external loading.[26] The technique involves placing a tourniquet cuff around a proximal muscle group and inflating the cuff to 100mmHg whilst the athlete completes an unloaded strengthening drill.

The process is thought to work in part through the generation of an anaerobic metabolic pathway, resulting in a lactate rich environment (a key cellular driver of the anabolic process) and type-II muscle tissue preferential activation. Whilst optimal pressures and loading characteristics are variable within the literature, consistent improvements are reported, often more than a match for traditional hypertrophy models.[26]

The following protocol would be considered appropriate to use in F+A rehabilitation with the aim being to increase the strength of the surrounding muscles without applying excessive load through the repairing joints.

- 20 per cent one repetition maximum (1RM) load split stance calf raise
- 1.3 x systolic pressure (cuff applied to upper thigh)
- 3 sets to failure (cuff to be worn throughout session)

Occlusion training has the potential to reduce overall load demand through the affected structures, whilst developing tissue characteristics important to explosive sport and bears consideration in the rehabilitation process.

## Volume/load consideration

Inevitably at this stage of any rehabilitation plan, the athlete will be exposed to an increase in the volume/load of training. This represents a significant increase in foot contacts and articular loading. In an isolated lateral ligament sprain, this is of little concern, but in a larger grade injury (greater shear forces), or injuries with a concomitant medial talar dome chondral irritation, this would be a significant consideration. Again, success in this regard will be ensured with good interdisciplinary communication, sound programme planning and accurate monitoring.

> Evidence of deterioration through escalating effusion or pain and decreasing markers of functional performance would alert the medical team to the potential for harm and may prompt a reduction in on-feet volume /load or regression back through to an earlier phase of rehabilitation

## Functional performance tests

Progression through this phase will require completion of several validated functional performance tests to gauge limb symmetry dynamically. Previous research has highlighted the use of the three-hop distance test and adapted crossover tests in lower-limb injuries to gauge functional progression and are worthwhile tests to employ in F+A rehabilitation.[27]

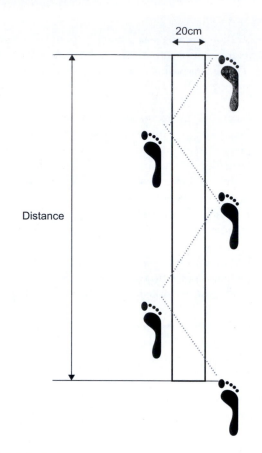

*Figure 26.3* Adapted cross over test

In terms of measuring linear qualities of force absorption, production and confidence in the whole kinetic chain, these tests are a useful component of a well-considered rehabilitation plan. We would traditionally expect a limb symmetry index (LSI) of 90 per cent as a good predictor of functional performance and recovery.

### Return to high-speed running

Once the athlete demonstrates good kinetic and kinematic qualities in limb deceleration, good reactivity in low-force bounding drills and 90 per cent limb symmetry in FPT, there is a strong indication that they are ready for a return to higher-intensity linear running.

From an articular loading perspective, greater vertical ground reaction forces are reported in slower-speed jogging than high-speed accelerations.[28] This may be due to the change in foot strike from heel to forefoot and altered neuromuscular characteristics previously described.

It is good practice (particularly for multidirectional athletes) to run with intent over small, confined spaces before running for extended distances due to the reduction in relative joint demands. This is of more importance in higher-graded lower-limb injuries, where the practitioner may be more concerned with aberrant effects of joint compression and shear, resulting in the potential for loss of homeostasis and muscle reflex latency through effusion increase.

An alternative strategy in higher-grade injuries where joint compression is a significant concern is the use of backward running, wherein previous research has also highlighted a significant reduction in vertical GRF.

Alternative options now include the use of anti-gravity treadmills, which reduced body weight and therefore weight force on impact in running. This has been demonstrated to promote early return and maintenance of high running volume in joint-compromised athletes.[29]

In terms of running, it is appropriate that attention initially be focused on regaining acceleration and deceleration quality and performance. As such, running distances would be limited to 20–30 metres to prevent the athlete from moving into maximal velocity running. Once satisfied that the athlete could tolerate repeated maximal acceleration/deceleration training, a progression into larger running distance is appropriate. Additional exit criteria in the completion of this phase may include repeated shuttle tests or sprint tests and comparison with pre-injury data.

---

In sports that require high-level foot and ankle function but do not involve significant amounts of running (such as martial arts, table tennis or fencing), the focus would be mainly on increasing the velocity and number of foot contacts on the ground (or, in the case of kicking sports such as taekwondo, pads) at various and increasingly demanding angles.

---

## Agility

Once comfortable in linear running, deceleration and dynamic lateral balance training, the final aspect of this stage involves the development of multidirectional qualities.

As with all aspects of rehabilitation, the specific drills are dependent on the athlete, their individual qualities, their position and the sport in question. Irrespective of this, however, the pathway must be methodical in its composition, with consideration given to:

- Tissue lines of stress
- Pace
- Coordinative complexity
- Surface
- Footwear
- Predictability
- Repetition
- Fatigue
- Sports specificity.

It is reasonable to initially use predictable, short-excursion drills, building the pace, complexity and distance, before introducing athlete decision making/unpredictable position-specific scenarios with and without central fatigue.

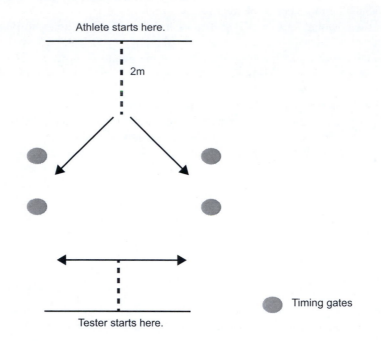

Figure 26.4 Reactive agility test

Previous studies have highlighted the significant role of athlete decision making in agility performance.[30] This should be considered in latter-stage drills, in sports where these qualities are important. The use of the *reactive agility test* (RAT) which incorporates decision making into a lateral agility/stepping task could represent a useful component of the exit criteria for this stage of rehabilitation (Figure 26.4).[30] For this to be valid and reliable component of objective testing, however, requires pre-injury baseline data.

In the absence of the RAT, once the athlete can freely demonstrate visibly symmetrical agility mechanisms in complex and unpredictable scenarios under the influence of fatigue, they are well equipped to return to light skill based training with activity restriction (a common example would be the use of a red bib to alert all other players and coaches of their limitations).

To allow progression to phase 4 of rehabilitation, we suggest the following exit criteria are passed:

90 per cent baseline or limb symmetry in FPT
Maximal intensity acceleration, deceleration and maximal velocity running
Completion of lateral and multidirectional running (predictable and unpredictable)
Reactive agility testing
No reaction to rehabilitation.

---

### Considerations in the progressive functional loading phase

1 Landing, deceleration and acceleration, quality and symmetry of motion
2 Neuromuscular pathways and optimal movement strategies
3 Contractile tissue qualities and endurance
4 Balance, control and optimal motor function whilst metabolically fatigued
5 Progressive acceleration, deceleration and maximal velocity running.

---

## Phase 4: High-level loading/return to competition

A successful return to competition requires the athlete to demonstrate that they can comfortably cope with their pre-injury training volume and intensity, without irritation to the injury. From a qualitative perspective, the athlete and management team must be satisfied that the injury has been overcome and the athlete is both physically and psychologically ready to return to match play. This is a pragmatic process, requiring good interpretation of training data, pertinent functional measures and injury monitoring.

The athlete must also be able to repeat training efforts on sequential days without loss of performance or injury irritation. This represents a far better strategy than an isolated 'fitness test'.

## S+C: return to performance

By this stage, the athlete has returned to non-contact training and full and unrestricted strength and conditioning package. To best ensure the athlete's previous level of performance has been regained or indeed surpassed, we require referral to baseline data of strength, power and endurance capabilities. Success in this regard would serve to build athlete confidence and become an objective measure of readiness to return to competition.

Dependent on the sport, such performance indices may include:

- Running speed over 10, 20, 40 meters for explosive running sports
- Vertical hop tests for jumping/bounding sports such as basketball or volleyball
- Validated endurance tests – for example Maximal Aerobic Speed or Interval field Test[31]
- Single-leg strength and rate-of-force development testing (to maximize validity in weight-bearing sports this should be done in closed chain).

In terms of functional rehabilitation, the outstanding areas of concern would now be:

- Specialist skills such as kicking (ball or opponent dependent on the sport) and tackling,
- Collision/evasion training (for contact sports)
- High-speed landing training (for sports such as netball and gymnastics)
- Return to full training +/- partial match play.

Load, volume and performance of specialist skills and collisions are best determined through previous competition data, and as previously stated, the inclusion of a specialist coach is crucial to ensure appropriate technical skills are regained. To further expose the athlete, rehabilitation would always now take place in a pre-fatigued state, either at the close of field training or weight sessions. This could include:

- Execution of kicks from either foot to specified targets, whilst under pressure for footballers
- Progressive exposure to contact (both tackling and being tackled), with a graded increase in external load (opponent momentum) and repetition and a decrease in predictability in contact sports
- Repeated backtracking smashes in sports such as badminton
- Sparring in martial arts
- Competitive drills in field sports such as hockey, handball or lacrosse.

> Once the athlete has completed these specific skills and returned to their normal training volume/load without any adverse reaction, they would be considered fit for the demands of competition.

## Taping

The use of rigid taping is commonplace in expediting return to play following injury. Whilst it often provides the athlete with confidence and may improve afferent information and even provide some short-lived mechanical support, it should not be used to cloud the true functional ability of the injury. In truth, the mechanistic benefits of taping have not been conclusively determined. Several studies have reported favourable results in preventing first-time injury rates and improving neuromuscular characteristics in previously injured ankles.[32] Therefore it may represent a useful adjunct in the final stages of rehabilitation.

Of note, there is some evidence demonstrating an increase in joint loading forces on landing in a taped ankle.[33] This may preclude its use in instances of articular injury or restricted dorsiflexion, although it should be remembered that there is a wide variation in strapping technique and strategy.

> **Match play**
>
> Depending on the severity of injury, it might be prudent to include completion of a partial match in this process. As previously described, fatigue is considered a significant risk factor in injury occurrence. In the absence of normative motion analysis/GPS data demonstrating conclusively that pre-injury intensity and volume has been regained, this will serve as a final demonstration of fitness to the management team and player.
>
> To allow exit from the rehabilitation process, we suggest the following exit criteria are passed:
>
> Baseline fitness, speed and lower limb strength
> Baseline training volume, intensity + quality (GPS determined)
> Completion of full contact training without reaction and with clear confidence
> Completion of partial match/match intensity.

This is certainly not the end of the process, however, as now attention inevitably moves towards injury prevention and ongoing foot/ankle conditioning.

---

**Considerations in this phase**

1 High-intensity multidirectional training under fatigue
2 Return to normal training sessions
3 Completion of return to special skills, for example kicking and collision training
4 Limb symmetry in single-leg loaded drills

---

## Foot and ankle injury prevention

Previous injury remains the strongest predictor of future pathology, and this is certainly true of the foot and ankle, where recurrence rates are consistently high in athletic populations. The failure to resolve the mechanical and neuromuscular sequelae from the initial injury (discussed at discussed at length through the earlier sections of this chapter) is undoubtedly the principle reason for this. To truly manage any injury, therefore, training that seeks to ensure the re-establishment and development of motor pathways, contractile qualities and tissue capabilities is necessary.

We know that functional recovery occurs well before physiological healing. We therefore have a duty of care to ensure that we continue to monitor the injury and pursue ankle conditioning until the athlete can demonstrate return to pre-injury risk values. In cases of significant injury or multiple previous injuries to a site, clinicians may choose to continue this process for the remainder of the athlete's career.

In a professional team set-up this can be well facilitated with regularly scheduled preventative sessions, either in small groups or individually attended. When delivering a prevention program it is important to consider the desired training stimulus and functional outcomes.

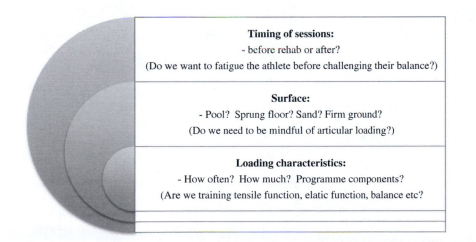

**Timing of sessions:**
- before rehab or after?
(Do we want to fatigue the athlete before challenging their balance?)

**Surface:**
- Pool? Sprung floor? Sand? Firm ground?
(Do we need to be mindful of articular loading?)

**Loading characteristics:**
- How often? How much? Programme components?
(Are we training tensile function, elatic function, balance etc?)

*Figure 26.5* Prevention considerations

This may involve manipulation of any of the variables discussed through the rehabilitation process to ensure that we consider the needs of the individual:

As with any form of athletic training the stimulus needs to be variable to maximize player interest, compliance and adaptation.

## Summary

Foot and ankle injuries are prevalent in all weight-bearing sports. Success in both the rehabilitation and prevention of these injuries requires a thorough understanding of normal anatomy and function and a clear and criteria-driven rehabilitation model.

## Notes

1  Doherty, C., Delahunt, E., Caulfield, B., Hertel, J., Ryan, J., & Bleakley, C. (2014). The incidence and prevalence of ankle sprain injury: A systematic review and meta-analysis of prospective epidemiological studies. *Sports Medicine*, *44*(1), 123–140.

2  Malliaras, P., Cook, J. L., & Kent, P. (2006). Reduced ankle dorsiflexion range may increase the risk of patellar tendon injury among volleyball players. *Journal of Science and Medicine in Sport*, *9*(4), 304–309.

3  Perry, J., & Davids, J. R. (1992). Gait analysis: Normal and pathological function. *Journal of Pediatric Orthopaedics*, *12*(6), 815.

4  Hicks, J. H. (1954). The mechanics of the foot: II. The plantar aponeurosis and the arch. *Journal of anatomy*, *88*(Pt 1), 25.

5  Sawicki, G. S., & Ferris, D. P. (2009). Powered ankle exoskeletons reveal the metabolic cost of plantar flexor mechanical work during walking with longer steps at constant step frequency. *Journal of Experimental Biology*, *212*(1), 21–31.

6  Murphy, A. J., Lockie, R. G., & Coutts, A. J. (2003). Kinematic determinants of early acceleration in field sport athletes. *Journal of Sports science & Medicine*, *2*(4), 144.

7  Gazendam, M. G., & Hof, A. L. (2007). Averaged EMG profiles in jogging and running at different speeds. *Gait & Posture*, *25*(4), 604–614.

8  Lichtwark, G. A., Bougoulias, K., & Wilson, A. M. (2007). Muscle fascicle and series elastic element length changes along the length of the human gastrocnemius during walking and running. *Journal of Biomechanics*, *40*(1), 157–164.

9  Kelly, L. A., Kuitunen, S., Racinais, S., & Cresswell, A. G. (2012). Recruitment of the plantar intrinsic foot muscles with increasing postural demand. *Clinical Biomechanics*, *27*(1), 46–51.

10  Docherty, C. L., & Arnold, B. L. (2008). Force sense deficits in functionally unstable ankles. *Journal of Orthopaedic Research*, *26*(11), 1489–1493.

11  Hertel, J. (2008). Sensorimotor deficits with ankle sprains and chronic ankle instability. *Clinics in sportsMmedicine*, *27*(3), 353–370.

12  Dayakidis, M. K., & Boudolos, K. (2006). Ground reaction force data in functional ankle instability during two cutting movements. *Clinical Biomechanics*, *21*(4), 405–411.

13  Drewes, L. K., McKeon, P. O., Casey Kerrigan, D., & Hertel, J. (2009). Dorsiflexion deficit during jogging with chronic ankle instability. *Journal of Science and Medicine in Sport*, *12*(6), 685–687.

14  Konradsen, L. (2002). Sensori-motor control of the uninjured and injured human ankle. *Journal of Electromyography and Kinesiology*, *12*(3), 199–203.

15  Hopkins, J. T., & Palmieri, R. (2004). Effects of ankle joint effusion on lower leg function. *Clinical Journal of Sport Medicine*, *14*(1), 1–7.

16  Bleakley, C. M., McDonough, S. M., & MacAuley, D. C. (2006). Cryotherapy for acute ankle sprains: a randomised controlled study of two different icing protocols. *British Journal ofSsportsMmedicine*, *40*(8), 700–705.

17 Pounder, N. M., & Harrison, A. J. (2008). Low intensity pulsed ultrasound for fracture healing: a review of the clinical evidence and the associated biological mechanism of action. *Ultrasonics*, *48*(4), 330–338.

18 Järvinen, T. A., Järvinen, T. L., Kääriäinen, M., Kalimo, H., & Järvinen, M. (2005). Muscle injuries biology and treatment. *The American Journal ofSsportsMmedicine*, *33*(5), 745–764.

19 Crewther, B., Cronin, J., & Keogh, J. (2005). Possible stimuli for strength and power adaptation. *Sports Medicine*, *35*(11), 967–989.

20 Hopkins, J. T., & Stencil, R. (2002). Ankle cryotherapy facilitates soleus function. *Journal of Orthopaedic & Sports Physical Therapy*, *32*(12), 622–627.

21 McHugh, M. P., Tyler, T. F., Mirabella, M. R., Mullaney, M. J., & Nicholas, S. J. (2007). The effectiveness of a balance training intervention in reducing the incidence of noncontact ankle sprains in high school football players. *The American Journal of Sports Medicine*, *35*(8), 1289–1294.

22 Olmsted, L. C., Carcia, C. R., Hertel, J., & Shultz, S. J. (2002). Efficacy of the Star Excursion Balance Tests in detecting reach deficits in subjects with chronic ankle instability. *Journal of AthleticTtraining*, *37*(4), 501.

23 Unger, C. L., & Wooden, M. J. (2000). Effect of foot intrinsic muscle strength training on jump performance. *The Journal of Strength & Conditioning Research*, *14*(4), 373–378.

24 Fiolkowski, P., Bishop, M., Brunt, D., & Williams, B. (2005). Plantar feedback contributes to the regulation of leg stiffness. *Clinical Biomechanics*, *20*(9), 952–958.

25 Sankey, R. A., Brooks, J. H., Kemp, S. P., & Haddad, F. S. (2008). The epidemiology of ankle injuries in professional rugby union players. *The American Journal of Sports Medicine*, *36*(12), 2415–2424.

26 Wernbom, M., Augustsson, J., & Raastad, T. (2008). Ischemic strength training: A low-load alternative to heavy resistance exercise? *Scandinavian Journal of Medicine & Science in Sports*, *18*(4), 401–416.

27 Clark, N. C., Gumbrell, C. J., Rana, S., Traole, C. M., & Morrissey, M. C. (2002). Intratester reliability and measurement error of the adapted crossover hop for distance. *Physical Therapy in Sport*, *3*(3), 143–151.

28 Keller, T. S., Weisberger, A. M., Ray, J. L., Hasan, S. S., Shiavi, R. G., & Spengler, D. M. (1996). Relationship between vertical ground reaction force and speed during walking, slow jogging, and running. *Clinical Biomechanics*, *11*(5), 253–259.

29 Wilk, B. R., Muniz, A., & Nau, S. (2010). An evidence-based approach to the orthopaedic physical therapy: Management of functional running injuries. *Orthopaedic Physical Therapy Practice*, *22*, 213–216.

30 Sheppard, J. M., Young, W. B., Doyle, T.L.A., Sheppard, T. A., & Newton, R. U. (2006). An evaluation of a new test of reactive agility and its relationship to sprint speed and change of direction speed. *Journal of Science and Medicine in Sport*, *9*(4), 342–349.

31 Buchheit, M. (2008). The 30–15 intermittent fitness test: accuracy for individualizing interval training of young intermittent sport players. *The Journal of Strength & Conditioning Research*, *22*(2), 365–374.

32 Dizon, J.M.R., & Reyes, J.J.B. (2010). A systematic review on the effectiveness of external ankle supports in the prevention of inversion ankle sprains among elite and recreational players. *Journal of Science and Medicine in Sport*, *13*(3), 309–317.

33 Riemann, B. L., Schmitz, R. J., Gale, M., & McCaw, S. T. (2002). Effect of ankle taping and bracing on vertical ground reaction forces during drop landings before and after treadmill jogging. *Journal of Orthopaedic & Sports Physical Therapy*, *32*(12), 628–635.

# Part 5

# Managing the training athlete

# Chapter 27

# Managing pre-season and in-season training

*Raphael Brandon*

## Introduction

The following guide to planning pre-season and in-season training is based upon underlying physiological principles and training research data. As individual sports have different length pre- and in-season periods, some with single and others multiple seasons across the year, this chapter is unable to detail specific plans for each. Therefore, the aim is to provide a framework in which the practitioner may plan and execute effective training, regardless of the sport. The discussion separates training in terms of periods of development versus maintenance. To begin, a brief overview of training adaptation and detraining is given, detailing important background knowledge for the following pre- and in-season training recommendations.

## Developmental training stimuli and de-training timescales

Development of a physical quality requires training sessions to be of significant stimulus, with a progressive overload of volume and/or intensity. Strength-and-power training results in a neuromuscular adaptation, specifically greater activation of the motor units and reduced reflex inhibition, resulting in greater force generation capacity.[1,2] These changes occur within two to three weeks of two to three sessions per week of high-intensity resistance exercise. Strength training also leads to a muscle hypertrophy adaptation. This requires progressive overload and sufficient time-under-tension (TUT) or session volume. Hypertrophy begins to occur after a few weeks of regular sessions,[3] with significant gains possible in three months. Unfortunately, after 8–12 weeks of no strength training, the increases in activation will return to pre-training levels,[4,5] and the majority of the gains in muscle size (especially fast-twitch fibre) are lost following 10 days of complete detraining.[5]

Energy system training (metabolic conditioning) results in greater ability of the muscles to generate ATP with and/or without oxygen.[6] To develop the cardiac output (i.e. oxygen delivery), high-intensity training is considered important.[7] Significant positive improvements are possible within 6–8 weeks of regular (three per week) aerobic interval training. To develop the muscle's ability to utilize oxygen requires consistent long-term training. Similar to strength, complete detraining results in a reversal of the improvements in aerobic capacity within 6–8 weeks. For example elite endurance athletes require continual high-intensity and high-volume aerobic training to develop and maintain optimal performance. Interestingly, the current recommendations for training 'taper' prior to competition comprise reduced volume for only two weeks, with maintained frequency and intensity.[8] Similar to strength training, it seems that the aerobic system requires continual training to be maintained, and reduced training volume results in reduced fitness within weeks.

Adaptations of the anaerobic energy systems occur within the muscle, including greater fuel supply, faster breakdown of energy and greater tolerance of fatigue-inducing metabolic changes. Anaerobic adaptation relies solely upon training intensity and can be optimised within 6–8 weeks of regular, high-intensity interval training. The metabolic adaptations are possibly maintained for months before returning to pre-training levels.[9,10] However, high-intensity or repetitive sprint performance is likely to reduce without regular high-intensity training, possibly due to aerobic system detraining.

In summary, strength and power may be developed through long-term hypertrophic adaptations, if this is desirable, or enhanced within weeks due to neural changes. Aerobic and anaerobic capacity may be optimized 6–8 weeks of high-intensity and high-volume training for most athletes, except the endurance specialists. It is essential to always base the developmental training upon the principles of adaptation and time-scales. These adaptations will typically occur during pre-season, where more time is available.

Competitive athletes never fully de-train (complete rest) during the in-season. However, it is likely that there may be in-season periods where there is no training with optimal intensity, volume or frequency to provide a stimulus for adaptation. Therefore, maintenance training is required to prevent the likely decline in a physical quality. Maintenance training is an applied concept. Little research has been directed towards understanding the volume and intensity required. One recent study showed development of strength in endurance runners over 14 weeks (with increased neuromuscular activation) was not maintained with a further 14 weeks of twice weekly, but reduced volume strength training.[11] However, another showed that one session per week, with similar session volume from pre-season levels, maintained strength levels for 12 weeks during a soccer competitive season.[12] This illustrates the challenge for the practitioner is to learn what combination of volume, frequency and intensity of training is required for each physical quality. This requirement is also likely to differ between sports.

## Balancing training and recovery during pre-season and in-season training

Developmental training by necessity, results in acute fatigue post session, and often involves accumulative fatigue across a training cycle. In a sense, fatigue is desirable as an indicator of sufficient stimulus for adaptation. The skill of the coach or sport scientist is to organize the training appropriately, providing overload whilst not causing injury or over-training. Training volume is a key requirement, but also a major risk factor for injury.[13] In elite sport, optimizing performance may require pushing athletes to the point where injury risks are also high.

In-season programmes require the recovery between training sessions and preceding competition to be complete. However, for in-season periods longer than a few weeks, it is difficult to achieve complete recovery and maintenance of physical qualities. The more recovery, the more de-training occurs. Paradoxically, the short-term benefit of enhanced competition performance may lead to reduced fitness, which in turn leads to greater recovery required from competition and training. Therefore, practitioners may need to be prepared to 'push' athletes in-season, especially in sports with prolonged competition periods.

Understanding post-exercise fatigue is important for the practitioner to make informed training program decisions. Post-exercise fatigue has different components, which have different recovery time-scales. Exercise induces a reduction in performance due to metabolic and neuromuscular fatigue. Metabolic primarily involves impaired or reduced energy supply, e.g. muscle glycogen stores. Neuromuscular fatigue refers to reduced activation (central fatigue) and impaired muscle contraction (peripheral fatigue). High-intensity and/or high-volume endurance training involves both metabolic and neuromuscular fatigue.[14] In contrast, sprint, strength and power training primarily involves peripheral neuromuscular fatigue immediately following the training.[15,16] Except after extremely strenuous sessions, neuromuscular fatigue typically recovers within 4–24 hours. All exercise results in some degree of inflammatory response (free radical release) and muscle damage. Dynamic eccentric contractions and impact exercise (e.g. running) are usually associated with greater muscle damage. Unaccustomed exercise such as novel exercises are also likely to result in greater inflammatory response. The post-exercise impairments resulting from inflammatory and damage responses are delayed and prolonged, possibly lasting two days. Therefore, this component of fatigue needs to be limited in-season.

The undesirable inflammatory/damage response post training explains why incorporating recovery-enhancing modalities, e.g. cold-water-immersion, are beneficial in-season. This is in contrast to developmental periods, where anti-inflammatory methods may limit adaptation mechanisms.[17]

For the coach and practitioner, neuromuscular fatigue and inflammatory-/damage-related impairments are the main concerns for planning effective training. This is based on the assumption that metabolic fatigue is readily recovered with appropriate time and nutrition between sessions. Both can be managed by limiting training volume, and the latter can be limited by ensuring no unaccustomed exercises or training intensities are performed. Therefore, it is possible to perform strength or endurance training in-season and ensure recovery between training days and/or pre-competition. Strategies for planning appropriate strength-and-power sessions are discussed below. For endurance training, research suggests maximal-intensity and low-volume (e.g. 8 x 30s) sprint interval sessions provide the best balance between stimulus and recovery.[18] Interestingly, a review of elite soccer training found evidence of improved in-season performance with high-intensity interval training.[19] For running-based athletes, the author also recommends a regular but small volume of sprint training in-season, to ensure this specific physical quality is always maintained for performance and injury-prevention reasons.

> For the coach and practitioner, neuromuscular fatigue and inflammatory-related impairments are the main concerns for planning effective training during the season.

The following is a guide to designing pre- and in-season training for most team and technical sports:

### Developmental training

- Aerobic system training – frequent (3–6/week), mix of high-intensity interval + high-volume continuous training
- Anaerobic system training – frequent (2–3/week) of high-intensity interval training
- Strength and power training – frequent (2–3/week) of progressive volume and intensity
- Recovery modalities – limited (0 or 1/week)
- Plan for 2–3 weeks of progressive volume interspersed with a reduced volume (recovery) week to avoid excess accumulation of fatigue that may inhibit training adaptation.

*Maintenance training*

- Aerobic/anaerobic system training – frequent high-intensity, low-volume interval training only (2–3/week)
- Strength and power training – (1–2 week) reduced volume, maintained intensity
- Recovery modalities – frequent (2–3/week)
- Organize training to ensure full days of active or passive recovery to allow for complete neuromuscular and inflammatory recovery following maintenance training.

## Strategies for effective in-season strength and power training

As discussed, the challenge of planning in-season strength training is to limit the post-exercise fatigue but at the same time provide sufficient neuromuscular stimulus. If programmes comprise accustomed exercises and intensities, then athletes should be able to include strength and power training in-season, without excessive muscle damage impairments. For example this author found very little post-session neuromuscular fatigue following 5 sets x 5 reps of heavy squat or deadlift exercise in a group of recreational weightlifters.[20] Furthermore, the lifters did not suffer with any muscle soreness the following day. This is a useful finding, as 5 x 5 is well established as an effective strength stimulus. Therefore, practitioners can be confident that well-trained athletes are able to perform five sets of a heavy whole-body resistance exercise without negative recovery implications.

In contrast, another study assessing elite track and field athletes found a high-volume session of barbell lifting (3 exercises x 4 sets x 5 reps) resulted in significant post-exercise neuromuscular fatigue (–12 per cent reduced force). Interestingly, there were large inter-individual differences in post-session fatigue (0–25 per cent reduced force), and 50 per cent of the athletes had not fully recovered force 24 hours post-session. These findings show that a typical volume of strength training used in developmental training phases may induce very little or substantial fatigue which impacts upon recovery, depending upon the individual's response. Therefore, the practitioner must tailor strength sessions for each individual carefully in-season, as they do for pre-season training blocks. Careful monitoring of session responses and recovery is also recommended, e.g. daily muscle soreness ratings.

Another approach to planning strength and power sessions whilst limiting recovery time could be to select or perform exercises that involve shorter time under tension (TUT). Strength session volumes are typical calculated as *load x reps completed*. This is a crude measure of work done and does not factor muscle contraction time as a component of exercise volume. For example split squats and step-ups usually involve comparable loads. However, the TUT of split-squat repetition performed with a controlled eccentric ≈ 3s, compared to a step-up TUT ≈ 1s, which is primarily a concentric-only movement. Therefore, estimated volume load would be equal, but more (metabolic) work is done during split squat.

Explosive or power type exercises (with moderate load) also have short TUT (< 1s). Sessions comprising explosive exercises have been shown to result in less post-session fatigue, but similar activation levels to heavy exercise sessions (with longer TUT).[15] Therefore, designing sessions that mix heavy with explosive/power exercises may reduce the overall fatigue impact of the session. In fact, mixed strength/power sessions have been shown to be highly beneficial in volleyball athletes during the competitive season, in comparison to sessions comprising heavy exercises only.[21,22] The practitioner may be tempted to use only explosive exercises during in-season, based on this information. However, in order to maintain (or optimize) strength and power, the inclusion of some heavy exercises is probably important.[23] Neural activation may be adequately maintained with explosive, moderate load exercises performed with maximal intention. However, a certain volume of heavy loads and high TUT may be required to ensure muscle fibre size (especially of fast-twitch) does not detrain.

> During the season, designing strength and power training with a mix of heavy and explosive exercises reduces the overall fatigue impact of the session, but provides enough stimulus to maintain strength adaptation.

Retrospective analysis of Olympic-level track and field athlete training diaries revealed that 50–60 per cent of the combined heavy and explosive lower-limb exercise volume load achieved during the pre-season was sufficient to maintain strength and power across a three-month in-season. For example, if athletes had built up to 10,000kg volume load of lower-limb exercises pre-season, then 5,000kg of lower-limb training was performed in-season. Five thousand kilograms may be a large stimulus for some individuals, but *relatively* easy in this hypothetical case. This example introduces the strategy of progressive accumulation of volume pre-season, in order that sufficient volume to elicit a strength-and-power stimulus may be performed in-season. The relative reduction in loading for the individual ensures that little post-session fatigue and recovery impairments occur.

This relative unloading approach is also useful for maintaining strength in specific muscle groups. This may be important for protecting against injury. For example heavy (eccentric bias) hamstring exercises are recommended to protect against hamstring strain.[24] If the pre-season strength program progressed up to two hamstring exercises, three sets each, twice each per week, then the in-season program may include one hamstring exercise, three sets, twice a week, without recovery issues.

The relative unloading strategy is dependent upon two conditions to be effective. First, sufficient volume must be accumulated during pre-season in order for a valid relative reduction that still counts as a training stimulus. Second, intensity of loads and explosive execution must be maintained relative to pre-season levels. In practical terms, this means at least one set per session is performed at a pre-season load, so that repetition maximum intensity does not also reduce as well as volume.

## Summary

Development of physical qualities requires progressive overload of sufficient stimulus to obtain an adaptation. Detraining results in reversal of the positive training effect. In particular, strength and aerobic capacity seems to require frequent and high-intensity training stimulus to prevent detraining. Unfortunately, less research exists to describe the volume and intensity of training required to maintain physical qualities. However, practitioners are recommended to combine (relatively) low volume with high-intensity training (for strength-and-power and energy-system sessions) in order to maintain performance levels, whilst limiting fatigue and recovery impairments.

## Notes

1 Aagaard, P., Simonsen, E., Andersen, J. L., Magnusson, S. P., & Dyhre-Poulsen, P. (2002). Increased rate of force development and neural drive of human skeletal muscle following resistance training. *J Appl Physiol, 93*, 1318–1326.

2 Jensen, J. L., Marstrand, P. C., & Nielsen, J. B. (2005). Motor skill training and strength training are associated with different plastic changes in the central nervous system. *J Appl Physiol, 99*(4), 1558–1568.

3 Holm, L., Reitelseder, S., Pedersen, T. G., Doessing, S., Petersen, S. G., Flyvbjerg, A., . . . Kjaer, M. (2008). Changes in muscle size and MHC composition in response to resistance exercise with heavy and light loading intensity. *J Appl Physiol, 105*(5), 1454–1461.

4 Andersen, L. L., Andersen, J. L., Magnusson, S. P., Suetta, C., Madsen, J. L., Christensen, L. R., & Aagaard, P. (2005). Changes in the human muscle force–velocity relationship in response to resistance training and subsequent detraining. *J Appl Physiol, 99*(1), 87–94.

5 Jespersen, J. G., Nedergaard, A., Andersen, L. L., Schjerling, P., & Andersen, J. L. (2011). Myostatin expression during human muscle hypertrophy and subsequent atrophy: Increased myostatin with detraining. *Scand J Med Sci Sports, 21*(2), 215–223.

6 Spurway, N. C. (1992). Aerobic exercise, anaerobic exercise and the lactate threshold. *Br Med Bull, 48*(3), 569–591.

7 Daussin, F. N., Ponsot, E., Dufour, S. P., Lonsdorfer-Wolf, E., Doutreleau, S., Geny, B., . . . Richard, R. (2007). Improvement of VO2max by cardiac output and oxygen extraction adaptation during intermittent versus continuous endurance training. *Eur J Appl Physiol, 101*(3), 377–383.

8 Mujika, I. (2009). *Tapering and peaking for optimal performance*. Champaign, IL.: Human Kinetics.

9 Linossier, M. T., Dormois, D., Geyssant, A., & Denis, C. (1997). Performance and fibre characteristics of human skeletal muscle during short sprint training and detraining on a cycle ergometer. *Eur J Appl Physiol Occup Physiol, 75*(6), 491–498.

10 Linossier, M. T., Dormois, D., Perier, C., Frey, J., Geyssant, A., & Denis, C. (1997). Enzyme adaptations of human skeletal muscle during bicycle short-sprint training and detraining. *Acta Physiol Scand, 161*(4), 439–445.

11 Taipale, R. S., Mikkola, J., Nummela, A., Vesterinen, V., Capostagno, B., Walker, S., . . . Hakkinen, K. (2010). Strength training in endurance runners. *Int J Sports Med, 31*(7), 468–476.

12 Ronnestad, B. R., Nymark, B. S., & Raastad, T. (2011). Effects of in-season strength maintenance training frequency in professional soccer players. *J Strength Cond Res, 25*(10), 2653–2660.

13 Gabbett, T. J., & Jenkins, D. G. (2011). Relationship between training load and injury in professional rugby league players. *J Sci Med Sport, 14*(3), 204–209.

14 Bentley, D. J., Smith, P. A., Davie, A. J., & Zhou, S. (2000). Muscle activation of the knee extensors following high intensity endurance exercise in cyclists. *Eur J Appl Physiol, 81*(4), 297–302.

15 Brandon, R., Howatson, G., Strachan, F., & Hunter, A. M. (2014). Neuromuscular response differences to power vs strength back squat exercise in elite athletes. *Scand J Med Sci Sports*, July 4. doi: 10.1111/sms.12289. [Epub ahead of print]

16 Perrey, S., Racinais, S., Saimouaa, K., & Girard, O. (2010). Neural and muscular adjustments following repeated running sprints. *Eur J Appl Physiol, 109*(6), 1027–1036.

17 Yamane, M., Teruya, H., Nakano, M., Ogai, R., Ohnishi, N., & Kosaka, M. (2006). Post-exercise leg and forearm flexor muscle cooling in humans attenuates endurance and resistance training effects on muscle performance and on circulatory adaptation. *Eur J Appl Physiol, 96*(5), 572–580.

18 Iaia, F. M., Hellsten, Y., Nielsen, J. J., Fernstrom, M., Sahlin, K., & Bangsbo, J. (2009). Four weeks of speed endurance training reduces energy expenditure during exercise and maintains muscle oxidative capacity despite a reduction in training volume. *J Appl Physiol, 106*(1), 73–80.

19 Iaia, F. M., Rampinini, E., & Bangsbo, J. (2009). High-intensity training in football. *Int J Sports Physiol Perform, 4*(3), 291–306.

20 Brandon, R. (2011). *Investigations of the neuromuscular response during and following elite maximum strength and power type resistance exercise* (Unpublished doctoral dissertation). University of Stirling, Scotland. Retrieved from http://hdl.handle.net/1893/3655

21 Marques, M.C., Tillaar, R., Vescovi, J.D., & Gonzalez-Badillo, J.J. (2008). Changes in strength and power performance in elite senior female professional volleyball players during the in-season: a case study. *J Strength Cond Res, 22*(4), 1147–1155.

22 Newton, R.U., Rogers, R.A., Volek, J.S., Hakkinen, K., & Kraemer, W.J. (2006). Four weeks of optimal load ballistic resistance training at the end of season attenuates declining jump performance of women volleyball players. *J Strength Cond Res, 20*(4), 955–961.

23 Newton, R. (2012). Combined strength and power Training for optimal performance gains. *Paper presented at the International Conference of Strength Training, Oslo, Norway.*

24 Askling, C., Karlsson, J., & Thorstensson, A. (2003). Hamstring injury occurrence in elite soccer players after preseason strength training with eccentric overload. *Scand J Med Sci Sport, 13*, 244–250.

# Chapter 28

# Monitoring training load

*Stuart Cormack and Aaron Coutts*

## Introduction

The development of effective training and rehabilitation programs for high-performance athletes is an intricate process. There are often multiple physical capacities that must be well-developed, along with the prioritisation of training towards developing technical and tactical elements, all of which requires large volumes and intensities of training. As a result, there is a need to effectively prescribe training/rehabilitation and monitor the athlete's responses to this training so that unplanned fatigue does not occur.

Whilst frequent competition is common in high-performance sport, inappropriately high loads from both training and competition can increase the likelihood of both injury and illness. In addition, the magnitude of the increment in training load from week to week, as much as the absolute load, is also likely to be important.[26] Despite this, the degree of planning applied to rehabilitation loads is sometimes less than optimal, and this can compromise adaptation and the rehabilitation process. Such unplanned fatigue states may not only lead to underperformance, but also to significant negative psychological, illness and injury issues.

Optimising the organisation of the training stimulus requires us to find the balance between fatigue and recovery. There are many factors that influence this dose-response relationship; key to this are the individual characteristics of the athlete. Whilst individualisation of the training stimulus should be an outcome of any load and fatigue monitoring program, this requires the use of valid and reliable tools to allow an objective assessment of athlete status. Therefore, the aim of this chapter is to provide a summary of the important scientific and practical aspects involved in monitoring training and rehabilitation load and fatigue.

## Training dose-response relationship

Programs that lead to improvements in performance are a function of completing stressful overload training doses matched with appropriate recovery. It is during the return to homeostasis that physiological adaptations (referred to as *supercompensation*) are made. Adaptations made by the athlete during the recovery period mean that a greater stimulus is then required to disrupt homeostasis in the future.

Although balancing the appropriate doses of training and recovery is a foundation of improving athletic performance, there are multiple factors that influence the athlete's response. These include a combination of physiological and psychological traits and issues related to the specifics of the training and competition environment. Due to this, it is unlikely that universal predictions regarding the impact of a given training load on performance, fatigue, injury or illness are possible. The likelihood of highly individual responses to the training process requires coaches and scientists to understand that these responses should be considered on a continuum.

## The fatigue continuum

Whilst fatigue is often perceived as a negative response, it is, in fact, a required component of the training process and can be considered on a continuum that ranges from fatigue from a single session, through to overtraining, via overreaching.[17] Acute fatigue from individual training sessions dissipates within hours or days when appropriate periods of recovery are provided; however 'overreaching' may develop when intensified training continues without appropriate unloading.[17] Interestingly, some scientists and practitioners distinguish between *functional overreaching*, which occurs in response to deliberate overload training, and *non-functional overreaching*, which results in unplanned fatigue that can persist for several weeks.[22] If chronic performance decrements persist (coupled with a negative psychological state) despite large reductions in training load and the absence of a diagnosable pathology, the athlete may be suffering from *overtraining syndrome*. It should be noted that these unplanned fatigue states are not only possible in healthy athletes, but also in athletes undergoing long-term high-load rehabilitation programs.

## Quantifying training, rehabilitation and competition load

Arguably, the first step in understanding the link between training, rehabilitation and competition load and the fatigue response in athletes is the quantification of load. This primarily relates to the type, volume, intensity and frequency of each training or competition stimulus. It is likely that, even though the exercise mode may be the same, the response to stress arising from competition or training will be quite different. Variables such as duration, speed, distance and other metrics are referred to as measures of *external load*. Quantification, and therefore control of the external load, can now be done very precisely with the use of various tools such as global positioning systems (GPS), accelerometers and power meters, which are commonplace in high performance sport.

> Although external load is increasingly easier to measure, it is the physiological stress or *internal load* resulting from this external load that determines adaptation.[31]

From this, it can be seen that many objective and subjective methods are available to measure internal load, including heart rate, blood lactate and the perception of effort. However, the utility of each method is probably dependent on the exercise mode, and it is unlikely that a single measure will provide all the information required.

## Objective measures of internal load: Heart rate

Arguably, the most commonly utilised measure of internal load is heart rate (HR). The use of HR as a measure of exercise intensity is based on the linear relationship between HR and the volume of oxygen consumed over a wide range of steady-state workloads.[1]

> The use of HR to assess internal load may be limited in intermittent sports, as the HR response may not provide an accurate reflection of intensity during short, high-intensity efforts, and as such may be most useful in continuous activities. The same can be said for the monitoring of blood lactate levels in intermittent sports.

The desire to condense the evaluation of training intensity into a single arbitrary unit has led to the development of the Training Impulse (TRIMP) concept. The TRIMP score is calculated from the mean HR during a session to which a 'weighting' factor to account for the relatively greater stress of higher intensity training is applied.[24] There are many modifications of the TRIMP method, but irrespective of which method is employed, there are potential practical limitations when dealing with large squads of athletes who complete multiple training sessions per week.

## Subjective measures of internal training load: Rating of perceived exertion

An athlete's perception of effort is a practical and valid tool for assessing exercise intensity and, when assessed properly, can reflect the inputs from multiple biological systems.[2] Ratings of perceived exertion (RPE) can be assessed using various scales but is most often assessed with the 15-point (i.e. 6–20) or category ratio 10-point (CR-10) scale.

Although no single RPE scale can be considered optimal in all environments, category-ratio scales are well suited to high-intensity exercise environments, such as team sports that are associated with non-linear physiological responses. Combining perception of effort with other measures (e.g. duration) provides additional information, and an extensively used scale for this purpose is the session-RPE (s-RPE) method.

## The session-RPE method

Using an RPE scale and multiplying the score (typically recorded 10–30 minutes post exercise) by training duration in minutes allows calculation of 'load', representing the internal load for each session.[16] In addition to the calculation of load from a single training or competition session, these values can be added for a day or week. Whilst calculation of weekly load (or other duration) is most common, determining variables such as *monotony* and *strain* may also be useful. *Monotony* refers to the variation in training load during a week and is calculated as daily mean load divided by daily load standard deviation, whilst *strain* (representing the overall stress on the individual) is the product of monotony and load. Calculation of these variables may provide valuable insight, as periods of training characterised by high monotony and strain predispose athletes to a greater risk of injury and illness.[15,26]

> Ideally, RPE should be collected 10–30 mins after the end of the session. It is critical that the athlete's rating is aligned to the verbal anchors of the scale and that they rate the intensity of the entire session.

## Other perceptual tools

In addition to s-RPE, various questionnaires can be useful tools in detecting mood disturbance in athletes. This is helpful, because disturbances in mood can be early indicators of overreaching and overtraining syndrome and have become popular tools for monitoring athletes. The Profile of Mood State Questionnaire is a useful tool and it is easy to implement, even with large groups of athletes, and offer a low-cost assessment of an athlete's status.

## Other 'wellness' inventories

It is common for athletes to complete 'wellness' questionnaires requiring them to provide a rating on categories, such as overall well-being, sleep, muscle soreness, fatigue and training quality. Acute and chronic changes in these wellness domains are often useful to track and can provide a context for both conversations with the athlete and coaching staff and interventions should the athlete(s) perceive a deterioration in their own wellness.

## Objectives markers of fitness and fatigue

Whilst subjective markers of fatigue and wellness are valuable, a mixed-methods approach using a combination of subjective and objective tools may provide the most insight. Many of the physical performance tests that are available to assess athletes' training status are not useful for regular monitoring due to aspects such as their fatiguing nature, logistical difficulties dealing with large numbers of athletes, the need for specialised equipment and issues associated with validity and reliability. Physiological, biochemical and neuromuscular parameters can, however, be relatively easily measured and give valuable insight into the status of an individual athlete during training or rehabilitation.

## Physiological markers

The physiological response to *submaximal* protocols is both practical and effective for monitoring an athlete's fitness/fatigue status. Submaximal HR during a standard bout of exercise has been reported to reflect changes in fitness and performance, whilst the rate of HR recovery (HRR) and heart rate variability (HRV) measures following these bouts also has shown to be related to fitness.[5]

### Heart rate recovery (HRR)

Autonomic nervous system (ANS) monitoring may give us an insight into an athlete's current status in terms of how they are tolerating training load. The ANS is divided into two parts: the sympathetic nervous system (commonly thought to be the 'activating', or 'fight or flight' system) and the parasympathetic nervous system (the 'recovery', or 'rest and digest' system). At the cessation of exercise, there is a reduction in sympathetic drive and parasympathetic reactivation that results in a reduction in HR.[3] There is therefore potential to use measures of heart rate recovery in order to reflect autonomic nervous system status. Indeed, improvements in HRR following a standard bout of exercise have occurred in parallel with improvements in fitness and training load tolerance ,whilst reduced HRR rate may suggest detraining or increased fatigue.[5]

## Heart rate variability (HRV)

Another method of measuring ANS status that is becoming increasingly widely used is heart rate variability. HRV represents the normal variation in beat-to-beat intervals and could be a useful tool because autonomic control of HR may be disrupted in overtraining states. The direction of shift towards sympathetic or parasympathetic dominance is unclear and may be individual-dependent. For example we might normally expect that athletes who are coping with training to have a powerful sympathetic response to training and parasympathetic dominance during recovery (high HRV), whilst those undergoing excessive stress may exhibiting low

HRV. However, these trends are not always evident.[6] In addition, increased HRV is not always reflected in field performance.[4] Therefore, despite increasing popularity in field settings, as with all monitoring tools, specific issues of validity and reliability should be considered.

> In a rehabilitation setting, we could measure HRR and HRV (amongst other variables, such as neuromuscular status) in athletes recuperating from long-term injuries, such as an ACL reconstruction, to ensure that they are tolerating the training load without undergoing excessive fatigue, as this would be counter-productive to the motor control aims of the rehabilitation process.

## Biochemical markers

Whilst numerous hormones and other markers from blood, saliva and urine have been used to assess the response to training, research findings are far from consistent, and there are substantial limitations to the use of biochemical markers on a regular basis in the practical setting.

## Muscle damage

It is well documented that high intensity eccentric exercise (particularly, unaccustomed) results in trauma known as exercise-induced muscle damage, and a number of enzymes, such as creatine kinase (CK), myoglobin, troponin, urea, uric acid, and ammonia, have been shown to reflect this damage.[19,28,29] CK is suggested to represent acute muscle damage, although elevations in CK have also been seen in overreached and over-trained athletes.[21] It has been reported that elevated CK may provide an indication of recovery status, elevated training loads and possibly even elevated injury risk.[7,18,20] Therefore, regular monitoring of CK is now a relatively common measure in athlete monitoring systems, as it provides objective feedback on the level of muscle damage resulting from training and competition. However, more work is required to establish the cost-benefit of regular assessment of CK, and if it provides any additional information beyond that provided by perceptual measures.

## Cortisol

Cortisol (C) is a glucocorticoid released from the adrenal cortex in response to both physical and mental stress and is often thought to represent a catabolic marker, although its suitability for regular use in sporting environments is unclear. Cortisol is frequently reported to elevate during periods of high training and competition loads.[13,14] However, low values have also been seen during long competition phases compared to pre-season values and may also be a reflection of suppression of the hypothalamic-pituitary adrenal axis due to severe overtraining.[27]

## Testosterone

Testosterone (T) is an anabolic hormone and generally increases following short, high-intensity exercise,[10,11] but decreases have been shown with prolonged strenuous exercise.[11,12] In addition, the T response during competitive seasons can be highly variable and may not necessarily be predictive of physical performance.[9]

Potentially confounding responses in both cortisol and testosterone levels to training loads suggest that neither should be used as independent indicators of training load or fatigue status.

## Testosterone/cortisol ratio

Due to the respective anabolic and catabolic properties of T and C, the ratio of T:C may be a reflection of overall anabolic:catabolic balance and therefore a good indicator of athlete status. Indeed, it has been suggested that a reduction in T:C of 30 per cent is representative of a catabolic or maladaptive state.[13] It has also been shown that the T:C decreases in response to high-intensity, long-duration exercise, as well as during periods of high-intensity training and competition.[30] However, since both psychological and physiological stress can impact C, and therefore the T:C, it can be difficult to determine if alterations in T:C are mediated through training or non-training factors.

### Salivary vs. blood markers

A major limitation to the use of biochemical markers as regular fatigue monitoring tools is the invasive nature of blood sampling. However, strong relationships exist between serum and salivary levels of various hormones, which makes frequent sample collection less onerous and the preferred option in field settings. In addition, technological advances now allow immediate analysis of some markers in saliva, which substantially reduces the cost and time lag between data collection and analysis. However, given the complexity and costs associated with these markers, their value needs to be carefully considered prior to their implementation in rehabilitation settings.

## Neuromuscular fatigue

There is currently great interest in the assessment of neuromuscular fatigue in athletes, particularly via results from performance tests. Importantly however, the validity of many of these inferences is questionable. A particular type of neuromuscular fatigue, known as low frequency fatigue (LFF) is of specific interest, as it results from high-intensity, repetitive-eccentric or stretch-shortening cycle activities and is long lasting. Whilst the 'gold standard' method of LFF assessment is via muscle or nerve stimulation, due to the limitations of these techniques in the field there is value in the potential for single or repeated jumps to assess this response. This could be particularly useful in the rehabilitation process, as the athlete is likely to undergo periods of substantial neuromuscular load.

### Countermovement jumps (CMJ)

Whilst both single and multiple jumps potentially provide valuable information, single repetitions may be more efficient. Although the use of CMJ performance as a measure of neuromuscular status has been extensively adopted, the validity of this approach is not always apparent. This is because not all variables are sensitive to either previous training or competition stress, nor are decrements indicators of reduced subsequent performance.[8,9,23] In many cases, simple outcome variables (e.g. height) are not useful because athletes modify their movement strategy to achieve a certain outcome. It is critical that practitioners investigate the validity of these measures as indicators of neuromuscular status (i.e., in this case, a return to normal function from an injured state) in their particular sport.

## Interpreting the data to gain meaningful information

We have presented numerous tests in the preceding sections, but the key with any test is to ensure that the results yield *information* that can be used to improve the training/rehabilitation process. Central to this is the process of the administration of the tests themselves, as well as how results are interpreted. This can sometimes be overlooked in the desire for a single measure of fitness or fatigue.

### Validity and reliability of measures

A critical aspect of the fatigue and load monitoring process is the use of valid and reliable tools, and the importance of these aspects continues to grow as more and more data can be collected in high-performance settings.

Prior to embarking on the collection of any fatigue and load monitoring variable with the intent to utilise this for informing future training, practitioners must consider the validity and reliability of the tools they are using. In many cases, validity and reliability information on particular tools is available in the published literature. In the absence of this, small-scale in-house projects can provide invaluable information. For example before concluding that an athlete is not fatigued because there has been no change in CMJ height, it must first be determined that this measure is in fact sensitive to competition and/or training stress in a given environment.

> Tests with good reliability allow confidence that variations in performance and due to biological change, rather than inherent error in the measurement process.
>
> Validity is comprised of various elements, critical of which is whether the variable actually measures what it is suggested to measure in a specific environment. For example does the 'field test' measure compare favourably to the 'gold standard' laboratory measure?

### Baseline values

Once validity and reliability of a measure have been established, the next step is to decide on a baseline value against which subsequent data can be compared. This becomes critical as the magnitude of change, and its practical importance may depend on the relevance of the baseline value. Whilst a myriad of baseline values can be calculated, the most important aspect is that it allows a meaningful comparison. For example a baseline value calculated during a general preparation phase of training may be largely irrelevant as a comparison for competition phase values. The baseline value should also represent a relatively 'fatigue-free' state so that changes in status can be clearly determined.

## Acute and chronic variations

The frequency of training load and fatigue data collection often varies depending on the measure. For example s-RPE is generally collected on a daily or sessional basis whilst biochemical markers may be collected less frequently. Regardless of collection frequency, consistency in both timeframe and mechanics of the collection procedures must be highly consistent and analysis considered on both an acute (e.g. weekly) and more chronic (e.g. monthly) basis.

Variables such as neuromuscular, biochemical, perceptual wellness scores and exercise intensity are often collected very frequently (e.g. weekly or even multiple times per week) and benefit from comparison on a week-to-week basis and where relevant to baseline values. Sometimes, more detailed psychometric inventories are used less frequently (e.g. monthly) but can be compared from one point to the next and against baseline values regardless of frequency.

Although, the frequency of collection to some extent dictates the approach taken in analysing the data, there may be value in determining the pattern of response over different periods (e.g. monthly). The use of monthly 'rolling averages' may provide significant insight where weekly values could represent 'fatigue' and monthly averages, 'fitness'. From this type of calculation it might be possible to determine that, although and athlete seems to be tolerating training on an acute basis, the chronic value suggests they may not be adapting as expected.

## Data analysis

The ever-increasing availability of training and competition data in high performance sport settings through devices such as micro-technologies, force-plates and position transducers necessitates familiarity with statistical techniques capable of determining the importance of derived values. Contemporary statistical techniques allow for identification of small but important changes. For example changes in excess of the error of the test (i.e. the reliability value) are likely to represent biological variation that may have implications for program prescription (e.g. a change of 10 per cent in a test with an error of 5 per cent is likely to be a 'real' change). More complete approaches are also possible, including determination of the 'smallest worthwhile change', which represents the smallest important change in performance.

An often overlooked aspect of data analysis are the issues associated with determining important change in self-reporting inventories such as wellness questionnaires. Issues can arise because athletes are required to respond relative to specific anchors (e.g. normal), which can sometimes result in an automated response, that do not provide a true indication of current status. Similarly, some athletes routinely rate themselves 'high' or 'low' on particular categories. A solution to overcoming these limitations is to determine not only the degree of change relative to a standardised verbal anchor, but also to what the individual athlete 'normally' rates. An example of a useful technique is a modified standard difference score.[25] Acutely, this can be calculated as:

(Current score − baseline score)/SD of individual baseline*
* = standard deviation of baseline scores (e.g. 4 scores collected from a pre-season cup competition phase).

This calculation converts the raw score to a standard deviation from baseline. Determining the level of variation required to be important is challenging. However, values of 0.5

to 2.0 are often set as thresholds. Lower values can potentially result in 'false negatives', although this should be balanced against the possibility of missing small but important changes by using higher thresholds. Another method of determining individual change would be to calculate the typical error (TE) to represent the 'normal' individual variation in a score (rather than as a measure of reliability from a test-retest trial involving multiple athletes). In this case, a variation in a score from one time point to the next that exceeds the TE may be considered 'important'. Regardless of the method employed, this process is likely to be critically important in rehabilitation, as closely monitoring the change in an athlete's status can maximise the opportunity for recovery and adaptation via appropriate training program manipulation.

### Other comparisons

In order to optimise individual training program design, it is critical to analyse changes in load and fatigue variables on both a within and between individual basis (i.e. compared to the group). This is because a lack of change, or change in a different direction from the majority of a squad, may suggest an inappropriate response to the stress of training and competition. For example if the average group response suggests a reduction in fatigue following an unloading phase, yet there is a minimal improvement in an individual for the same time comparison, it could be that this lack of change actually means the athlete has failed to respond as planned.

## Day-to-day application

The value of assessing training/rehabilitation load and fatigue lies in the ability to use valid and reliable data to effectively manipulate the training process. The effectiveness of a program is likely to be highest with the use of minimally invasive tools and without requiring a specific session devoted to data collection (particularly if the data collection involves the accumulation of further load).

> Unfortunately, although perhaps understandably, there is a desire in many high-performance sport settings to use a single variable or value as a 'silver bullet' marker of athlete status. To date, no such variable has been discovered, and it appears unlikely that this will occur. Equally, the use of warnings based on secret algorithms from commercially available computer software should also be viewed somewhat sceptically.

We recommend the adoption of a 'mixed methods' approach. This should involve the use of objective and subjective measures of both internal and external load that display acceptable levels of validity and reliability. Table 28.1 provides a summary of the measures that we recommend for monitoring of training and rehabilitation load in team sports.

When combined with the 'art' of coaching, this seems to provide the most effective intervention. The use of graphical methods to display data that highlight important aspects (e.g. traffic light system) are of great value when reporting information to athletes and coaches. In addition, reporting change as a percentage can also be easily understood, although this should occur relative to the error in a test so that the importance of a change can be identified.

*Table 28.1* Example monitoring system for high-performance team sports.

| Variable | Collection Frequency | Statistical Analysis Technique | Practical Value |
|---|---|---|---|
| **RPE** | every session | Modified standard difference score. Intra- & inter-individual comparisons. | Critical |
| **Load** | weekly | As above | Critical |
| **Monotony** | weekly | As above | Important |
| **Strain** | | As above | Important |
| **Wellness Questionnaire** | 2–4 x per week | As above | Critical |
| **Training & Competition Intensity** | Every session | Change relative to reliability value. Week-to-week and chronic variation. | Very important |
| **Psychological Inventory** | Weekly – monthly | As above + psychologist interpretation. | Very important |
| **Biochemical/ Neuromuscular/ Autonomic NS markers (HRV)** | Weekly | Change relative to reliability value. Week-to-week and chronic variation. | Important but can be expensive and require specialised equipment. |
| **Other markers (e.g. sleep)** | As needed | Change relative to reliability value. Week-to-week and chronic variation. | Very important but rely on specific equipment and expertise. |

## Summary

The desire and, in fact, requirement to accurately assess athlete responses to the training and competition stress are likely to increase. Performing this task effectively begins with accurately quantifying the training or rehabilitation load. Although the use of valid and reliable objective variables can undoubtedly be beneficial, there is growing interest supported both practically and by research, in the use of subjective tools. These tools have the advantage of low cost and ease of implementation, and when combined with appropriate objective markers (i.e. mixed methods approach) are likely to provide the most useful information. Regardless of the objective or subjective nature of the variable, appropriate statistical analysis is inherently critical.

## Notes

1 Åstrand, P. O., & Rodahl, K. (1986). *Textbook of work physiology*, New York, McGraw Hill.
2 Borg, G. (982). Psychophysical bases of perceived exertion. *Medicine and Science in Sports and Exercise*, *14*, 377–381.

3   Bprresem, J., & Lambert, M. I. (2008). Autonomic control of heart rate during and after exercise: Measurements and implications for monitoring training status. *Sports Medicine, 38,* 633–646.

4   Boullosa, D. A., Abreu, L., Nakamura F. Y., Muñoz, V. E., Domínguez, E., & Leicht, A. S. (2012). Cardiac autonomic adaptations in elite Spanish soccer players during pre-season. *International Journal of Sports Physiology and Performance, 8*(4), 400–409.

5   Buchheit, M. (2014). Monitoring training status with HR measures: Do all roads lead to Rome? *Frontiers in physiology, 5,* 73.

6   Buchheit, M., Racinais, S., Bilsborough, J. C., Bourdon, P. C., Voss, S. C., Hocking, . . . Coutts, A. J. (2013). Monitoring fitness, fatigue and running performance during a pre-season training camp in elite football players. *Journal of Science and Medicine in Sport, 16,* 550–555.

7   Coelho, D. B., Morandi, R. F., Melo, M.A.A.D., & Silami-Garcia, E. (2011). Creatine kinase kinetics in professional soccer players during a competitive season. *Revista Brasileira de Cineantropometria & Desempenho Humano, 13,* 189–194.

8   Cormack, S. J., Newton, R. U., & McGuigan, M. R. (2008). Neuromuscular and endocrine responses to an elite Australian rules football match. *International Journal of Sports Physiology and Performance, 3,* 359–374.

9   Cormack, S. J., Newton, R. U., McGuigan, M. R., & Cormie, P. (2008). Neuromuscular and endocrine responses of elite players during an Australian rules football season. *International Journal of Sports Physiology and Performance, 3,* 439–53.

10  Crewther, B., Cronin, J., Keough, J., & Cook, C. (2008). The salivary testosterone and cortisol response to three loading schemes. *Journal of Strength and Conditioning Research, 22,* 250–255.

11  Cumming, D. C., Wheeler, G. D., & McColl, E. M. (1989). The effects of exercise on reproductive function in men. *Sports Medicine, 7,* 1–17.

12  Elloumi, M., Maso, F., Michaux, O., Robert, A., & Lac, G. (2003). Behaviour of saliva cortisol [C], testosterone [T] and the T/C ratio during a rugby match and during the post-competition recovery days. *European Journal of Applied Physiology, 90,* 23–28.

13  Filaire, E., Bernain, X., Sagnol, M., & Lac, G. (2001). Preliminary results on mood state, salivary Testosterone:Cortisol ratio and team performance in a professional soccer team. *European Journal of Applied Physiology, 86,* 179–184.

14  Filaire, E., Lac, G., & Pequignot, J. M. (2003). Biological, hormonal, and psychological parameters in professional soccer players throughout a competitive season. *Perceptual and Motor Skills, 97,* 1061–1072.

15  Foster, C. (1998). Monitoring training in athletes with reference to overtraining syndrome. *Medicine and Science in Sports and Exercise, 30,* 1164–1168.

16  Foster, C., Florhaug, J. A., Franklin, J., Gottschall, L., Hrovatin, L. A., Parker, S., . . . Dodge, C. (2001). A new approach to monitoring exercise training. *Journal of Strength and Conditioning Research, 15,* 109–115.

17  Halson, S. L., & Jeukendrup, A. E. (2004). Does overtraining exist?: An analysis of overreaching and overtraining research. *Sports Medicine, 34,* 967–981.

18  Hunkin, S. L., Fahrner, B., & Gastin, P. B. (2013). Creatine kinase and its relationship with match performance in elite Australian rules football. *Journal of Science and Medicine in Sport, 17*(3), 332–336.

19  Kirwin, J. P., Costill, D. L., Houmard, J. B., Mitchell, J. B., Flynn, M. G., & Fink, W. J. (1990). Changes in selected blood measures during repeated days of intense training and carbohydrate control. *International Journal of Sports Medicine, 11,* 362–366.

20  Lazarim, F. L., Antunes-Neto, J. M., Da Silva, F. O., Nunes, L. A., Bassini-Cameron, A., Cameron, L.-C., . . . De Macedo, D. V. (2009). The upper values of plasma creatine kinase of professional soccer players during the Brazilian National Championship. *Journal of Science and Medicine in Sport, 12,* 85–90.

21  Lehmann, M., Dickhuth, H. H., Gendrisch, G., Lazar, W., Thum, M., Kaminski, R., . . . & Keul, J. (1991). Training-overtraining: A prospective, experimental study with experienced middle-and long-distance runners. *International Journal of Sports Medicine, 12,* 444–452.

22  Meeusen, R., Duclos, M., Foster, C., Fry, A., Gleeson, M., Nieman, D., . . . American College of Sports. (2013). Prevention, diagnosis, and treatment of the overtraining syndrome: Joint consensus

statement of the European College of Sport Science and the American College of Sports Medicine. *Medicine and Science in Sports and Exercise, 45,* 186–205.

23 Mooney, M. G., Cormack, S., O'Brien, B. J., Morgan, W. M., & McGuigan, M. (2013). Impact of neuromuscular fatigue on match exercise intensity and performance in elite Australian football. *The Journal of Strength & Conditioning Research, 27,* 166–173.

24 Morton, R. H., Fitz-Clarke, J. R., & Banister, E. W. (1990). Modeling human performance in running. *Journal of Applied Physiology, 69,* 1171–1177.

25 Pettit, R. W. (2010). The Standard Difference Score: A new statistic for evaluating strength and conditioning programs. *Journal of Strength and Conditioning Research, 24,* 287–291.

26 Rogaliski, B., Dawson, B., Heasman, J., & Gabbett, T. J. (2013). Training and game loads and injury risk in elite Australian footballers. *Journal of Science and Medicine in Sport, 16,* 499–503.

27 Steinacker, J. M., Lormes, W., Reissnecker, S., & Liu, Y. (2004). New aspects of the hormone and cytokine response to training. *European Journal of Applied Physiology, 91,* 382–91.

28 Stone, M. H., Keith, R. E., Kearney, J. T., Fleck, S. J., Wilson, G. D., & Triplett, N. T. (1991). Overtraining: A review of the signs, symptoms and possible causes. *Journal of Applied Sport Science Research, 5,* 35–50.

29 Stray-Gundersen, J., Videman, T., & Snell, P. G. (1986). Changes in selected objective parameters during overtraining. *Medicine and Science in Sports and Exercise, 18,* s54–55.

30 Urhausen, A., Gabriel, H., & Kindermann, W. 1995. Blood hormones as markers of training stress and overtraining. *Sports Medicine, 20,* 251–276.

31 Viru, A., & Viru, M. (2000). Nature of training effects (pp. 67–95). In W. E. Garret & D. T. Kirkendall, (Eds.), *Exercise and sport science.* Philadelphia: Lippincott Williams and Wilkins.

Chapter 29

# Optimising athlete recovery

*Christian Cook, Liam Kilduff and Blair Crowther*

## Introduction

Athletes prepare for competition through a complex training process where the physiological objective is to improve function, optimise performance and reduce the risk of injury.[25] Training induces considerable stress on our physiological systems, including energy substrate depletion, neuromuscular fatigue, hormonal modifications, oxidative stress, muscle damage and inflammation.[16] Depending on the exercise stimulus, one may expect to see a reduction in physical performance ranging from several hours to days.

Given that these responses can compromise training and competition, there is significant interest in developing recovery strategies to restore physical performance.[1,6,16,20,24] These strategies include 'active' approaches, such as light exercise and stretching, and 'passive' approaches, such as cold-water immersion (CWI) and/or hot water immersion (HWI), compression garments, nutritional and psychological strategies. Approaches that focus on soft-tissue injuries (e.g. massage, foam rolling) are also common.

This chapter will examine the activation, integration and restoration of the physiological systems during post-exercise recovery. We will also address the link between psychological and physiological recovery, and review some common recovery strategies and their potential application in sport. A resistance exercise model will be used throughout to give the reader context around this complex topic.

## Responses to resistance exercise

### Neuromuscular system

As with other exercise modalities, resistance exercise can induce a state of fatigue lasting several hours and perhaps longer, depending on workout design.[17,18] This fatigue response is characterised by increases in blood lactate, a decrease in muscle electromyographic activity and force produced, a shift in the force-velocity relationship and the depletion of metabolic resources (e.g. glycogen stores in liver and muscle).

Resistance exercise also places mechanical stress on the contractile and non-contractile components of the neuromuscular system, which can lead to muscle damage.[3] The net result is an increase in muscle soreness, tenderness and swelling, and ultimately a decrease in physical performance. Determining the mechanism/s of fatigue is crucial for understanding the recovery processors after exercise and the effective implementation of any recovery strategy thereafter.

## Endocrine system

Testosterone (T) and cortisol (C) help to support energy release, protein metabolism and muscle repair.[10] Traditionally, T and C are viewed as being anabolic and catabolic to muscle growth, respectively, but their training roles may involve several neuromuscular mechanisms (e.g. intracellular signalling, behaviour, neural function). Growth hormone (GH) has also been linked to the secretion of T and other growth factors.[10]

Hypertrophy workouts can increase T, C and GH concentrations, and more so than maximal strength and/or power workouts,[10] due to greater mechanical and metabolic strain. Thus, exercise selection, lifting technique, training volume and intensity are important moderators of these hormonal outcomes. Overall, the GH increases (up to 200-fold) are considerably greater than T (up to 72 per cent) and C (up to 175 per cent),[10] but the temporal responses are somewhat similar, increasing mid- to post-workout before returning to baseline levels within 1–2 hours of exercise.

The catecholamine's epinephrine (EP) and norepinephrine (NOR) also stimulate various metabolic functions important for exercise.[28] Catecholamine secretion occurs within a few seconds of exercise and can increase by several-fold from baseline.[28] Overall, these hormonal changes play a key role in preparing individuals for, and responding to, exercise stress in order to restore homeostasis.

## Immune system

The immune system plays a major role in defending the integrity of an organism against foreign proteins and microorganisms.[21] Exercise provides a stress stimulus that can activate an inflammatory response via innate and adaptive cells, although the innate cells show more consistent responses to resistance exercise.

As with the hormonal systems, workout design can influence the temporal pattern and/or magnitude of leucocytosis,[14] Generally, leukocyte subpopulations increase after resistance exercise and decrease up to 90 minutes in the recovery period. Conversely, natural killer (NK) cells exhibit an early increase followed by a rapid return to baseline or below.[14]

Cytokine release at the inflammation site is another important recovery signal, producing an influx of lymphocytes, neutrophils, monocytes, and other cells to participate in antigen clearance and tissue healing.[23] From an exercising viewpoint, the immune system essentially works to protect the body from pathogens and other harmful cells that arise from homeostatic changes.

# Interplay between the neuro-endocrine and immune systems

## Physiological interactions

The recovery phase can be characterised by one or more overall lapping processes of neuromuscular fatigue, muscle damage, increased hormonal activity, inflammation and immune activity, depending on the exercise protocols performed. There is evidence of complex interplay between the physiological systems.

Changes in hormone levels may influence immune activity including T-lymphocyte selection, splenic lymphocyte release, and intercellular mediators (see Table 29.1),[13,21] Specifically, the rapid exercise increases in catecholamine concentrations can contribute to leukocytosis, whereas the slower steroid and peptide hormones responses could be important for maintaining neutrophilia and lymphopenia.

*Table 29.1* Hormonal influences on immune function.

| Hormones | Effects on the immune system |
| --- | --- |
| Testosterone | Inhibit IL-2, IL-4, IL-10, TNF, IFN$_\gamma$ secretion |
| | Enhance IL-12- and IL-1$\beta$-producing monocytes |
| Cortisol | Enhance leukocyte liberation from bone marrow |
| | Mediate lymphocyte distribution |
| | Inhibit T-cell proliferation |
| | Inhibit IL-1, IL-2 production |
| | Enhance IL-4 production |
| Growth hormone | Promote T-cell generation |
| Catecholamines | Via $\beta$-adrenoreceptors: induce leukocytosis |
| | May reduce endothelial adhesion of leukocytes to vessel walls |
| | Enhance the proliferation of CD3$^+$, CD4$^+$ and CD8$^+$ cells (by $\beta$-adrenergic stimulation) |
| | Inhibit the proliferation of CD4$^+$ and CD8$^+$ cells (by $\beta$-adrenergic stimulation) |
| | Inhibit the degranulation of mast cells and basophilic granulocytes |

Regular exercise training can improve immune function by potentially modulating neutrophil, eosinophil and basophil counts, where heavy intense training can suppress several parameters of the immune response.[21]

### Physiological and psychological interactions

Recent studies have linked changes in athlete physiology to behaviour and physical performance. For instance, exposing male athletes to different biofeedback strategies (e.g. video footage, coach feedback) was found to influence T levels, the hormonal responses to a stressor and/or physical performance several hours to days later.[8,9] This physiological link could provide an additional avenue for improving athlete recovery.

The rationale for biofeedback interventions is based on the psycho-physiological principle that a physiological response is accompanied by a concomitant change in emotional and behavioural state. It is important to acknowledge that a change in thoughts, feelings and emotions can itself modify an individual's physiology.

## Recovery strategies

### Light exercise

Light exercise is widely used as a recovery strategy and often integrated into a warm-down after training or competition. Proposed benefits include enhanced lactate removal, a smoother decline in temperature and blood flow, a dampening of nervous system activity to promote sleep and improved ratings (e.g. soreness) of recovery.[6,24]

Recent work reported similar effects on repeated cycling performance using either active or passive recovery strategies, although the active strategy was superior to a combined method.[11] Exercise in the form of games can also be prescribed to provide psychological benefits. As a recovery strategy, exercise should be used judiciously after activities that promote extreme glycogen depletion or muscle damage.

Deep-water running is often prescribed as a recovery session immediately after, or the day after, competition and for rehabilitation from injury.[24] This approach prevents soft tissue injury, minimises physiological effort, and reduces loading on the joints and musculature.

## Stretching

Stretching is also integrated within training and recovery in either static, dynamic or pre-contraction forms, and generally held for 10 to 30 seconds.[22] In rehabilitation, stretching is prescribed to increase muscle length and range of motion or align collagen fibres during muscle healing, with possible pain relieving benefits.[22] Other benefits include a reduction in muscle tension, postural enhancement and relaxation.

All types of stretching are effective for increasing range of movement, but pre-contraction methods (e.g. proprioceptive neuromuscular facilitation) appear to be the most effective,[22] since they activate both the structural and reflex components of muscle.

A post-exercise programme could involve the prescription of static stretches for relevant muscle groups, each held for 6–10 seconds. This could compliment an additional programme that focuses more on development stretches (each held for 30–180 seconds), partner-assisted stretches and proprioceptive neuromuscular facilitation techniques.

## Soft tissue therapies

Sports massage is commonly used for rehabilitation and injury prevention, as well as being an adjunct warm-up procedure. Positive outcomes include improved blood flow and greater lactate clearance, a more relaxed state and mood improvements.[2] Other psychological effects include a decrease in soreness perception.

Despite its wide use, evidence has yet to conclusively demonstrate that a massage can enhance functional performance or recovery markers. This could be due to differences in the massage technique and treatment time, and who is administering the massage (Table 29.2), as reviewed by Brummitt.[2]

Foam rolling can also be employed to improve range of motion and myofascial restrictions, and to decrease pain.[19] This method utilizes the concept of autogenic inhibition to improve soft tissue extensibility, thereby relaxing the muscle and activating the antagonist

*Table 29.2* Research examining the effect of sports massage on recovery from exercise and competition.

| Techniques used | Treatment times | Administered by |
| --- | --- | --- |
| Effleurage | Continuous and intermittent protocols of varying duration, ranging from 5 to 30 minutes | Physical therapist |
| Petrissage | | Athletic trainer |
| Tapotement | | Certified masseur |
| Mixture of the above techniques | | Massage therapist |
| | | Physiotherapist |

muscle. The process involves rolling the foam roller under each muscle group until a tender area is found, and maintaining pressure on the tender area for 30–60 seconds.

Ultrasound, electrical nerve stimulation and hyperbaric oxygen therapy offer additional treatments for soft tissue injuries, although their efficacy for improving muscle function, soreness or related symptoms is still unclear.

## Cold and/or hot water immersion

A range of cooling methods can reduce skin or core temperature, such as showers, ice-baths, cold rooms, vests, sprays and fans.[12] Pre- and post-exercise cooling may lower internal thermal load and facilitate the activation and recruitment of muscle force, thereby aiding performance and recovery.[12]

Water immersion techniques can also relax gravitational muscles, conserve energy, and may reduce pain perception.[12] A recent meta-analysis reported that cold water immersion (CWI) can improve power recovery during SSC activities, but has little effect on strength.[16] Post-exercise cooling may also aid endurance or prolonged high-intensity exercise performance in short (1–2 hrs) or intermediate (24 hrs) time frames.[12]

Hot water immersion (HWI) works by increasing tissue temperature and local blood flow, thereby enhancing muscle elasticity and local vasodilation.[27] The effects of CWI and HWI could also be combined to improve recovery. The recovery protocols involve alternating hot (37–43°C) and cold (10–15°C) water treatments using a 3:1 or 4:1 time ratio.[7] Hot and cold showers may be used when baths are not available.

## Compression garments

Compression garments are widely used by recreational and competitive athletes as a recovery tool. Reported benefits include a reduction in muscle damage, swelling and muscle soreness, improved lactate clearance, an increase in vitality and performance restoration.[20] The wearing of a compression garment may also offer psychological benefits for the user through a placebo effect.

Many styles of garments exist, including stockings (knee length, thigh length), sleeves, upper-body garments (covering the torso and the upper limbs in full or part) and lower-body garments (from the waist with full or part covering).[20]

A review of compression garment use did report limited physiological or performance effects.[20] One issue is the amount of pressure needed to elicit a beneficial effect, due to individual differences in body size and shape, as well as the fabric properties and structure.

## Nutrition

Nutritional intake can influence many steps involved in training adaptation and recovery. Post-exercise carbohydrate (CHO) consumption can restore glycogen levels and attenuate lymphocytosis.[5,15] Foods containing CHO that are rated high (>85) to moderate (60–85) in the glycaemic index are ideal for rapid replenishment of glycogen stores and should be consumed within 30–60 minutes of exercise completion. Combining CHO with protein (PRO) can facilitate protein accretion.

Post-exercise CHO and PRO requirements differ across athletic groups, but there are general guidelines for endurance (CHO 7–10 g/kg of bodymass, PRO 1.2–1.8 g/kg of body mass) and strength athletes (CHO 10–12 g/kg of bodymass, PRO 1.6–2.0 g/kg of body mass). Given that strenuous exercise can suppress appetite, concentrated CHO and/or PRO drinks may prove useful during recovery.

Athlete rehydration is also important to exercise performance, especially in humid environments. Fluid lost during training and competition should be replaced with water or a sports drink with electrolytes, notably sodium, to facilitate absorption.[24] Additional salt added to food or drinks may be needed for individuals incurring high salt losses.

Other supplements used to enhance performance and/or recovery include non-steroidal medications, creatine, caffeine, amino acids, antioxidants, pyruvate and β-hydroxy-β-methylbutyrate, but their ergogenic effects appear to be exercise- and individual-dependent. Still, these strategies could be trialed within a wider nutritional programme.

### Psychological

A number of different psychological recovery techniques are currently available, including meditation, muscle relaxation and autogenic training, imagery, and breathing exercises. Music can also be used as a recovery- or performance-enhancement tool, by manipulating mood state to generate optimal arousal or relaxation, synchronizing movements to music, or by diverting the mind from fatigue sensations.[26]

Again, using biofeedback strategies in pre-or post-competition settings can potentially modify athlete behaviour, stress resilience, and enhance performance.[8,9] Where possible, other relaxing activities (e.g. watch a movie, read a book, socialize) should be encouraged outside of normal training and recovery programmes to improve mood, aid in emotional recovery, and reduce stress.

## Prescribing a recovery programme

Although a resistance model was emphasized in this chapter, many of the reported outcomes could be extrapolated to other forms of exercise and competition. The prescription of a recovery programme will depend on the physiological outcomes of exercise, which could include one or all of the following;

*   Restoration of peripheral or central fatigue
*   Manufacturing muscle protein and other components (cellular and hormonal) as part of the repair and adaptation process
*   Refueling muscle and liver glycogen stores
*   Replacing fluid and electrolytes lost in sweat
*   Allowing the immune and endocrine systems to handle the exercise stressors, subsequent damage and inflammation
*   Addressing soft tissue injuries
*   Psychological recovery and possible endocrine influences.

The evidence for some recovery approaches is inconclusive or unclear; however, given the marginal gains needed to succeed in sport, a holistic approach that combines one or more tools may give better responses than isolated strategies.[7] The symptoms of exercise-induced muscle damage are arguably similar to that of an injured muscle, so the same treatment modalities and protocols could be used.

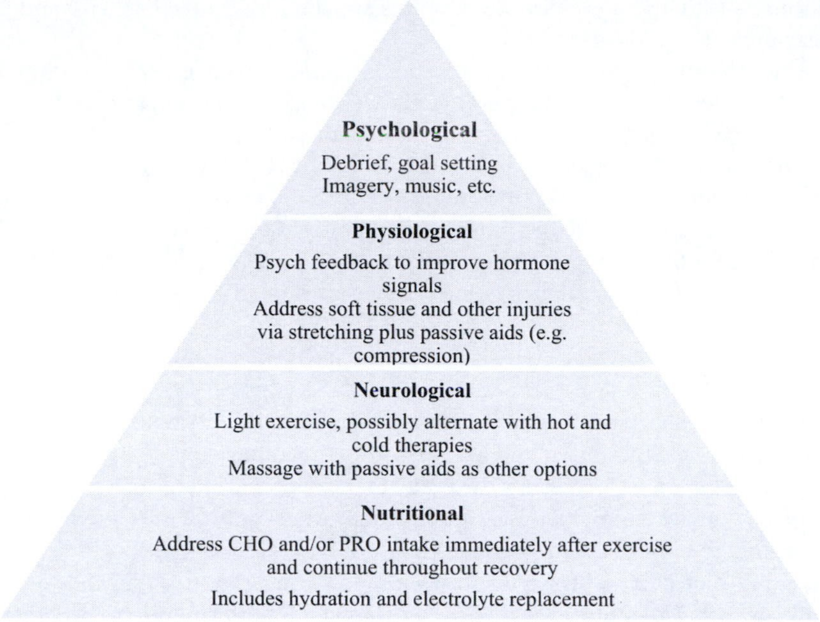

*Figure 29.1* Pyramid for recovery tools

A ranking system may be employed by coaches and trainers to identify which fatigue components or sites are most stressed from different training sessions, using the broad definitions of nutritional, physiological, neurological and psychological.[4] The most appropriate recovery tools may then be prescribed and tailored to meet the specific needs of an individual. The different components of recovery (using the definitions above) may be addressed with one or more strategies (Figure 29.1).

It is important to recognise that exercise-induced increases in catabolic hormones, muscle damage and the inflammatory response are possible precursors to the signalling mechanisms, which initiate the repair and growth of cells. Therefore, implementing one or more recovery strategies may be detrimental to some longer-term adaptations. This trade-off should be recognised when employing a recovery programme.

When the goal of training is to adapt to stress and improve performance capacity over time (e.g. off-season), then emphasis should be placed on good management practices, including adequate sleep, rest and relaxation techniques. If the training goal is to maximise the expression of performance on a continual basis (e.g. competition season), then other recovery techniques can be employed.

## Summary

Post-exercise recovery can be characterised by overall lapping processes of increased hormonal activity, fatigue, muscle damage and inflammation. The exercise protocols are key determinants of these responses and moderated by factors such as training experience, age and gender. A number of active (e.g. light exercise, stretching) and passive (e.g. massage, foam rolling, CWI, HWI, contrast therapy, compression garments, nutritional intake) strategies are currently used to facilitate athlete recovery. A holistic approach that combines one or more recovery tools and is tailored for the individual athlete would be worthwhile, given the marginal gains needed to succeed in sport.

## Notes

1  Barnett, A. (2006). Using recovery modalities between training sessions in elite athletes. Does it help? *Sports Med, 36*(9), 781–796.
2  Brummitt, J. (2008). The role of massage in sports performance and rehabilitation: Current evidence and future direction. *N Am J Sprts Phys Ther, 3*(1), 7–21.
3  Byrne, C., Twist, C., & Eston, R. (2004). Neuromuscular function after exercise-induced muscle damage: Theoretical and applied implications. *Sports Med, 34*(1), 49–69.
4  Calder, A. (1995). Accelerating adaptation to training. Paper presented at the Australian Strength and Conditioning Association National Conference and Trade Show, Gold Coast, Queensland.
5  Carlson, L. A., Headley, S., DeBruin, J., Tuckow, A. T., Koch, A. J., & Kenefick, R. W. (2008). Carbohydrate supplementation and immune responses after acute exhaustive resistance exercise. *Int J Sport Nutr Exerc Metab, 18*(3), 247–259.
6  Cheung, K., Hume, P., & Maxwell, L. (2003). Delayed onset muscle soreness: Treatment strategies and performance factors. *Sports Med, 33*(2), 145–164.
7  Cochrane, D. J. (2004). Alternating hot and cold water immersion for athlete recovery: A review. *Phys Ther Sport, 24*(5), 26–32.
8  Cook, C. J., & Crewther, B. T. (2012). Changes in salivary testosterone concentrations and subsequent voluntary squat performance following the presentation of short video clips. *Horm Behav, 61*(1), 17–22.
9  Crewther, B. T., & Cook, C. J. (2012). Effects of different post-match recovery interventions on subsequent athlete hormonal state and game performance. *Physiol Behav, 106*(4), 471–475.
10  Crewther, B. T., Keogh, J., Cronin, J., & Cook, C. (2006). Possible stimuli for strength and power adaptation: acute hormonal responses. *Sports Med, 36*(3), 215–238.
11  De Pauw, K., De Geus, B., Roelands, B., Lauwens, F., Verschueren, J., Heyman, E., & Meeusen, R. R. (2011). Effect of five different recovery methods on repeated cycle performance. *Med Sci Sports Exerc, 43*(5), 890–897.
12  Duffield, R. (2008). Cooling interventions for the protection and recovery of exercise performance from exercise-induced heat stress. *Med Sport Sci, 53*, 89–103.
13  Fragala, M. S., Kraemer, W. J., Denegar, C. R., Maresh, C. M., Mastro, A. M., & Volek, J. S. (2011). Neuroendocrine-immune interactions and responses to exercise. *Sports Med, 41*(8), 621–639.
14  Freidenreich, D. J., & Volek, J. S. (2012). Immune responses to resistance exercise. *Exerc Immunol Rev, 18*, 8–41.
15  Koch, A. J., Potteiger, J. A., Chan, M. A., Benedict, S. H., & Frey, B. B. (2001). Minimal influence of carbohydrate ingestion on the immune response following acute resistance exercise. *Int J Sport Nutr Exerc Metab, 11*(2), 149–161.
16  Leeder, J., Gissane, C., van Someren, K., Gregson, W., & Howatson, G. (2012). Cold water immersion and recovery from strenuous exercise: A meta-analysis. *Brit J Sport Med, 46*(4), 233–240.
17  Linnamo, V., Häkkinen, K., & Komi, P. V. (1998). Neuromuscular fatigue and recovery in maximal compared to explosive strength loading. *Eur J Appl Physiol Occ Physiol, 77*(1–2), 176–181.
18  Linnamo, V., Newton, R. U., Häkkinen, K., Komi, P., Davie, A., McGuigan, M., & Triplett-McBride, T. (2000). Neuromuscular responses to explosive and heavy resistance loading. *J Electromyogr Kinesiol, 10*(6), 417–424.
19  MacDonald, G. Z., Penney, M. D., Mullaley, M. E., Cuconato, A. L., Drake, C. D., Behm, D. G., & Button, D. C. (2013). An acute bout of self-myofascial release increases range of motion without a subsequent decrease in muscle activation or force. *J Strength Cond Res, 27*(3), 812–821.

20  MacRae, B. A., Cotter, J. D., & Laing, R. M. (2011). Compression garments and exercise: garment considerations, physiology and performance. *Sports Med, 41*(10), 815–843.

21  Natale, V. M., & Shephard, R. J. (2000). Interrelationships between acute and chronic exercise and the immune and endocrine systems. In M. P. Warren and N. W. Constantini (Eds.), *Sports Endocrinology* (pp. 281–302). New Jersey: Humana Press Inc.

22  Page, P. (2012). Current concepts in muscle stretching for exercise and rehabilitation. *Int J Sports Phys Ther, 7*(1), 109–119.

23  Pedersen, B. K., & Hoffman-Goetz, L. (2000). Exercise and the immune system: Regulation, integration, and adaptation. *Physiol Rev, 80*(3), 1055–1081.

24  Reilly, T., & Ekblom, B. (2005). The use of recovery methods post-exercise. *J Sports Sci, 23*(6), 619–627.

25  Smith, D. J. (2003). A framework for understanding the training process leading to elite performance. *Sports Med, 33*(15), 1103–1126.

26  Terry, P. C., & Karageorghis, C. I. (2006). Psychological effects of music in sport and exercise: An update on theory, research and application. Paper presented at the Joint Conference of the Australian Psychological Society and the New Zealand Psychological Society – Psychology bridging the Tasman: Science, culture and practice, Melbourne, Australia.

27  Wilcock, I. M., Cronin, J. B., & Hing, W. A. (2006). Physiological response to water immersion: A method for sport recovery? *Sports Med, 36*(9), 747–765.

28  Zouhal, H., Jacob, C., Delamarche, P., & Gratas-Delamarche, A. (2008). Catecholamines and the effects of exercise, training and gender. *Sports Med, 38*(5), 401–423.

# Chapter 30

# Environmental stress – heat and altitude

*Chris R. Abbiss*

## Introduction

Numerous factors may influence the stress and, as a result the adaptations, that are induced by training. It's not just the training and competition stress that influence the development of fatigue, cell signalling responses and adaptations to an exercise task. Indeed, the environment in which we train or compete can have a significant influence on our physiological responses, metabolic function, fatigue and adaptations to exercise. Of these environmental conditions, high altitude exposure and hot/humid environmental conditions considerably influence the stress response to exercise, reduce performance and place us at increased risk of illness and injury. This chapter will examine the physiological responses to exercise in such environmental conditions and the most effective strategies of dealing with them.

### Exercise and heat

#### Physiological responses to exercise at extreme temperatures

When exercising, a considerable amount of energy is liberated as heat. Metabolic heat production during high-intensity exercise can increase core body temperature by approximately 1°C every 5–7 minutes.[1,2,3] However, core body temperatures in excess of 40°C cannot be tolerated for prolonged periods and it is therefore important that the body dissipates the majority of this heat.

Heat created within the body is transferred to environment via a number of mechanisms which involve convection, conduction, radiation and evaporation (Figure 30.1). In hot and humid environmental conditions, the body's ability to liberate heat is reduced, resulting in elevated body temperatures. Under such conditions, exercise capacity is compromised and people are placed at a greater risk of hyperthermic-induced illness or complications.

Interestingly, the detrimental effects of hyperthermic-induced fatigue are often only considered when athletes are performing prolonged exercise (i.e. marathon running, triathlon or cycling) in hot and humid environmental conditions. However, well-trained athletes are capable of exercise at extremely high workloads, thereby producing a great deal of metabolic heat. This, coupled with reduced capacity to dissipate heat due to protective clothing (i.e. NFL, motor racing) and/or low wind flow observed in a number of sports (i.e. combat sports, tennis), may result in body temperatures that compromise performance and can result in heat-related illness (40–42°C),[4] even in temperate environmental conditions (16–25°C)[5] and during relatively short bouts of physical activity.

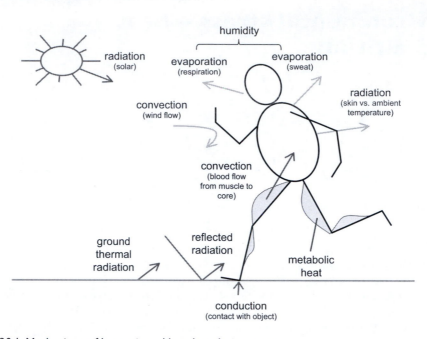

*Figure 30.1* Mechanisms of heat gain and heat loss during exercise

While the precise mechanisms responsible for the reduction in exercise capacity in hot environmental conditions are unclear, it appears that the attainment or anticipation of critically high core body temperatures results in a down-regulation of skeletal muscle drive. Within this hypothesis, the hypothalamus and brain regulate central neural drive and autonomic processes responsible for heat removal (i.e. onset of sweating, sweat rate and blood flow) in order to control total heat balance within the body.[6] These mechanisms usually reduce our exercise performance before we hit critically high core body temperatures.[5,7] It has been suggested that this down-regulation and altered pacing strategy occurs in response to the rapid rate of rise in core body temperature and high thermal sensations experienced early in the exercise task.[6]

In addition to altering central neural drive, exercise in heat and humidity may also compromise muscle and brain blood flow.[8] As body temperature rises, blood flow is redistributed towards the skin in order to assist in convective cooling, creating competition for blood flow demands with contracting muscle. Altered blood flow and thus oxygen delivery to contracting muscle can influence muscle metabolism. Indeed, exercise in the heat has been shown to result in greater muscle glycogen utilisation, which may also contribute to earlier or more pronounced fatigue during exercise in the heat. As such, athletes are likely to benefit from altering their nutritional strategies and consume more simple carbohydrates during exercise in the heat.

As well as a competition for blood flow with the skin, brain blood flow during exercise in the heat may be reduced due to hyperventilation-induced reductions in arterial carbon dioxide ($PaCO_2$) and resulting cerebral vasoconstriction.[9,10] The influence of this reduced brain blood flow during exercise is currently not well understood but may be associated with reduced substrate delivery and a decline in cognitive function (i.e. decision making). It is therefore possible that athletes may be more likely to make technical and tactical errors when competing in hot and humid conditions. Strategies that aid to assist with dealing with hyperthermic-induced fatigue (discussed later in this chapter) may reduce such declines in cognitive function during exercise in the heat.

## Illness, injury and performance risks from exercise at extreme temperatures

Heat illness is a spectrum of heat-related disorders resulting from elevated body temperature and include heat cramps, syncope, heat exhaustion and heat stroke. *Heat cramp* is the term given to brief muscle cramps or spasms that may occur during or following strenuous exercise in the heat. The precise mechanisms responsible for heat cramps are not clear but are probably associated with imbalances in intra- and extracellular concentrations of electrolytes and minerals, such as sodium, potassium, calcium and magnesium. These electrolytes and minerals are important in muscular contraction and transported to different compartments within the body through active transport (i.e. requiring ATP). It is therefore possible that cramps may be caused by insufficient transport of these molecules, rather than insufficient dairy intake or excessive loss due to sweating. Reduced cerebral blood flow and high core body temperature during exercise in the heat may result in dizziness (syncope) and nausea.

Prolonged or severe exposure to the heat may result in heat exhaustion. Signs and symptoms of heat exhaustion include profuse sweating, dizziness, shallow breathing, rapid pulse, dry clammy skin, nausea and a possible loss of consciousness. Heat stroke is a more severe heat illness, which is often characterised by dysfunction in our ability to control body temperature. Signs and symptoms include a reduction in or lack of perspiration, flushed skin, rapid pulse, high body temperatures and ratings of thermal sensation ranging from cool to very hot. If untreated, heat stroke may lead to multiple organ failure, loss of consciousness and death.

## Dealing with the stresses of exercise at extreme temperatures to reduce illness, injury and performance risks

The most important treatment for heat-related disorders is to reduce body temperature. Mild heat illnesses may be treated by ceasing exercise and moving to a well-ventilated shaded area. However, more severe forms of heat illness may require active means of cooling with the use of fans, water or ice (described below). Where dehydration is expected, ad libitum fluid ingestion may be beneficial. However, fluid loss of approximately 2–3 per cent is not uncommon and appears to have little influence on exercise performance. Furthermore, it should be noted that excessive or forced fluid ingestion may result in dangerous electrolyte imbalances (e.g. hyponatremia).[11]

A number of strategies can be employed to reduce the incidence of heat illness and improve performance of athletes competing in the heat. These strategies typically aim to either: i) improve our tolerance to the heat, or ii) rapidly reduce body temperature to prevent or treat hyperthermia.

## Heat acclimation

Heat acclimation is an important strategy that has been shown to reduce the incidence and severity of heat-related illnesses and improve performance. Heat acclimation involves regular exposure to hot environmental conditions resulting in a number of physiological adaptations, which primarily improve our ability to dissipate heat. Adaptations to heat exposure may include an increase in plasma volume, earlier onset of sweating, reduced electrolyte concentration in sweat and increased skin blood flow, reduced oxygen consumption for a given workload and improved myocardial efficiency.[12,13] Many of these adaptations are relatively rapid and occur within 10–14 days of heat exposure with some adaptations (i.e. plasma volume expansion, altered skin blood flow) sometimes occurring within the first five days.[12] These adaptations have been shown to improve performance, not only in hot and humid environmental temperatures, but also in cool or temperate 10–20°C environments. The plasma volume expansion that occurs with heat acclimation increases stroke volume and cardiac output may result in a slight improvement in maximal aerobic uptake ($VO_{2max}$).[14] Heat acclimatisation may therefore be used as a method of fast-tracking adaptation early in a competitive season or to improve performance prior to important competitions.

Since the primary stimulus for many of these adaptations is an increase in body temperature, acclimation may be accomplished by either passive (i.e. hot bath, sauna) or active (i.e. exercise) heat exposure. However, it appears that active heat exposure involving moderate, strenuous or intermittent exercise performed for periods long enough to result in elevated body temperatures (>30 minutes) results in the most favourable adaptive response. In addition, deliberately compromising heat dissipation by exercising in hot and humid conditions, limiting wind movement (i.e. no fan) and/or overdressing can increase heat gain resulting in adaptation.

## Body cooling

Pre-, mid- and post-exercise cooling techniques have gained increasing interest as strategies that may assist in reducing heat illness and improving exercise performance in the heat. These strategies aim to rapidly remove heat from the body using a number of different techniques. These techniques typically involve external or internal exposure to cold air, water, ice or a combination of these strategies.[15] Furthermore, cooling may be localised to a specific region of the body or, as in the case of whole body water immersion, may involve cooling the majority of the body. Since the application, effectiveness and location of cooling differ among cooling methods, the practical application and best use of these strategies will differ depending on the goal of the cooling and characteristics of an event or individual athlete.[15]

In general, pre- and mid-exercise cooling are often performed in order to reduce body temperature with the aim of increasing the athlete's ability to store heat and thus increase exercise performance (Figure 30.2). Such cooling is therefore important immediately prior to or during athletic competition.[15] Post-exercise cooling, however, is usually conducted in order to rapidly reduce body temperature (Figure 30.2), enhance recovery and improve performance during subsequent bouts of exercise.[16] Whilst studies have shown that post-exercise cooling may result in improved same-day or subsequent-day performance, the ability to facilitate local muscle recovery is controversial, with studies showing improved,[17] unchanged[18,19] or impaired[20,21] recovery of neuromuscular function and/or indirect muscle damage markers (i.e. muscle soreness, creatine kinase). Furthermore, evidence has recently been provided to suggest that localised post-exercise cooling may both enhance[22] and compromise[23] muscle

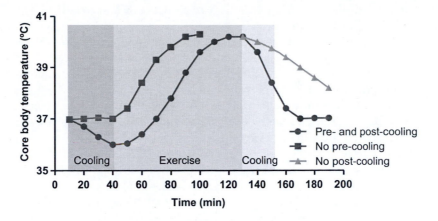

*Figure 30.2* Schematic representation of alterations in core body temperature with whole body cooling prior to (pre-cooling) and following (post-cooling) prolonged exercise in the heat

metabolic and cardiovascular adaptations to exercise. Clearly, strategic planning and thought
should precede the use of pre-, mid- and post-cooling strategies within a periodised competition and training program.

Furthermore, some methods of cooling may place participants at risk. For instance, methods such as whole body ice immersion may result in rapid alterations in blood distribution,
elevating central blood pressure and increasing the risk of adverse cardiovascular events. It
has also been hypothesised that internal cooling or selective brain cooling may trick the hypothalamus into believing that body temperature is lower than it actual is, thereby overriding
the body's normal regulatory mechanisms of exercise intensity and resulting in greater risk
of heat illness.[24] However, further research is needed to confirm or refute these hypotheses.

## Thoughts on heat stress and the use of pre-, mid- and post-cooling

The most effective method of improving our tolerance to the heat is to acclimate. As a
result, athletes competing in hot and humid conditions will usually benefit from prior
acclimation. Under ideal circumstances, athletes should be exposed to similar conditions to the competition for 2–7 days per week in the 2–6 weeks prior to competition.
However, many adaptations to the heat are extremely rapid and can occur within a
few days of exposure. During such exposure the most important factor to consider is
that internal body temperature is elevated (38–40°C) for a prolonged period of time
(15–60 min). This is often accomplished through prolonged moderate-intensity exercise or repeated high-intensity exercise.

One of the most important factors to consider when deciding whether or not to
cool an athlete and, if so, what method(s) to employ is the primary purpose or goal
of the cooling. This may seem a relatively basic concept, but if the purpose is to alter
muscle blood flow in order to aid recovery, then strategies that rapidly reduce muscle

temperature are likely to be best. Whole-body or partial-body immersion in cold water (~8–15°C) for 10 to 15 min has been shown to be extremely effective in lowering core and muscle temperature. Colder temperatures and longer periods often result in a high degree of discomfort and may decrease athletes' desire to use such strategies, whereas, warmer temperatures may take considerable time to significantly reduce temperatures.

Often, the primary purpose of pre- and mid-cooling is to reduce body temperature in order to allow greater capacity for heat storage (Figure 30.2). Under such conditions, a variety of cooling strategies can be successfully implemented, with the best strategy often dependant on the activity, environment and practical constraints. Internal cooling with use of as little as 300–400 millilitres of ice-slushy consumed 30–60min prior to exercise may be effective in lowering body temperature and improving performance. However, the optimal volume to improve performance is likely to be dependent on the sport and subsequent exercise task. When the primary goal of cooling is to lower body temperature, a combination of strategies (i.e. internal and external) may be most beneficial.

## Exercise and altitude

As we climb to high and higher altitudes, barometric pressure declines because each litre of air contains fewer and fewer gas molecules. While the percentages of $O_2$, $CO_2$ and $N_2$ remain unchanged, the decrease in barometric pressure at altitude results in a reduction in the partial pressure of each gas. A significant reduction in the partial pressure of oxygen ($PO_2$) with altitude reduces haemoglobin saturation and therefore compromises oxygen transport. Haemoglobin saturation decreases from approximately 96–98 per cent at sea-level to only 85 per cent at 2,500m. This exponential decline in haemoglobin saturation with increasing altitude means that most of us will experience symptoms of altitude sickness at altitudes above 3,000–4,000m. The reduction in $PO_2$ is referred to as hypoxia and results in numerous acute responses and long-term adaptations within the body.

An important primary response to acute altitude exposure is an increase in our ventilation rates both at rest and during exercise. This increase is important in order to maintain oxygen delivery to cells in the body. However, as we breathe off carbon dioxide, this hyperventilation also results in a decrease in arterial partial pressure of carbon dioxide ($PCO_2$; hypocapnia) and an associated elevated blood pH (alkalosis). The kidneys compensate for this elevated pH by secreting bicarbonate ion and increasing urine output. This, coupled with respiratory fluid loss from hyperventilation, may result in dehydration and ultimately a low body fluid volume (hypohydration) at altitude. The consequential reduction in plasma volume may cause diminished venous return, often resulting in a reduction in maximal stroke volume.[25] As a result, maximal cardiac output may be compromised in the days following exposure to at altitude (Figure 30.3). However, the decrease in plasma volume increases haemoglobin concentration (Hb) and haematocrit (Hct), resulting in an increase in oxygen-carrying capacity per litre of blood.[26] Regardless, the dramatic reduction in cardiac output decrease the ability to supply sufficient blood to working muscles and, as a result, aerobic exercise capacity (i.e. $VO_{2max}$) is often reduced, especially within the first few days of altitude exposure.

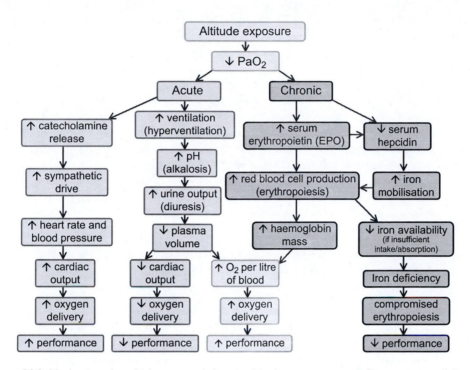

*Figure 30.3* Mechanisms by which acute and chronic altitude exposure may influence oxygen delivery and exercise performance

Despite reductions in plasma volume with acute altitude exposure, changes in cardiac output are inconsistent, since the reduction in $PO_2$ may also result in elevated submaximal blood pressure and heart rates, associated with altered catecholamine release (Figure 30.3). Irrespective of changes in cardiac output, a reduction in the haemoglobin saturation with altitude reduces arterial oxygen content and thus oxygen delivery. Consequently, aerobic exercise performance is reduced at altitude. Such reductions in aerobic performance have been observed as low as 600m above sea-level.[26] Altered catecholamine release upon acute exposure to altitude may also alter metabolism by increasing the reliance on carbohydrates (glycolysis) for energy production. As a result, careful consideration may be required to ensure athletes consume sufficient carbohydrates when training or competing at altitude.

## Illness, injury and performance risks from exercise at altitude

Acute exposure to altitude may lead to a number of conditions of varying severity including acute altitude or mountain sickness (AMS), high altitude pulmonary edema (HAPE) and high altitude cerebral edema (HACE). Acute mountain sickness is the most common altitude sickness encountered, with symptoms such as headache, fatigue, dizziness and difficulties sleeping typically observed 6–10 hours following ascends greater than 2,000m. Increased arterial and capillary blood pressures and hypoxic-induced vasoconstriction can lead to fluid build-up, known as oedema, in different regions of the body. The accumulation of fluid within the lungs (pulmonary oedema) or brain (cerebral oedema) can be life-threating, with symptoms becoming evident within the first two to four days of altitude exposure. Symptoms for pulmonary oedema include difficulties breathing, persistent cough, congestion and tightness of the chest, whereas cerebral oedema may result in loss of coordination, disorientation, loss of memory and irregular behaviour.

Following prolonged exposure to altitude, a number of chronic adaptations will occur which allow the body to acclimatize and better cope with the reduced $PO_2$. While numerous physiological adaptations occur, the most important appear to be haematological changes, which enhance oxygen delivery. Hypoxia stimulates transcription of erythropoietin (EPO), which enhances the production of red blood cells (erythropoiesis). This increase in red blood cell mass increases oxygen-carrying capacity of the blood, which may enhance performance and reduce the risk of altitude-related illnesses. However, an increase in erytheropoisis requires iron, and if insufficient iron is available, then a reduction in serum ferritin levels may result in iron deficiency and compromised adaptations to altitude.

## Dealing with the stresses of exercise at altitude to reduce illness, injury and performance

Acclimatisation is the most important process to improve tolerance to altitude, reduce the risk of illness and improve performance both at altitude and sea-level. The duration and level of exposure required for full altitude acclimatisation has been debated, with some reports stating that individuals may adapt within 12–14 days, and others indicating that favourable adaptations may require several of months of exposure. Discrepancies among studies may occur because numerous factors influence our adaptive response to altitude, including the total duration of exposure, total elevation,[27] characteristics of the individual,[28] model of exposure (live high or live low) and the type of exposure (hypobaric vs. normobaric).[29] Generally, it is believed that elevations above 1,500–2,000m are required in order to observe meaningful haematological improvements. Furthermore, athletes are required to spend at least 12 hours per day at these elevations for a period of three to four weeks to observe improvements in haemoglobin mass, $VO_{2max}$ and aerobic performance.[27,30,31,32] However, not all athletes respond to altitude exposure, and instead, altitude exposure may result in little change or even decrements in performance in some athletes.[33] Indeed, altitude exposure may result in an increase in red blood cell mass, which will increase oxygen delivery but also cause a decline in plasma volume, which may decrease oxygen delivery (Figure 30.3). Since heat acclimation may increase plasma volume, it has recently been proposed that the combination of altitude acclimatisation and heat exposure may assist in maximising haematological adaptations, oxygen delivery and thus aerobic exercise performance. However, to date, there is limited research examining the combination of heat and altitude exposure. Such programs should be implemented with caution, since the combined physiological stress of altitude, heat and training load may place athletes at increased risk of illness and/or over-reaching.

## Models of altitude acclimation

To date, a number of models of altitude exposure have been established with varying advantages and disadvantages. Classic altitude exposure, whereby people travel to areas of moderate or high altitude (2,000–3,500m) in order to live and train, has been shown to result in significant haematological and performance improvements within two to three weeks.[26]

A benefit of classic altitude exposure is that athletes will be exposed to a hypoxic environment for 24 hours a day, resulting in considerable erythropoietin signalling and improvements in endurance exercise performance, especially at altitude. However, as mentioned previously, exercise capacity may be reduced at altitude, thereby compromising other important neuro-muscular adaptations that would usually occur with high-intensity exercise at sea-level. Consequently, despite numerous studies observing an increase in sea-level exercise performance there is a risk that classic altitude training may result in little or no change in performance.[34] Instead, classic altitude training is probably most beneficial in improving performance of athletes who have to compete at altitude.

Due to the reduced exercise capacity at altitude, many recommend the use of live-high/train-low.[34,35] This model of hypoxia involves sleeping and living at altitude but training at sea-level. Natural hypoxic environment which allow athletes to perform live-high/train-low exposure are often impractical. As such, simulated normobaric hypoxic exposure is often used. As opposed to hypobaric hypoxia, which reduces $PO_2$ through a reduction in total barometric pressure, normabaric hypoxia refers to a reduction in $PO_2$ resulting from nitrogen dilution or buffering of oxygen. In order to ensure benefits from live-high/train-low altitude training, it is accepted that participants are required to spend sufficient time in altitude (at least 12–16 hours per day) but also train low enough to maintain intensity during high-intensity exercise.[30,31,32]

An alternate model of altitude exposure involves acute intermittent hypoxic exposure during rest (intermittent hypoxic exposure) or exercise (intermittent hypoxic training, also referred to as live low/train high). Due to the limited time spent in hypoxia, it is unlikely that intermittent hypoxia will provide a sufficient stimulus for an increase in erythropoiesis and associated increases in endurance performance.[30,31,32] However, it has been suggested that exposure to altitude may results in non-haematological adaptations that may improve athletic performance (i.e. altered metabolic responses).[36,37] A further possible benefit of training in hypoxia is that the increased metabolic stress, and therefore cell signalling, may occur at slightly lower exercise intensities, and therefore, athletes can train at a lower total training load (i.e. speed or power output). However, the reduced exercise intensity observed in hypoxia will also alter neuromuscular adaptations and thus may compromise performance. Clearly, further research examining the influence of intermittent hypoxic exposure and intermittent hypoxic training is needed.

## Nutritional considerations during altitude training

Due to the increased erythropoitic activity that occurs with chronic altitude exposure, many athletes may be required to increase iron consumption through diet or supplementation (Figure 30.3). This is especially important in athletes at an increased risk of anaemia, such as endurance athletes, vegetarians, females and those participating in activities with repetitive foot strike with hard surfaces, which can damage red blood cells. It is best practice to measure athlete's iron status prior to and during chronic altitude exposure to determine athletes that may be at need of supplementation. It is important to note that altitude exposure in itself results in considerable physiological stress. This, coupled with reduced sleep quantity and quality that can occur at altitude, increases the physiological load on athletes. It is therefore important that careful consideration is made when structuring training programs for athletes undergoing prolonged altitude exposure. It is possible that some athletes may be required to reduce training load at least for the first few weeks of exposure.

---

**Thoughts on use of altitude training**

The major factor influencing the method of altitude exposure is access and practicality. Aerobic adaptations appear to be best when athletes are exposed to altitude for prolonged periods of time, such as during *live-high/train-low* or *classic* altitude exposures. When using these methods, it is recommended that athletes spend approximately 16 hours or more per day above 2,000m. Such a commitment can be demanding and difficult, and as such the training load, physiological stress and well-being of athletes should be carefully monitored.

Acute models of altitude exposure may be more beneficial in adding variability to training and thus altering the physiological stress induced by an exercise session.

---

## Summary

Exercise capacity is reduced at altitude and in hot and humid environmental conditions. Even minor alterations in elevation, ambient temperature or humidity may significantly influence an individual's physiological stress, placing them at greater risk of various illnesses. However, a number of strategies may be employed to reduce such risk and improve athletic performance. Most importantly, with repeated or prolonged exposure to high body temperatures or hypoxia, the human body will better cope with the harsh environmental conditions. Exercise in the heat results in adaptations, such as an increase in plasma volume, altered blood flow and an earlier onset of sweating, which improve heat loss capacity and exercise performance in not only hot but also cool conditions. Following prolonged exposure to a hypoxic environment, adaptations include, but are not limited to, an increase in haemoglobin mass resulting in subsequent improvements in the oxygen carrying capacity of the blood.

## Notes

1  Armstrong, L.,E., & Maresh, C. M. (1998). Effects of training, environment, and host factors on the sweating response to exercise. *International Journal of Sports Medicine, 19*, S103–5.
2  Abbiss, C. R., & Laursen, P. B. (2008). Describing and understanding pacing strategies during athletic competition. *Sports Medicine, 38*(3), 239–252.
3  Cheuvront, S. N., & Haymes, E. M. (2001). Thermoregulation and marathon running: biological and environmental influences. *Sports Medicine, 31*(10), 743–62.
4  Gonzalez-Alonso, J., et al. (1999). Influence of body temperature on the development of fatigue during prolonged exercise in the heat. *Journal of Applied Physiology, 86*(3), 1032–39.
5  Peiffer, J. J., & Abbiss, C.R. (2011). Influence of environmental temperature on 40 km cycling time-trial performance. International Journal of Sports Physiology and Performance, 6(2), 208–20.
6  Tucker, R. The anticipatory regulation of performance: The physiological basis for pacing strategies and the development of a perception-based model for exercise performance. *British Journal of Sports Medicine, 43*(6), 392–400.
7  Tucker, R., et al. (2004). Impaired exercise performance in the heat is associated with an anticipatory reduction in skeletal muscle recruitment. *European Journal of Physiology, 448*, 422–30.
8  Nybo, L., et al. (2002). Effects of hyperthermia on cerebral blood flow and metabolism during prolonged exercise in humans. *Journal of Applied Physiology, 93*(1), 58–64.

9  Nybo, L., & Nielsen, B. (2001). Hyperthermia and central fatigue during prolonged exercise in humans. *Journal of Applied Physiology, 91*(3), 1055–60.

10  Abbiss, C. R., Nosaka, K., & Laursen, P. B. (2007). Hyperthermic-induced hyperventilation and associated respiratory alkalosis in humans. *European Journal of Applied Physiology, 100*(1), 63–69.

11  Draper, S. B., et al. (2009). Overdrinking-induced hyponatraemia in the 2007 London Marathon. *BMJ Case Rep*. doi:10.1136/bcr.09.2008.1002. [Epub]

12  Armstrong, L. E. (1998). Heat acclimatization. In T. D. Fahey (Ed.). *Encyclopedia of sports medicine and science.* Retrieved from http://sportsci.org.

13  Lorenzo, S., et al. (2010). Heat acclimation improves exercise performance. *Journal of Applied Physiology, 109*(4), 1140–47.

14  Coyle, E. F., Hopper, M. K., & Coggan, A. R. (1990). Maximal oxygen uptake relative to plasma volume expansion. *International Journal of Sports Medicine, 11*(2), 116–19.

15  Ross, M., et al. (2013). Precooling methods and their effects on athletic performance: A systematic review and practical applications. *Sports Medicine, 43*(3), 207–25.

16  Peiffer, J. J., et al. (2010). Effect of a 5-min cold-water immersion recovery on exercise performance in the heat. *British Journal of Sports Medicine, 44*(6), 461–65.

17  Vaile, J., et al. (2008). Effect of hydrotherapy on the signs and symptoms of delayed onset muscle soreness. *European Journal of Applied Physiology, 102*(4), 447–55.

18  Pointon, M., et al. (2011). Cold application for neuromuscular recovery following intense lower-body exercise. *European Journal of Applied Physiology, 111*(12), 2977–86. doi: 10.1007/s00421-011-1924-1

19  Peiffer, J.J., et al. (2009). Effect of cold-water immersion duration on body temperature and muscle function. *Journal of Sports Sciences, 27*(10), 987–93.

20  Peiffer, J. J., et al. (2009). Effect of cold water immersion after exercise in the heat on muscle function, body temperatures, and vessel diameter. Journal of Science and Medicine in Sport, *12*(1), 91–6.

21  Pointon, M., et al. (2011). Cold water immersion recovery following intermittent-sprint exercise in the heat. *European Journal of Applied Physiology, 111*(12), 1–12.

22  Ihsan, M., et al. (2013). Post-exercise cold water immersion enhances gene expressions related to mitochondrial biogenesis and vascular remodelling (p. 193). In *Proceedings from the 18th Annual Congress of the European College of Sports Science* . Barcelona, Spain.

23  Ihsan, M., et al. (2013). Influence of regular post exercise cold water immersion on skeletal muscle microvascular function assessed by near infrared spectroscopy (p. 194). In Proceedings from the 18th Annual Congress of the European College of Sports Science. Barcelona, Spain.

24  Siegel, R., et al. (2010). Ice slurry ingestion increases core temperature capacity and running time in the heat. *Medicine & Science in Sports & Exercise, 42*(4) 717–25.

25  Alexander, J. K., & Grover, R. F. (1983). Mechanism of reduced cardiac stroke volume at high altitude. *Clinical Cardiology, 6*(6), 301–3.

26  Hahn, A. G., & Gore, C. J. (2001). The effects of altitude on cycling performance. *Sports Medicine, 31*(7), 533–557.

27  Clark, S. A., et al. (2009). Time course of haemoglobin mass during 21 days live-high:train-low simulated altitude. *European Journal of Applied Physiology, 106*(3), 399–406.

28  Garvican, L. A., et al. (2007). Variability of erythropoietin response to sleeping at simulated altitude: A cycling case study. International Journal of Sports Physiology and Performance, *2*(3), 327–31.

29  Millet, G. P., Faiss, R., and Pialoux, V. (2013). Evidence for differences between hypobaric and normobaric hypoxia is conclusive. *Exercise and Sport Science Reviews, 41*(2) 133.

30  Saunders, P. U., Pyne, D. B., & Gore, C. J. (2009). Endurance training at altitude. *High Altitude Medicine & Biology, 10*(2), 135–48.

31  Rusko, H. K., Tikkanen, H.O., & Peltonen, J. E. (2003). Oxygen manipulation as an ergogenic aid. *Current Sports Medicine Reports, 2*(4), 233–38.

32  Levine, B. D., & Stray-Gundersen, J. (2006). Dose-response of altitude training: how much altitude is enough? *Advances in Experimental Medicine and Biology, 588*, 233–47.

33 Robach, P., et al. (2006). Living high-training low: Effect on erythropoiesis and maximal aerobic performance in elite Nordic skiers. *European Journal of Applied Physiology* , *97*(6), 695–705.

34 Bonetti, D. L., & Hopkins, W. G. (2009). Sea-level exercise performance following adaptation to hypoxia: a meta-analysis. *Sports Medicine, 39*(2), 107–27.

35 Levine, B. D., & Stray-Gundersen, J. (1997). 'Living high–training low': Effect of moderate-altitude acclimatization with low-altitude training on performance. *Journal of Applied Physiology, 83*(1), 102–12.

36 Millet, G. P., et al. (2010). Combining hypoxic methods for peak performance. *Sports Medicine, 40*(1), 1–25.

37 Holliss, B. A., et al. (2013). Influence of intermittent hypoxic training on muscle energetics and exercise tolerance. *Journal of Applied Physiology, 114*(5), 611–19.

# Part 6

# Special considerations

# Chapter 31

# The developing athlete

*Ian Jeffreys*

## Introduction

Competitive youth sports are commonplace in most countries and are generally accepted as playing a positive role in the development of the youth as both an athlete and a person. This has led to the development of intricate competition structures, allowing a youth athlete to participate in sport at a range of levels and, via which, a select few athletes are able to develop through to the highest levels of sport. Traditionally, the development of performance has taken a sport-specific route, with the vast majority of focus being on the development of the technical and tactical skills associated with particular sports. However, the physical preparation of young athletes for sports performance has not met with such universal agreement, and much debate still exists regarding appropriate training interventions with the youth population. The cost of this is that, in many instances, key physical capacities required for optimal performance are not addressed, thus leaving the athlete unable to fully maximise their potential, while also placing them at greater risk of injury. What is needed is a long-term athlete development structure in which all aspects of performance are appropriately addressed.

## The nature of optimal sports performance

Optimal sports performance depends upon the interaction of a wide range of factors and cannot be determined by skill alone; simply playing the game will not enable a youth athlete to maximise their performance in the short- or long-term. Instead, what is required is a programme of development that addresses as many aspects of performance as possible.

Ideally, this process should contain a staged progression, with advanced skills and abilities based upon appropriate mastery of basic skills and capacities. This has led to an increased interest in the concept of long-term athlete development (LTAD), where sequential systems and methods are put in place that address as many of these critical factors as possible, ultimately maximising the chances of an athlete achieving their full potential. In this way, all of the following need to be a part of an effective long-term athlete development programme:

1   the development of physical capacities
2   the development of psychological capacities
3   the development of technical skill
4   the development of tactical ability
5   the development of decision making capacities
6   the development of lifestyle management capabilities.

Unfortunately, while there are no shortages of competitive sports opportunities, these often focus on short-term results rather than long-term preparation, and the provision of appropriate long-term development programmes is rare. This focus on short-term performance is often exacerbated by selection processes happening at increasingly younger ages, further shifting the focus onto getting an athlete to perform in the short-term in order to gain selection for elite teams/squads, etc.

> It should always be remembered that a youth's talent potential is not a stable innate trait, but rather is constantly transforming during the maturation process, and that full potential will require a great deal of time before it can be assessed.[1]

Maximising an athlete's full potential necessitates sophisticated planning and the integration of inputs from a range of sources, working harmoniously with the aim of optimising athletic performance over the long-term. This chapter will focus on the development of physical capacities; however, coaches are advised to look at methods by which these capacities can be combined with the other areas highlighted above to ensure the optimal development of athletic performance.

## The rationale for long-term athlete development

It can be argued that without the correct experience and opportunity, optimum performance will never be achieved. However, in many sports systems, focus in the youth years has often been on achieving short-term results, using periodised programmes built around adult models of peaking for competitions, rather than on maximising long-term development and future potential.

Unfortunately, this short-term approach to training and performance can be detrimental to the long-term development of youth athlete, as focus will naturally shift towards the physical parameters that can enhance performance in the short-term, rather than ensuring that physical capacities that ultimately underpin performance in the long-term are prioritised. In this way, many youth athletes may demonstrate what appear to be high levels of sporting prowess, but in reality, may lack competency in key physical parameters. If these deficiencies are not addressed, the athlete may not be able to reach their full athletic potential, and may be more susceptible to injury.[3]

To address this challenge, long-term athlete development models have been devised that take a much more strategic approach to the development of performance, with a greater emphasis on the achievement of performance over the longer term, rather than on the achievement of short-term goals. Although the concept of long-term athlete development is not novel, current models take a more scientific approach, often based upon the allocation of appropriate training stimuli stemming from the interaction between training and growth maturation processes,[4] with each stage of development related to the important biological, psychological and social development periods in the person's life.[5] These processes are, in turn, identified through objective physiological measures, such as peak height velocity and peak weight velocity. It is argued that through the identification of these phases, youth athletes can be trained according to their biological status as opposed to their chronological age.[6]

As well as a strong performance argument for long-term athlete development, there is also a strong injury reduction rationale for the implementation of an effective long-term programme. While no programme can totally eliminate the risk of injury, the model highlighted can help minimise the risk of injury to the athlete by directly addressing some of the key causes of injury in youth athletes. Typical causes of injury in youth athletes include:

- lack of physical competence in relation to the activities required in sports
- lack of variability in the training
- overuse
- inappropriate training volume or loads
- lack of mobility and/or balance across joints
- lack of appropriate strength or muscle balance.[3,7]

Through the application of an effective programme of long-term athlete development (outlined later), many of these potential risks can be effectively reduced. By establishing baseline movement and skill competencies, issues such as mobility imbalances and movement incompetencies can be resolved at source.

Similarly, the establishment of basic movement competency in skills such as jumping, landing, squatting, bracing, etc., ensure that the athlete is best prepared to deal with the stresses placed upon them during sports performance. As there is also a focus on the maintenance of these competencies throughout the process, the potential for imbalances to accrue through sports performance, especially of asymmetrical sports such as golf, tennis, etc., is also reduced. Another key feature of the system is that it is built upon staged progression, and thus volumes and intensities are progressively staged and based upon the demonstration of successful performance at a previous level. In this way, the likelihood of overuse injuries is greatly reduced.

It takes 8–12 years of training for a talented athlete to reach elite levels,[2] and therefore, focus within any athletic development programme for youth athletes should focus on laying the foundations for long-term performance.

One aspect of development that has received a great deal of attention is the adolescent growth spurt, during which there is a perceived increase in injury risk. However, whether this is due to a natural increase in injury risk or due to a lack of appropriate physical preparation and competence at a time when competition is often increasing is unclear. What is important is that the system outlined later allows for the establishment and, importantly, the maintenance of fundamental capacities throughout an athlete's development, so that many of the performance challenges associated with the growth spurt and adolescent awkwardness can be significantly reduced, thus reducing the potential for injury.

## Current models of long-term athlete development

While a number of long-term athlete development models exist, the most widely used is Balyi's LTAD model.[8,9] This model has been adopted in many sports organisations around the world and is the basis for a number of player development pathways. While often thought of as a single model, the model itself varies, depending upon whether sports can be classified as either early specialisation or late specialisation.

Early specialisation sports are characterised by the fact that peak performance is reached at a relatively young age. In these sports, such as gymnastics, diving, etc., early specialisation of training is required, as skill levels need to be optimised at a young age. Balyi[8] suggests that early specialisation sports should develop sport-specific models rather than generic models. Late specialisation sports, such as team sports, track and field, rowing, cycling, etc., typically see peak performance reached at a much later age, and therefore allow for a longer-term approach to training.

Within this late specialisation model, Balyi[8] suggests that there should be five phases of development, namely:

1 FUNdamental
2 Training to train
3 Training to compete
4 Training to win
5 Retirement/retaining.

The underpinning aims of each phase are outlined below, and generally, the LTAD model outlines a phased progression from the acquisition of general physical capacities, through to the development of specific physical capacities associated with high-performance in a particular sport.

### FUNdamental

In the FUNdamental stage, emphasis is on the overall development of fundamental movement skills and general physical capacities. Focus is on the ABCs of athleticism (agility, balance, coordination and speed), with emphasis on developing correct running, jumping and throwing techniques. Athletes at this stage are encouraged to participate in a range of sports, to enable the development of a wide range of sports-related skills. These activities are often delivered through open play, but with all programmes structured and monitored. Strength work during this phase includes exercises using the athlete's own body weight, together with medicine ball and Swiss ball exercises. This phase is normally delineated on an age basis, and is generally considered to happen between the ages of six and nine.

### Training to train

In this stage, athletes are essentially taught how to train and learn the basic skills of a specific sport. The aim is to enable youth athletes to undertake and understand basic training principles, such as warming up, preparing for competition, the need for recovery, etc. The major focus is on learning and preparation, rather than on competition, with ideally a 75:25 per cent ratio between training and competition. This stage addresses the critical or sensitive periods of physical and skill development,[8] which are fundamental features of the LTAD model. Indeed, Balyi[8] claims that the reason so many athletes plateau during the late stage of their careers is primarily because of an over-emphasis on competition instead of training during this period.

## Training to compete

This phase is introduced after the goals and objectives of the 'training to train' phase have been achieved. Here, the focus shifts more to competition, with the ratio of 50:50 between training and competition. It is hoped that athletes are now proficient at performing basic and sport-specific skills and can now learn to perform these in more intense competitive situations. Preparation programmes become increasingly individualised to address athlete strengths and weaknesses.

## Training to win

This is the final stage of athletic preparation, where the focus of training shifts to the optimisation of performance. Athletes should now have all the underpinning capacities required for optimal performance, and the aim is now to allow them to peak for specific competitions. The training to competition ratio is 25:75, with a competition ratio also including competition-specific training activities, such as practice games. Training is on a periodised basis, with periods of high-intensity high-volume interspersed with appropriate recovery protocols.

# The trainability of youth and the physiological basis for windows of opportunity

A key component of Balyi's model is the concept of windows of opportunity – times at which physical development of youth athletes can be accelerated and enhanced. This concept is based around exploiting natural physiological processes of growth and maturation. However, a number of recent papers suggest that there is a distinct lack of empirical data to support the concept of critical windows of opportunity, and whether the windows of opportunity actually raise the ceiling of the future potential or just allow an athlete to reach their potential at a younger age.[10,11] This requires an examination of the trainability of key fundamental components of fitness in the youth population.

## Motor skill development and physical literacy

The literature regarding the importance of developing physical literacy and motor skill fitness is limited.[12] However, studies of brain maturation show a series of peaks between the ages of six and eight up to twelve years of age.[11] These would fit in with the windows of opportunity for skill development highlighted in the LTAD model. However, the existence of these peaks does not necessarily demonstrate a greater sensitivity to training,[20] or evidence that failure to develop the skills at this age will by necessity limit overall development at a later age. While it would appear logical from the physiological and motor-control viewpoint to develop fundamental skills as early as possible, there is great inconsistency in the current literature surrounding the long-term effects of this type of training. While studies have shown that physical literacy can be improved in six- to nine-year-olds,[12] follow-up studies question the long-term effect of such programmes, without continued reinforcement and development of these skills.[13]

## Speed

Age and maturation have been shown to influence linear running speed. This is because speed will be affected by a range of factors, such as neural coordination, motor performance, muscle cross-sectional area, morphological alterations to muscle and tendon, etc. This makes it difficult to identify and predict a fixed window of opportunity for speed, as all of the above may be developing at different times. Natural speed development appears to reach a plateau after the age of 15 for boys and between 12 and 13 for girls. This supports the assertions that scores in motor performance, in the absence of training interventions, appear to plateau at the end of the peak height-velocity phase.[14,15] However, there is no evidence to demonstrate that speed cannot be developed by an appropriate intervention of training beyond these natural plateaus.[16,17] Indeed, the author has successfully increased speed in athletes pre-adolescent, adolescent and senior athletes, suggesting that speed can be increased with an appropriate training intervention at all stages of an athlete's career.

## Strength

It can be expected that healthy children will experience noticeable gains in muscle strength during the developmental years as a result of natural maturation.[18] The key question is whether training can augment this, and whether this augmentation is limited to specific windows of opportunity. Today, a compelling body of evidence indicates that children and adolescents can significantly increase their strength, over and above that resulting from growth and maturation alone, by following an appropriate resistance training programme.[7]

Whilst strength gains can be observed in both groups, the mechanisms of these increases are likely to be different. In pre-pubertal athletes, it is likely that adaptations to strength training will be predominantly neural in nature, including changes in motor unit recruitment, firing and coordination.[19,20] Post puberty, strength gains will be the result of a combination of neural and hypertrophic factors.[7] Resistance training programmes in youth athletes have been demonstrated to improve a range of tasks, including standing long jump, vertical jump, sprint speed and medicine ball toss.[7]

It would appear that gains in strength can be made at all ages, and these are not restricted to windows of opportunity. However, it is likely that the post-pubertal period, with an associated increase in hormonal concentrations, will offer a greater opportunity for overall strength and muscle mass gains. Given this potential for strength increases, and the role strength plays in other components of performance, such as speed, agility, coordination, etc., strength training should be a key aspect of the entire spectrum of a long-term athlete development model. What need to vary are the mechanisms of application, and this will be addressed later in the chapter.

## Aerobic endurance

Natural accelerated periods of development for aerobic endurance exist during maturation, although these may be highly individual.[12] However, we do not know whether these offer critical windows of opportunity, or whether they just represent times of accelerated development, and so there is no clear conclusion as to the trainability of aerobic fitness in the youth population. Given that many sports require a baseline aerobic fitness, it may be more appropriate to suggest that developing a suitable degree of aerobic fitness should be stressed throughout childhood and adolescence.[21]

Thus, it would seem that youth athletes show a degree of trainability in a wide range of fitness parameters across a wide range of ages. While it may be that sensitive periods exist, during which natural progression is at its greatest, this does not necessarily indicate that training adaptation will be automatically enhanced at these times. Similarly, the assertions that training outside of windows of opportunity will result in few, if any, training gains is unsupported and contrary to my experience in training athletes. Furthermore, the assertion that if participants do not utilise windows of opportunity they will never reach maximum athletic performance is unjustified.[12] This then opens up opportunities to deploy a range of development models by which to instigate an effective long-term athlete development system, and which can be tailored to the given situation faced by the coach.

## The sequential nature of skilled performance

While the concept of fixed windows of opportunity may be, to some extent, flawed, what is generally accepted is that there needs to be a sequential development of physical capacities, and that many advanced physical capacities depends upon fundamental skills and abilities. It is logical that high levels of sports skills are built on general athleticism and that we need to develop special skills on top of basic function.

Therefore, a simplistic approach, which targets a generic fitness capacity such as speed at a given time, is flawed, unless the fundamental techniques underpinning this capacity have already been introduced and developed. This requires the development of a programme by which underpinning physical competencies are first introduced, and which is progressively sequenced until physical performance can be maximised at a later date.

The fact that the majority of physical fitness capacities are trainable, regardless of age, means that the coach can implement an appropriately sequenced physical development programme at whatever point the youth athlete enters the programme. What is needed is a sequential plan through which an athlete can progress towards the highest levels of performance. This requires identification of key physical capacities that underpin effective performance and then the development of staged progression from these fundamentals. Essentially, this can be thought of as an athletic curriculum through which an athlete progresses, allowing for an accumulation of training over an extended period of time and ultimately leading to optimal performance.

In order to be able to set up an appropriate system of development, movement needs to be standardised and baselines for performance set.[8] Here the work of Cook[3,22] and Jeffreys[11,23,24,25] help identify key fundamental capacities that will underpin fundamental movement skills. Cook's fundamental movement screen (FMS) sets a baseline standard of competency of mobility and stability which can be seen to underpin performance, and without which any strength programmes will ultimately be limited. Similarly, my target Gamespeed movement syllabus provides a range of locomotive movements that underpin effective performance in a range of sports, while the target movement patterns provide models of performance within these movements via which performance can be qualitatively monitored. Together, these provide a comprehensive syllabus of fundamental movements which need to be mastered as a basis of any athlete development programme.

## A model for the individual application of LTAD methods

The following model is flexible and can be utilised by coaches at a range of levels and within a multitude of sport, and, while similar to the LTAD model in many respects, it differs markedly in that, rather than being based around critical windows of opportunity, it is instead based around basic movement competency and subsequent sequential development. This allows it to be utilised in a range of situations and also across a range of timescales, affording far more flexibility than traditional models. A critical aspect of the programme is the use of qualitative assessments of competency with progress based on achievements of set competencies, allowing skills to be appropriately sequenced based on motor learning principles. While a number of stages are outlined, there is no definite time period for the stages. Instead, an athlete will work on a specific skill or pattern until they demonstrate the appropriate competency to move to the subsequent stage:

Key stages:

- athletic foundation
- athletic development
- performance development
- performance actualisation.

Each stage is characterised by key training objectives rather than on a timescale. Here, the content of training sessions can be devised specifically to achieve given objectives. While ideally, the longer this process takes the more opportunity there is to establish stable skills and abilities, the model itself can be adapted to the unique situation facing us. For example the above model has been utilised by the author as a complete long-term athlete-development model (Future Champions) a six-year development cycle, a four-year quadrennial cycle and a three-year performance cycle.

This model can be likened to a typical education model, where an overall curriculum of development is first identified, based upon a clear picture of the physical skills and competencies required of the graduating athlete. This curriculum then outlines the overall journey from entry into the programme to graduation from the programme, and is designed to address all aspects that have the potential to impact upon athletic performance. Details of the key objectives of each stage are shown in Figures 31.1–31.4.

### *Athletic foundation*

This stage is based around the establishment of primary movement capacities that ultimately underpin effective performance, and the start of an accumulation of skill development which is essential to long-term performance. Focus at this time is on the establishment of fundamental standards of performance across the key critical capacities of mobility, stability and locomotion. Indeed, it is highly unlikely at this time that perfect performance on any of these patterns will be achieved. Instead, what is important is that baseline competencies need to be established,[8] without which there will always be a potential for breakdown later on in the athlete's development.

A key factor at this point is that the programme should be based around qualitative assessments, rather than quantitative assessments. For example the quality of an athlete's sprint needs to be assessed, rather than simply how fast they run. This places the emphasis on the attainment of a quality movement pattern, rather than on the attainment of performance which could be achieved despite an ineffective movement pattern, and which could limit performance moving forward. In this way, the programme goals will be process in nature, rather than performance goals, focussing on quality rather than quantity. This reinforces the fact that the critical aim at this stage is to ensure that all athletes have a baseline of fundamental movement competence, which will allow them to undertake more advanced training at a later age.

Unlike the LTAD model, the unique feature of the current model is that there is no fixed time duration or entry point. It is highly likely that the time spent in this phase of development will be highly individual. Some athletes will be able to demonstrate competency of the key components of the stage relatively rapidly, while for others it may take considerable time in order for these capacities to reach a level of competency-appropriate development to the next stage. Quite often with high-level athletes, specific capacities will often mask issues with fundamental capacities, and it is important that these are identified and addressed as soon as possible. So regardless of the situation, it is important that the athlete is able to demonstrate fundamental competencies before they are deemed able to progress to higher levels of training.

One of the key focuses at this stage of development is on the development of effective movement. Cook points out that normal motion does not guarantee normal movement; movement also requires motor control, which includes stability, balance, postural control, coordination and perception.[3] In this way, while mobility and stability will be a key focus, these must be trained and assessed as they relate to movement capacities and not as they relate to individual muscles or static postures.

What is important is that preparation takes precedence over performance, and that planning is built around the accumulation of training, rather than on preparation for competition. This also has beneficial effects on reducing the potential for injury. Key aspects of this phase are shown in Figure 31.1.

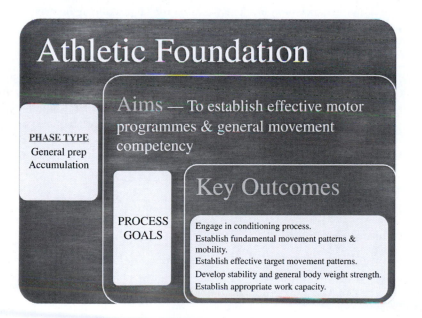

*Figure 31.1* Key aspects of athletic foundation

## Athletic development

All athletes entering this stage should now have fundamental movement and locomotor competencies. The aim at this stage is to develop these competencies and start to develop quantitative levels of performance onto these fundamental competencies. For example, in the athletic foundation stage, athletes will have demonstrated the capacities for squatting, lunging, etc. In this stage, low levels of load can start to be progressively placed on these movements, but with no compromise on technique. Indeed, resistance training for the youth athlete needs to be thought of as the development of movement under loads. This emphasises the fact that, as the athlete progresses through the programme, the development and preservation of effective movement patterns should be at the forefront of the coaches' thinking. Development of locomotor capacities should also progress to reflect more open and sport-generic situations.

Similar to the athletic foundation phase, the athletic development phase is also an accumulation phase, but with an emphasis on progressively developing the skills established in the previous phase. Here, the aim must be the establishment and development of sound fundamental capacities and sport-generic skills, and the introduction of training-generic skills (e.g. weight training techniques, plyometric techniques) that will allow for the maximisation of performance in the later stages. However, as an athlete at this stage has a greater training age than in the athletic foundation stage, more manipulation of the programme needs to be carried out to allow for a greater degree of variation in the means and methods utilised and in the intensity and volume of work allocated.

Critical throughout this phase, and indeed to all subsequent phases, is that, while the focus of training will shift to higher capacities, fundamental capacities are maintained. Young athletes will often go through growth spurts, and capacities such as mobility, stability and coordination can be negatively affected. Thus, this development must never be seen as linear; instead, an athlete will show phases of progression and also possible regression. The emphasis on the maintenance of competency is also crucial in reducing injury risks through the development process.

Processes must therefore be in place to ensure the maintenance of the quality of movements and capacities initially established. As a consequence, qualitative assessment methods must continue to be in place throughout this period, and ideally should take precedence over the quantitative methods that start to be introduced at this time. However, it is often useful to provide target scores for athletes to achieve towards the later stages of this phase to provide feedback to the athletes on their progress to date and on the standards required for them to move to the next stage of development. Scores can include speed scores, jump scores and strength-based scores. Coaches should be encouraged to integrate information from these systems to get a true evaluation of the athlete's capacities.

Key aspects of this phase are shown in Figure 31.2.

## Performance development

As the name of this phase suggests, focus now shifts from an establishment of basic athletic qualities, to the transference of these qualities into enhanced athletic performance, but whilst also continuing to emphasise the overall accumulation of training. This requires a shift from the *sport-generic* viewpoint to *sport-specific* viewpoint, and it is likely that athletes at this stage will be specialising in one or maybe two sports.

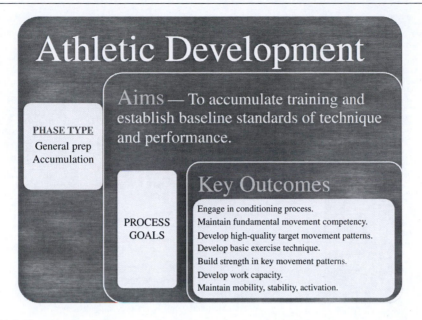

Figure 31.2 Key aspects of athletic development

Training objectives will therefore need to become more specific and relate to the key rate-limiting factors identified for each sport. For example rugby players will need to develop far greater muscle mass than football (soccer) players, and thus, at this stage, minimum performance standards can be set that relate to specific sports or specific sports groupings. For example targets can be set in exercises such as the squat that reflect the importance of strength to sports groupings, and these will vary among strength sports (throwing, weight-lifting, etc.), collision sports (rugby, American football, etc.), team sports (football, handball, etc.) and court sports (tennis, badminton, etc.). It is recommended that a range of tests be utilised that assess the fitness parameters required in sports or sport groupings, with appropriate targets set in each.

Similarly, more formally periodised programmes will start to be introduced, with focus starting to be paid to the level of athletic performance achieved. In this way, key competitions can be targeted where athletes will be able to test their levels of prowess and develop their abilities to peak and compete at higher levels. In essence, this phase is both an accumulation and a trans-mutational phase, where the generic capacities developed in the previous two stages start to be translated directly into enhanced performance, but while still developing key capacities that will ultimately determine the performance levels reached. This accumulation of training still needs to be emphasised, as often an athlete's physical capacities remain well short of that required at the highest levels of sport.

### Performance actualisation

Here, the focus shifts to maximising athletic performance. As an athlete should have established a large training history, then they will require the use of more advanced periodised models, planned around the maximisation of performance at key competitions. However, the

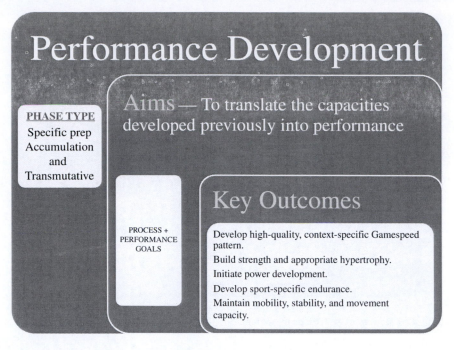

*Figure 31.3* Key aspects of performance development

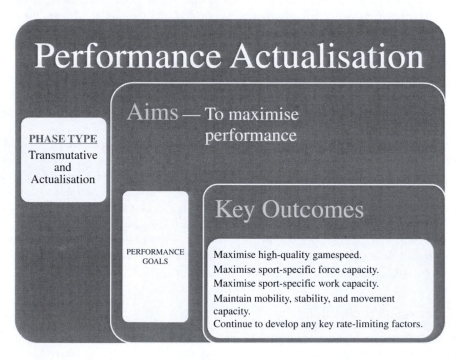

*Figure 31.4* Key aspects of performance actualization

accumulation of training and competencies in the previous stages ensures that the athlete is adequately prepared for this work. This phase will utilise a wider range of means and methods, and with the use of a greater degree of variation within the programme itself. However, while performance will be a focus, it is highly likely in a number of sports that an athlete may be some way from the elite level. This will require the identification of key strengths and weaknesses and the use of development programmes to ensure that the athlete is able to address these and maximise the likelihood of achieving optimal performance. Therefore, the start of the performance actualisation programme needs to reflect the type of sport played and the typical ages at which an athlete ultimately reaches their peaks. Indeed, this may also vary between sports, and even within sports, as certain positions may require the development of different physical capacities that will peak at different times. For example prop forwards in rugby may need more time in the performance-development stage, to develop the physical capacities to compete at elite level, than outside halves.

## Summary

Whether the focus of youth training is on performance or on the development of a healthy lifestyle, there is no doubt that the appropriate development of key physical capacities at a young age can significantly enhance the success of these aims. Whilst in the past, the physical training of young athletes has been the subject of much debate, it seems logical that the effective preparation of the youth athlete, via the application of appropriate physical training interventions, is crucial. As with any skills, physical development should entail a staged progression from general physical capacities through to sports performance. To achieve this, an appropriate long-term athlete-development model provides a structure around which to build an effective programme.

While the LTAD model has been universally accepted and can be applied in a range of situations wherein athletes' progress can be controlled from start to finish, it may not be easy for a coach to apply it in a situation where they only have athletes for a short period of time. Similarly, the fact that it is based around windows of opportunity and critical periods of physical development makes it difficult to apply for coaches working outside of these windows.

The objectives-based system outlined here provides a structure around which to instigate a long-term athlete development programme within a coach's own sphere of influence. This flexibility allows it to be applied to a wider range of situations, and, being objective-led, allows it to be modified to fit into the logistical constraints facing the coach. What is crucial is that progression through the system is based on competency rather than time, and athletes, regardless of their athletic prowess, have to demonstrate fundamental competency before advancing to the higher stages of training. This will ultimately ensure that they have all of the key physical competencies required to maximise performance and to reduce the risk of injury throughout the process.

## Notes

1 Wolstencroft, E. (Ed.). (2002). *Talent identification and development: An academic review.* Edinburgh: Sportscotland.
2 Bloom, B. (1985). *Developing talent in young people.* New York: Ballantine Books.
3 Cook, G. (2010). *Movement: Functional movement systems: Screening assessment and corrective strategies.* Aptos, CA: On Target Publications.

4  Lloyd, R. S., & Oliver, J. L. (2012). The youth physical development model: A new approach to long-term athletic development. *Strength and Conditioning Journal, 34*(3), 61–72.

5  Sportscotland. (2004). *Player improvement: A consultancy paper.* Edinburgh: SportScotland.

6  Balyi, I., & Hamilton, A. (2000). A key to success – long-term athlete development. *Sport Coach, 23*, 10–32.

7  Faigenbaum, A. D., Kraemer, W. J., Blimkie, C.J.R, Jeffreys, I., Micheli, L. J., Nitka, M., & Rowland, T. W. (2009). Youth resistance training: Updated position statement paper from the National Strength and Conditioning Association. *Journal of Strength and Conditioning Research, 23*(5), S60-S79.

8  Balyi, I. (2001). Sport system building and long term athlete development in British Columbia Canada. SportsMed BC. Retrieved from http://iceskatingresources.org/sportssystemdevelopment.pdf

9  Balyi, I. (2002). Long-term athlete development, the systems and solutions. *Faster Higher Stronger, 1*, 6–9.

10  Bailey, R. P., Collins, D., Ford, P. A., MacNamara, A., Pearce, G., & Toms, M. (2010). *Participant development in sport: An academic literature review.* Leeds, UK: Sports Coach UK.

11  Jeffreys, I. (2011). A task based approach to developing reactive agility. *Strength and Conditioning Journal, 33*(4), 52–59.

12  Ford, P., De Ste Croix, M., Lloyd, R., Meyers, R., Moosavi, M., Oliver., Till, K., & Williams, C. (2011). The long term athlete development model, physiological evidence and application. *Journal of Sport Sciences, 29*(4), 389–402.

13  Barnett, L. M., van Beurden, E., Morgan, P. J., Brooks, L. O., AvigdoeZask, A., and Beard, J. R. (2009). Six year follow up of students who participated in a school based physical activity intervention. A longitudinal cohort study. *International Journal of Behavioural Nutrition and Physical Activity, 6*(48), 1–8.

14  Graf, C., Koch., B., Falkowski, G., Jouck, S., Christ, H., Staudenmaier, K., et al. (2005). Effects of a school based intervention on BMI and motor abilities in childhood. *Journal of Sport Science and Medicine, 4*(3), 291–299.

15  Philippaerts, R. M., Vaeyens, R., Janssens, M., Van Renterghem, B., Matthys, D., Craen, R., Bourgois, J., et al. (2006). The relationship between peak height velocity and physical performance in youth soccer players. *Journal of Sports Science, 24*(3), 221–30.

16  Kotzamanidis, C. (2003). The effect of sprint training on running performance and vertical jump in preadolescent boys. *Journal of Human Movement Studies, 44*, 225–240.

17  Kotzamanidis, C., Chatzopoulos, D., Michailidis, C., Papaiakovou, G., & Patikas, D. (2005). The effect of a combined high-intensity strength and speed training programme on the running and jumping ability of soccer players. *Journal of Strength and Conditioning Research, 19*(2), 369–75.

18  Rowland, T. (2005). *Children's exercise physiology* (2nd ed.). Champaign, IL: Human Kinetics.

19  Ozmun, J., Mikesky, A., & Surburg, P. (1994). Neuromuscular adaptations following prepubescent strength training. *Medicine & Science in Sports & Exercise, 26*, 510–514..

20  Ramsay, J., Blimkie, C., Smith, K., Garner, S., Macdougall, J., & Sale, D. (1990). Strength training effects in prepubescent boys. *Medicine & Science in Sports & Exercise, 22*, 605–614.

21  Shephard, R. J. (1992). Effectiveness of training programmes for prepubescent children. *Sports Medicine, 13*(3), 194–213.

22  Cook, G. (2003). *Athletic body in balance.* Champaign IL: Human Kinetics.

23  Jeffreys, I. (2006). Motor learning: Applications for agility, Part 1. *Strength & Conditioning Journal, 28*(5), 72–76.

24  Jeffreys, I. (2008). Movement training for field sports: Soccer. *Strength & Conditioning Journal, 30*(4), 19–27.

25  Jeffreys, I. (2010). Gamespeed: *Movement training for superior sports performance.* Monterey, CA: Coaches Choice.

# Chapter 32

# The female athlete

*N. Travis Triplett and Margaret Stone*

## Introduction

It is well known that there are physical differences between the sexes, but there are existing questions regarding how these differences impact training and the risk of injury. It is therefore natural for us to consider specific variations that may need to be addressed when coaching the female athlete compared to coaching the male athlete. It is the intent of this chapter to address some of the specific challenges facing the female athlete, including training considerations, strength development and biomechanical and hormonal differences.

## Training considerations

In general, there are very few differences between males and females when structuring the training program. However, some differences do exist and may possibly have an impact on an athlete's potential for injury or maladaptation to the training. For example many female athletes enter a sport less conditioned than their male counterparts, and therefore a longer general preparation phase may be necessary to fully prepare the female athlete for future blocks of training.[15] Failure to address readiness for more advanced blocks of training could result in unplanned overreaching or overtraining, which would be detrimental to performance. An assessment of readiness, of course, must be carried out on an individual basis. Several other training considerations have been noted regarding the female athlete including:[15]

- Females vary in levels of absolute strength but the range is between 40 and 60 per cent of the strength levels of males in the upper body and 70–85 per cent of the strength levels of males in the lower body;
- The rate of force development (RFD) is lower in the average female than in the average male;
- Females generate less power absolutely, and there is some evidence indicating less power per unit of volume of muscle.

### Strength levels

Much of the strength difference between males and females is related to the distribution of muscle mass around the body.[7,16] For example males have more muscle mass in the upper body than females, irrespective of body size. The distribution of lower body muscle mass is more similar between the sexes. Thus, the ratio of strength to lean body mass is a more meaningful measure to use when comparing strength levels between males and females. Using these criteria, women are about equal to men in strength, especially in the lower body, with much smaller (but still existent) differences between strength levels in the upper body. When muscle tissue samples are extracted and force capabilities measured, determining whether the muscle is from a male or female is not possible without genetic analysis. Thus, the amount of muscle mass and how it is distributed on the body are the primary determinants of strength, and resistance training can enhance this.

### Rate of force development (RFD) and power

The ability to reach peak force quickly (RFD) and produce high levels of power is largely determined by neural factors.[14] Power is defined as the ability to perform work (produce force) in a short amount of time, so the neural factors relate more to the time component of power. Strength is directly related to force production and therefore the work component of power. Power outputs in females are thus influenced by their lower RFD and strength.

### Strength and muscle development

Planning a resistance training program to improve strength levels in a female is not really different from doing the same in a male. The basic principles of exercise choice (multi-joint, large-muscle group), loading (80 per cent 1RM or higher) and repetitions (8 or fewer), and training frequency (2–3 times per week) apply. However, to optimize strength development, it may be necessary to emphasize muscle development at some point in the training year, especially in the upper body, since females have much smaller amounts of muscle.

Although strength gains can be made at any time, maximizing strength levels will require some increases in muscle mass, especially as strength levels begin to plateau after longer-term training. Many females do not wish to have significant levels of muscle hypertrophy, which is generally not possible anyway without supplementing with anabolic substances, but increasing muscle mass can result in decreases in per cent of body fat, as well as increases in resting metabolism, both positive factors for overall body-weight control and performance.[5]

> The basic principles of exercise choice, loading, repetitions and training frequency are similar between males and females when planning a programme to focus on strength.

## Biomechanical considerations

Strength levels and movement mechanics are related because muscle weaknesses around a joint can alter proper movement patterns. One of the best examples is the knee position during squatting movements. Females have a much higher prevalence of knee valgus ('knock knees') when squatting, which reduces force production and results in greater potential for knee ligament injury. The most commonly injured knee ligament associated with female athletes is the anterior cruciate ligament (ACL), and prevalence in females ranges from 2–10 times that in males participating in the same sport (e.g. basketball, soccer).[12]

Although contact can be a factor, most female ACL injuries occur in non-contact situations – activities such as cutting, turning, pivoting and deceleration movements.[13] Furthermore, it is not uncommon for multiple injuries to happen to the structure of the knee, including the anterior cruciate and medial collateral ligaments, and lateral meniscus. These injuries are often referred to as the 'unhappy triad'.

There have been several proposed reasons for the increase in injury potential of the female athlete. These reasons include the different ratio of hip width to knee position, joint laxity issues, and the ACL thickness.[13] These issues seem to have been somewhat discounted, and more likely causes include:

- Rate of force development, as previously mentioned, where females take longer to develop the same relative force level as their male counterparts;
- Hamstring activation deficits which result in quadriceps-dominant knee function with a greater anterior translation;
- Greater ankle dorsiflexion, combined with valgus position of the knees and external rotation of the hip.

## Body positioning

These factors and the possibility that some female athletes do not position themselves the same as their male counterparts during single-leg movements such as cutting, or while squatting, may contribute to the potential for increase in the number of ACL injuries. However, the major contributing factor appears to be the lack of strength, both absolute and relative, due to the lower relative training status of the female athlete in comparison with her male counterpart.[4] Teaching the female athlete how to land properly and position the knee properly in cutting and turning movement would be beneficial. While strength training should occur prior to or concurrent with explosive training, since muscle weaknesses can impact technique, there are some basic technique points that can be emphasized, such as landing with the shoulders in line with the knees so the centre of gravity does not end up too far forward of the body. Change of direction involves a combination of deceleration and acceleration, so teaching the optimal amount of body lean (e.g. more with a smaller turning radius) and foot contact (e.g. cutting on a full foot) can also help to minimize injury risk separately from strength levels.[11]

## Hormonal considerations and the female athlete triad

Men have levels of testosterone, a hormone responsible for influencing strength and size gains, that are on average 10 times those of females.[17] Therefore, the fear many female athletes have of developing larger muscles is not justified because of the lower levels of testosterone. In addition, genetics, nutrition and program design also have a role in the amount of muscle mass that can be developed. The male's bigger skeleton also supports more lean body mass. Females have other hormonal considerations apart from males, primarily the menstrual cycle and the related hormones which can influence performance, but also musculoskeletal development and maintenance.

## The menstrual cycle

During a normal menstrual cycle, estrogen, progesterone and some other hormones (FSH, LH) fluctuate in a set pattern over the course of approximately 28 days. While these fluctuations are not a strong influence, both aerobic and anaerobic performance has been shown to vary at times throughout the normal menstrual cycle. For example some studies have shown both detrimental and enhanced performances during various phases of the menstrual cycle.[10] Constructing a training program with regard to the menstrual cycle of an athlete must be approached on an individual basis and may prove to be too labour-intensive. Although possible, the observation and subsequent recording of performances during a training phase and/or block of training to determine adaptations to the training programme, is essential if maximizing the athlete's performance in relation to the phases of the menstrual cycle is to be achieved. Of greater importance may be simply the monitoring of the athlete for disturbances in the menstrual cycle, which can have negative implications for healthy body weight, bone density, overall responses to training and injury potential, which will ultimately impact athletic performance.

## The female athlete triad

The female athlete triad describes a set of conditions that, when combined, predispose female athletes especially to greater risk of illness and injury. The female athlete triad is composed of three elements: disordered eating (including anorexia nervosa and bulimia nervosa), osteoporosis (loss of bone density) and amenorrhea (lack of menstrual cycle).[1,3] Bringing these elements together is heavy training (high volumes and/or intensities). This triad is often represented by the figure below:

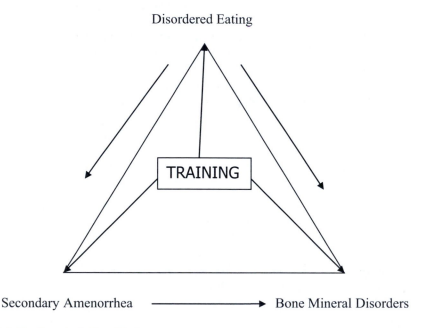

*Figure 32.1* The Female Athlete Triad

Heavy training and disordered eating can result in per cent body fat that is too low to be healthy, as well as amenorrhea. Heavy training, disordered eating and amenorrhea can result in osteoporosis. It is possible for an athlete to have only one or two of the triad elements, but having all three is especially detrimental to health and performance.

***Disordered eating:*** There is a range of conditions that can be classified under the broader term of disordered eating. An athlete may simply not get enough calories or nutrients to support the training being performed. More serious conditions such as anorexia nervosa or bulimia nervosa also can be classified as disordered eating.

Anorexia nervosa is an eating disorder that is identified by an athlete losing more weight than is considered healthy for their age and height. It is very commonly found in focused high achievers, and excessive exercise is often used as the vehicle for weight loss, as well as the use of laxatives or vomiting. Bulimia nervosa is an illness in which an athlete binges on food or has regular episodes of overeating and feels a loss of control. The person then uses different methods, such as vomiting or abusing laxatives, to prevent weight gain.

While many individuals with these conditions tend to show outward physical effects of the disease, some types of athletes may appear to have an eating disorder when none is present. These athletes include those in endurance sports, or diving and gymnastics, who are often extremely lean due to the training. Any type of athlete is at risk of using these methods as a means of weight management, although these conditions are more common in sports with body weight categories or where being very lean is advantageous. Nonetheless, any level of disordered eating can result in performance decrements or increased injuries, especially muscle cramping or other dehydration-related or electrolyte-deficit problems.[18]

***Amenorrhea:*** By definition, amenorrhea is the absence of menstrual periods. Amenorrhea or oligomenorrhea (irregular menstrual cycle) have detrimental effects, primarily on bone mineral density, which could elevate the incidence of stress fractures.[6] Primary amenorrhea is the failure of the onset of menses by the age of 16. Secondary amenorrhea is more common and refers to either the temporary or permanent cessation of menstrual periods in an athlete who has menstruated normally in the past. Many female athletes miss a period occasionally but amenorrhea is said to occur if an athlete misses three or more periods in a row.[6]

Key causes of these phenomena in athletes are training factors, including training at an early age, running volume, frequency, intensity and duration of training, although the presence of eating disorders is also a contributing factor. These training factors need to be adjusted according to the individual circumstances of the athlete, and can be anywhere for an extended period of time away from training completely, to minor adjustments in volume, intensity and/or frequency of training.[6]

***Osteoporosis:*** The word osteoporosis literally means 'porous bones'. It occurs when bones lose an excessive amount of their protein (collagen) and mineral content, particularly calcium.[2] As previously mentioned, all of the other components of the female athlete triad contribute to the development of osteoporosis. Over time, bone mass and therefore bone strength is decreased. Osteoporosis related to amenorrhea, eating disorders and heavy training in a young athlete is particularly bad because bone takes a long time to rebuild, and having a low bone density while young results in severe bone problems with aging. Osteoporosis can lead to stress fractures and shin splints and, if left unattended, a full fracture. In such cases the type, volume and intensity of training may need to be adjusted to address the injury potential, in addition to dietary adjustments to ensure that bone has the materials it needs to rebuild. This is discussed in more detail in chapter 16.

> The female athlete triad describes a set of conditions that, when combined, predispose female athletes especially to greater risk of illness and injury.

## Pregnancy and training

While low-to-moderate intensity and duration aerobic exercise has been recommended during pregnancy for many years, only recently has engaging in strength training during pregnancy become more common. Aside from any adjustments to exercise choice or technique that are necessary as the shape of the body changes, there are a few important concepts that are critical in maintaining a safe environment in which to strength train:[9]

- Avoid supine exercises later in pregnancy (>4th month) because of the pressure the uterus exerts on the blood vessels returning to the heart; upright or inclined exercise are acceptable;
- Avoid heavy resistances or ballistic movements later in pregnancy because of the increases in joint laxity throughout pregnancy;
- Avoid isometric movements or the Valsalva manoeuvre because of the accompanying elevations in blood pressure.

There are no specific recommendations for returning to exercise post-partum. since the time to return to exercise is highly dependent on the number of complications during the pregnancy and during labour and delivery. The general recommendation is that exercise can be resumed after vaginal bleeding has stopped and when the physician clears the individual to resume normal activity, which can take up to 10 weeks post-partum.[8]

## Summary

These sex differences highlight the importance of including strength and power training in the training regimen of female athletes, as well as monitoring the female athlete for factors that contribute to the female athlete triad. Focusing on strength and power development will improve performance and should contribute to reducing injury risk. The key to progress and success in resistance training is a well-planned and periodised program which manipulates volume and intensity over a specific time to enhance muscle tissue development, strength and power.

## Notes

1  Barrack, M. T., Ackerman, K. E., & Gibbs, J. C. (2013). Update on the female athlete triad. *Curr Rev Musculoskelet Med, 6*(2), 195–204.
2  Chen Y. T., Tenforde, A. S. & Fredericson, M. (2013). Update on stress fractures in female athletes: Epidemiology, treatment, and prevention. *Curr Rev Musculoskelet Med, 6*(2), 173–81.

3  Gibbs, J. C., Williams, N. I., & De Souza, M. J. (2013). Prevalence of individual and combined components of the female athlete triad. *Med Sci Sports Exerc, 45*(5), 985–96.

4  Haines, T. L., McBride, J. M., Triplett, N. T., Skinner, J. W., Fairbrother, K. R., & Kirby, T. J. (2011). A comparison of men's and women's strength to body mass ratio and varus/valgus knee angle during jump landings. *J Sports Sci, 29*(13), 1435–42.

5  Lemmer, J. T., Ivey, F. M., Ryan, A. S., Martel, G. F., Hurlbut, D. E., Metter, J. E., . . . Hurley, B. F. (2001). Effect of strength training on resting metabolic rate and physical activity: Age and gender comparisons. *Med Sci Sports Exerc, 33*(4), 532–41.

6  Manore, M. M., Kam, L. C., & Loucks, A. B. (2007). The female athlete triad: Components, nutrition issues, and health consequences. *J Sports Sci, 25*, 61–71.

7  Miller, A. E., MacDougall, J. D., Tarnopolsky, M. A., & Sale, D. G. (1993). Gender differences in strength and muscle fiber characteristics. *Eur J Appl Physiol Occup Physiol, 66*(3), 254–62.

8  Mottola, M. F., & Wolfe, L. A. (2000). The pregnant athlete. In B. Drinkwater (Ed.), *Women in sport* (pp. 194–207). Oxford, UK: Blackwell Science.

9  O'Connor, P. J., Poudevigne, M. S., Cress, M. E., Motl, R. W., & Clapp, J. F. (2011). Safety and efficacy of supervised strength training adopted in pregnancy. *J Phys Act Health, 8*(3), 309–20.

10  Oosthuyse, T., & Bosch, A. N. (2010). The effect of menstrual cycle on exercise metabolism: Implications for exercise performance in eumenorrhoeic women. *Sports Med, 40*(3), 207–27.

11  Plisk, S. S. (2008). Speed, agility, and speed-endurance development. In T.R. Baechle & R.W. Earle (Eds.), *Essentials of strength training and conditioning* (3rd ed.) (pp. 457–485). Champaign, IL: Human Kinetics.

12  Renstrom, P., Ljungqvist, A., Arendt, E., Beynnon, B., Fukubayashi, T., Garrett, W., . . . Engebretsen, L. (2008). Non-contact ACL injuries in female athletes: An International Olympic Committee current concepts statement. *British J Sports Med, 42*(6), 394–412.

13  Russell, K. A., Palmieri, R. M., Zinder, S. M., & Ingersoll, C. D. (2006). Sex differences in valgus knee angle during a single-leg drop jump. *J Athl Train, 41*(2), 166–71.

14  Ryushi, T., Hakkinen, K., Kauhanen, H., & Komi, P. V. (1988). Muscle fiber characteristics, muscle cross-sectional area and force production in strength athletes and physically active males and females. *Scand J Sports Sci, 10*(1), 7–15.

15  Stone, M. H., Stone, M. E., & Sands, W. A. (2007). Physical and physiological adaptations to resistance training. In M. R. Stone, M. Stone, & W. Sands (Eds.), *Principles and practice of resistance training* (pp. 211–13). Champaign, IL: Human Kinetics.

16  Vanderburgh, P. M., Kusano, M., Sharp, M., & Nindl, B. (1997). Gender differences in muscular strength: An allometric model approach. *Biomed Sci Instrum, 33*, 100–05.

17  Viru, A., & Viru, M. (2005). Resistance exercise and testosterone. In W. J. Kraemer (Ed.), *The endocrine system in sports and exercise* (pp. 319–338). Oxford, UK: Blackwell Science.

18  Zach, K. N., Smith-Machin, A. L., & Hoch, A. Z. (2011). Advances in management of the female athlete triad and eating disorders. *Clin Sports Med, 30*(3), 551–73.

Chapter 33

# The travelling athlete

*Shona Halson and Emidio Pacecca*

## Introduction

Travel is an inherent part of professional sport. In the 2013–14 season, the average team in North America's NHL travelled 41,390 miles (66,611km). This is the equivalent of travelling around the world more than 11 times. Tennis players are arguably the most travelled athletes, with players reported to have travelled 48,237 miles (77,600km) in a two-month period. Travel may take the form of long-haul international flights, shorter domestic flights or even hours spent on buses, trains or in cars.

As many people can attest, travelling is tiring, and so travel medicine and jet lag management are important to minimise the detrimental effects of travel, to optimise recovery and to maintain athletic performance.

This chapter discusses the effect travel has on athletic performance and illness and injury risk. It provides the basis for practical recommendations for athletes, coaches and performance support personnel that can be applied across a variety of sports.

## Jet lag and travel fatigue

Jet lag can be of particular concern to the elite athlete, so identifying practical and effective means of managing the resultant fatigue and potential performance decrements are extremely important.

Jet lag is described as a circadian desynchrony, or a mismatch between the timing of the internal body clock and the external environment.[1] There are a number of symptoms that are manifested by this desynchrony, including:

- fatigue and general tiredness
- sleep disruption
- loss of concentration
- loss of motivation
- gastrointestinal distress
- loss of appetite
- headaches
- general malaise.[2]

Travel fatigue is described as a more complex summation of physiologic, psychological and environmental factors that accrue during an individual trip and which accumulate over the course of a season,[3] The symptoms of travel fatigue may be persistent fatigue, recurrent illness, changes in behaviour or mood and a loss of motivation.[3] Therefore, it is important to manage jet lag and travel fatigue across a season. Importantly, travel fatigue results not simply from air travel, but also from travel in buses and cars and time spent at the airport (departure, stopovers and arrival).

The consequences of jet lag and travel fatigue may depend on a number of factors, including direction of travel, number of time zones crossed, frequency of travel and length of season.[3] Research has demonstrated that eastward travel may result in greater symptoms of jet lag than westward travel,[2] This is due to the fact that the body clock's rhythm is not exactly 24 hours in duration but closer to 25–26 hours.[2] Therefore, it appears to be easier to adapt to changes that lengthen the day, rather than shorten it.

## Effects of jet lag on performance

Given the above-mentioned symptoms of jet lag, it is not surprising that research has identified performance decrements associated with long-haul travel. The effect that jet lag may have on performance will depend on a number of factors. These include not only the previously mentioned number of time zones crossed and direction of travel, but also the type of activity performed and the time of day for optimal performance of that type of exercise.[4] Individual responses will likely also determine severity of performance decrements as well as the level of concentration and complex coordination required for optimal performance in specific sports.[4]

## Planning the travel

There are many variables that influence travel, and optimisation of such variables can reduce the physiological and psychological costs of travel. These elements encompass the time periods before, during and following travel and can be seen below. In order to formulate the best plan for dealing with the effects of travel, a number of practical suggestions should be followed.

### Pre-departure adjustment

Adapting to the new time zone before travel can be one of the best ways to minimise jet lag, but it is also one of the most difficult methods to achieve successfully. Pre-adjustment generally involves either light exposure or light avoidance (depending on direction of travel), ingestion of melatonin and altering eating and sleeping times. Adjustments of approximately one hour/day can be achieved by timing light exposure to either phase-advance or phase-delay the body clock. To achieve a phase delay, athletes should seek light exposure in the early evening hours (according to home time) and avoid exposure in the second half of the night and early morning. To phase advance, light exposure should be in the late evening or early morning (according to home time).[2]

Adjusting as much as possible to the new time zone can be effective; however, a large amount of time and commitment are required, and in our experience, pre-adjusting sleep-wake cycles of athletes may simply induce fatigue. Moreover, as light exposure is the most critical factor in this process, should the athlete be exposed to light at the incorrect time during pre-adjustment, then any possible benefits are negated. Therefore, this strategy is very difficult to perform from a practical perspective, particularly in athletes where training times may be set (especially those that compete in sports like swimming and rowing that have early starts). Finally, it is advisable to avoid fatigue as much as possible before departure, focusing instead on optimising sleep pre-departure.

### During travel

There are several modifiable elements to acknowledge when travelling. By optimising nutritional input and minimising musculoskeletal tightness, we can reduce the detrimental effects of travel. The main elements to consider are listed below.

### Nutrition and diet (meal timing, hydration)

Dehydration is a pertinent issue with long-haul flights due to the changes in cabin air pressure and air quality. Increased carbon dioxide concentration, increased ventilation rate, and a low relative humidity (10–20 per cent) with a subsequent reduction in ambient moisture have been demonstrated in commercial flights.[5] This results in an increased rate of evaporation of fluid from the upper respiratory tract. In combination with the increased ventilation rate, the increased fluid loss associated with evaporation needs to be replaced to prevent dehydration. It is advised that an 80kg male consume 100–150ml per hour. This can be in the form of water, energy drinks, fruit juice, soft drinks and hot drinks. Whilst it is preferable to use water as the main source of fluids, variety is also important to ensure adequate intake. Juices and sports drinks can contain high levels of sugar and are energy dense. Caffeinated drinks can affect sleep, so it is advised that this is taken into consideration in terms of timing. If, for example, it is late evening at the destination, having a coffee on the flight has the potential to inhibit sleep on the plane and can therefore delay the adjustment to local time.

### Strategies to prevent musculoskeletal tightness and minimise risk of thromboembolic events

Vascular thromboembolic events (VTE) are considered one of the major health problems that can be associated with flying.[6] Deep vein thrombosis (DVT) and pulmonary embolisms (PE) are the two most common VTEs. A number of risk factors for VTE relating to travel have been identified, including: the length of travel (2.3-fold risk with flights over 6 hours), age of 40 years or older, women who use oral contraceptive drugs, lower-limb varicose veins, obesity (BMI> 30) and genetic thrombophilia.[6]

Methods to prevent VTE during flights include: avoiding dehydration, improving sitting position (allowing for legs movement/exercises), activity on the aircraft, such as walking, and preventing venous blood stasis by wearing graduated compression stockings (GCS).[6] Pharmacological prophylaxis may be required in high-risk travellers.

Frequent movement of the ankles and knees assists in circulation to the lower limb. For long-haul travel we recommend that the athletes perform 5–10 mins of walking and stretching every 1–2 hours whilst awake. This reduces the risk of VTE and minimises post-travel tightness and stiffness.

Muscle/nerve stimulation devices have been suggested to increase venous velocity and blood flow in deep veins. Whilst no studies have demonstrated the positive effects on performance or reduction in VTE risk, any changes in blood flow may be of benefit.

Graduated compression stockings (GCS) have been shown to reduce the risk of VTE by almost 90 per cent in standard risk patients.[6] While many athletes like to wear full-leg compression tights, we recommend wearing properly fitted, below-knee GCS, providing 15–30mmHg of pressure at the ankle. It is possible that the full-leg compression tights that finish at the ankle may act as a tourniquet around the ankle if not fitted properly and thus may increase venous pooling.

> Compression garments can reduce the risk of DVT and reduce the swelling that can occur in the lower leg during travel.

## Upon arrival

In order to transition effectively into the time zone there are several considerations to be addressed, specifically regarding light exposure, sleep hygiene and nutrition.

### Light exposure or avoidance

Light is one of the most powerful means of altering circadian rhythms,[1] and strategic exposure to or avoidance of light at specific times can help speed resynchronisation of the body clock. A number of websites as well as smartphone applications are available to assist with making calculations regarding specific timing of light exposure or avoidance. Figure 33.1 is an example of a light-avoiding and light-seeking schedule for travel from Barcelona to Rio de Janeiro.

> Light exposure is one of the best ways to speed adaptation to the new time zone.

Artificial light can be particularly effective and seasonal affective disorder light devices (wavelength of 450–480nm) at approximately 1,500 lux are often utilised. Further, when it is difficult to avoid natural sunlight, light-blocking glasses designed to block 80–98 per cent of light in the blue range are recommended.[3]

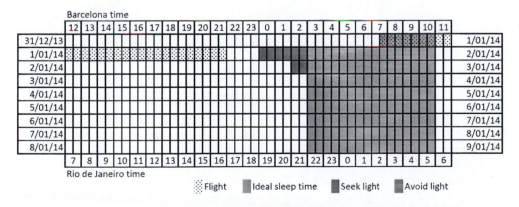

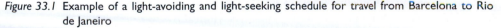

*Figure 33.1* Example of a light-avoiding and light-seeking schedule for travel from Barcelona to Rio de Janeiro

## Melatonin

Another powerful means of body clock adjustment is melatonin. Melatonin is a hormone which, when secreted endogenously, facilitates and reinforces sleep.[1] Exogenous melatonin influences the timing of the body clock and promotes sleepiness or sleep itself by providing a biological signal for night and day.[1] Melatonin aids phase advancement when taken in the evening (eastward travel) and phase delay when taken in the very late evening or morning (westward travel).[7]

A Cochrane Review from 2002[8] recommended that melatonin may be used in adults when travelling across five or more time zones and potentially when crossing as few as two. Doses of 0.5–5mg were similarly effective, though higher doses were more effective at inducing sleep. It is important that athletes seek medical advice before taking melatonin and that a WADA sanctioned product is taken to avoid an inadvertent positive doping test.

## Sleep hygiene

Sleep is an extremely important part of performance and recovery. It is essential that good sleep habits are maintained whilst travelling. Setting up an optimal sleep environment can ensure good sleep and assist in overcoming jet lag. The key points for an optimal sleep environment are:

- Darkness – ensure the windows are covered with block-out blinds. Eye masks are an alternative option.
- Noise – arrange a room where there is minimal outside noise (away from street traffic). Earplugs are also useful.
- Avoid stimulants such as caffeine in the hours prior to sleep, as well as excessive ingestion of fluid.
- Routine – perform a pre-sleep ritual to prepare your body for sleep. This may be as simple as reading a book for 10 mins and avoiding the use of computers and smart phones in the 30 minutes prior to sleep.

## Nutrition and hydration

Maintaining adequate dietary and fluid intake is important in minimising the detrimental effects of travel and ensuring a swift return to optimal performance levels. Challenges to this include:

- Reduced energy needs on transit days
- 'Downtime' with increased opportunity for 'boredom-eating'
- Altered training schedules and limited access to food (especially snacks)
- Different foods and language barriers
- Timing of training/competition and scheduling of meals.

Poor food choices whilst away from home can result in reduced energy levels, impair muscle repair and lead to muscle atrophy and strength decay, plus gains in body fat, compromised immunity and dehydration. Itineraries, changes in time zone, athlete appetite and accessibility to food can influence timing of meals whilst travelling.

*Table 33.1*  Practical recommendations for travel prior to, during travel and upon arrival

Practical Application
Key points for travel from Paris to Tokyo
(Flight time 12 hours West to East with +7-hour time change)

Prior to travelling:
- If possible, choose a departure time late afternoon/evening to arrive mid-afternoon in Tokyo.
- Prepare meal plan for flight.
- Purchase drinks once you have gone through security checks. You should be looking at drinking 2–3 litres during the 12-hour flight.

Flight: Departing Paris 18:00, arriving Tokyo 12:20 (+1):
- Put on compression socks.
- Change your watch forward 7 hours.
- Eat dinner shortly after take-off.
- Relax and try to go to sleep. Wear eye mask and earplugs if comfortable.
- After waking, walk around the cabin and perform some dynamic and static lower limb stretches for 5–10 mins. Stairs can be useful to allow a greater variety of stretches.
- Continue to walk and stretch for 5–10 mins every 1–2 hours for the remainder of the flight.
- Eat snacks until lunchtime.
- Continue snacking and hydrating for the remainder of the flight.

On arrival (14:20 local time):
- Exposure to sunlight is advised up until 6 p.m., so it is recommended to go for a walk or easy jog outside that afternoon. If there is access to a pool or beach, then some dynamic stretching and walking in the water is beneficial.
- Stay awake until 8 or 9 p.m.
- Continue to hydrate.
- Commence eating meals according to local time.

Following day:
- You may wake up early but try to stay in bed until daylight.
- Light exercise in the morning and afternoon.

As we have said, it is important to adjust to the new time zone as quickly as possible, and eating appropriate food types at appropriate times can assist with this. For example cereal for breakfast and a meal high in carbohydrates prior to sleeping can encourage a transition in time zone. Overall, it is important for the athlete to maintain sufficient nutritional input, so travelling with snacks is a useful idea. Cereal bars, fruit, sandwiches and nut mixes are good options, but care needs to be exercised to avoid boredom eating. Having a well-planned menu including snacks can help alleviate this issue.

Table 33.1 represents an example of advice for pre-travel, during travel and upon arrival.

## Medical considerations for travel

When travelling, there is an increased risk of infection due to a variety of issues including air quality on flights, fatigue and change of climate. There can be an increased risk of infection and exposure to diseases that may not be as prevalent as at home. Vaccinations are advisable prior to travelling. It is best to consult a doctor prior to departure to assess the individual risks for the athlete when travelling to specific countries. The current World Health Organisation (WHO) guidelines regarding vaccinations are as follows:

## Routine vaccination

• Diphtheria
• Hepatitis B
• Haemophilus influenza type b
• Human papillomavirus
• Seasonal influenza and influenza A (H1N1)
• Measles
• Mumps
• Pertussis
• Rubella
• Pneumococcal disease
• Poliomyelitis (Polio)
• Rotavirus
• Tuberculosis (TB)
• Tetanus
• Varicella.

## Selective use for travellers

• Cholera
• Hepatitis A
• Japanese encephalitis
• Meningococcal disease
• Rabies
• Tick-borne encephalitis
• Typhoid fever
• Yellow fever.

Prior to departing, it is important to have a concise history of athletes' past medical history, allergies and medication usage. It is also advisable to have next-of-kin details in case of medical emergency. Certain allergies may require the administration of an 'epipen' and a method of transporting and carrying the 'epipen' in proximity of the athlete.

Divulging relevant athlete medical history to coaches, team managers and fellow players is an ethical consideration. For example, if a player is diabetic or epileptic, it can be important that there is appropriate assistance provided in case of a seizure. Athletes are therefore encouraged to disclose such information in order to minimise risk of adverse reactions.

Adequate medical supplies should be prepared. Depending on location, it can be difficult to source certain supplies, so it is advised that doctors, therapists and trainers travel with a basic first aid kit comprising of disinfectant, plasters, scissors, bandages and paracetamol.

A sport-specific kit and equipment should be included. Table 33.2 below illustrates a list of basic stock and equipment. Additional sports-specific items should also be included, e.g. additional wound dressings for cycling.

Portable cryotherapy can vary from ice bags through to compression/cryotherapy units. These are particularly important in the acute management of injuries.

Medical practitioners travelling with athletes/teams need to consider travelling with medication. As different countries can have medications with different generic names, it can sometimes be difficult to correctly identify certain medications, especially in countries with foreign

*Table 33.2* Example of medical travel kit and supplies

| Kit and Supplies | | |
| --- | --- | --- |
| Strapping tape | Scissors | Treatment table |
| Adhesive Spray | Tape remover | Crutches |
| Massage cream | Hand sanitiser | Cryotherapy/heat apparatus |
| Acupuncture needles | Gauze | Blister care |
| Compressive stockings | Petroleum jelly | Assorted splints/slings |
| Medicines | Gloves | Self-treatment items (massage balls, stretch bands, foam rollers, resistance tubing) |

languages. This can raise issues concerning anti-doping. It can be advisable that medical practitioners travel with a certain amount of medication to avoid such issues.

Different countries have varying laws, rules and regulations regarding importation and traveling with prescription and non-prescription medication. As all countries have different laws and regulations, it is strongly advised that the appropriate local authorities are contacted prior to travelling. Most will require a detailed inventory of medications being carried and limitations of amounts and types.

> Always pay careful attention to the laws and regulations of other countries when travelling abroad.

## Registration and insurance

Prior to travelling, it is advisable that practitioners check with relevant authorities concerning the local registration laws and insurance implications. Countries will vary on what treatment they allow visiting practitioners to perform. Contacting relevant providers in the intended travel areas can assist with this. It is useful to travel with a list of local hospitals, radiology departments, pathology services and dentists in case they are required. Contacting the event organisers prior to departure can be of assistance in providing these contacts.

It is advised that the travelling practitioner contact their specific professional indemnity insurance provider to obtain a geographical extension to cover treatment of athletes in different countries. Relevant registration boards should also be contacted to confirm registration requirements for practicing within that country for short or long periods of time. For athletes, it is encouraged that they are aware of their travel or health insurance so that they are aware of what it covers in terms of injury and illness.

## Summary

Travel is an unavoidable aspect of sport for most athletes. Minimising the detrimental effects of travel is imperative to optimising performance. By understanding the effects of travel on performance and following these practical recommendations, the athlete can be adequately prepared to perform at their best, whilst reducing the risk of injury and illness.

## Notes

1 Arendt, J. (2009). Managing jet lag: Some of the problems and possible new solutions. *Sleep Med Rev*, *13*, 249–56.
2 Leatherwood, W. E., & Dragoo, J. L. (2013). Effect of airline travel on performance: A review of the literature. *Br J Sports Med*, *47*, 561–7.
3 Samuels, C. H. (2012). Jet lag and travel fatigue: A comprehensive management plan for sport medicine physicians and high-performance support teams. *Clin J Sport Med*, *22*, 268–73.
4 Forbes-Robertson, S., Dudley, E., Vadgama, P., Cook, C., Drawer, S., & Kilduff, L. (2012). Circadian disruption and remedial interventions: Effects and interventions for jet lag for athletic peak performance. *Sports Med*, *42*, 185–208.
5 Giaconia, C., Orioli, A., & Di Gangi, A. (2013). Air quality and relative humidity in commercial aircrafts: An experimental investigation on short-haul domestic flights. *Building and Environment*, *67*(9), 69–81.
6 Gavish, I., & Brenner, B. (2011). Air travel and the risk of thromboembolism. *Intern Emerg Med*, *6*, 113–6.
7 Lee, A., & Galvez, J. C. (2012). Jet lag in athletes. *Sports Health*, *4*, 211–6.
8 Herxheimer, A., & Petrie, K. J. (2002). Melatonin for the prevention and treatment of jet lag. *Cochrane Database Syst Rev*, *2*, CD001520.

# Index

ABCDE method 26, 28
acceleration: throwing 141
Achilles tendon 117, 210; tendinopathy 116, 199–200, 202, 203–4, 207–9
acid/base balance: nutrition, 34
adductors 72–3, 90, 109–10, 112–13, 115, 199, 203, 315–16, 318
Ader, Robert 23
aerobic and anaerobic energy system assessment 102
aerobic endurance: athlete development 420–1
afferent input: foot and ankle 352, 360
agility 101–2; foot and ankle 363–4
altitude: acclimation models 408–9; acute and chronic exposure 407; exercise and 406–10; illness, injury and performance risks 407–8; landings 133–6; nutrition 409; training 409, 410
amenorrhea: female athlete 432, 433
amino acids: rehab shake 35
ankle: brain response to sprained 224; landing technique 125–6; see also foot and ankle
anorexia nervosa 433
anterior cruciate ligament (ACL): case study of rehabilitation of 17–20; core stability 153; injury 5–6, 12, 63; landing injury 129; neuromuscular control during landing 127–8; rehabilitation 9
anti-catabolic agents: healing 37, 38
arginine 35, 37, 38, 39, 40
arm: throwing pain 139–40
arm cocking: throwing 140, 141
arrhythmogenic right ventricular cardiomyopathy (ARVC) 52, 53
arthrogenic muscle inhibition (AMI) 5–6, 9
asymmetries: kinetic chain 88–90, 91
athlete recovery 392, 398–9; cold-water immersion (CWI) 392, 396, 399; compression garments 396; endocrine system 393, 394; hot-water immersion (HWI) 392, 396, 399; immune system 393,

394; light exercise 394–5; neuromuscular system 392; nutrition 396–7; physiological interactions 393–4; prescribing recovery programme 397–8; pyramid of tools 398; resistance exercise 392–3; soft tissue therapies 395–6; stretching 395
athletes: circulation and vasodilation 36–7; designing a landing training program 130–6; de-training timescales 373, 374; female 429–34; immune function 37; injury equation 63–4; injury-specific supplementation 39; management of bone stress 220–1; monitoring the returning 240; neck pain 246–7; nutrition for stabilising 32–6; pain and chronically injured 228; rebuilding 36–9; regeneration 37; returning to sport 27–8; stretching training 169, 176–7; targeted spine conditioning 301; travelling 436–43; see also long-term athlete development (LTAD)
athlete sustainability program (ASP) 6
athlete triad: female 432–4
athletic development 6–7, 424, 425
athletic foundation: long-term athlete development (LTAD) 422–3
athletic kinetic chain 77–8
athletic qualities: aerobic and anaerobic energy system assessment 102; agility 101–2; jump and hop assessment 98–9; maximal power 97–8; maximal strength 96; profile, 95; rate of force development 96–7; sprinting speed 100

balance performance: foot and ankle, 356–7
basal metabolic rate (BMR) 33, 38
biomechanical analysis: kinetic chain 82
biomechanical overload syndrome: anterior 338, 341–2; centre of mass 340; extrinsic risk factors 338; features of 337–8; kinetics 340; posterior 338, 342–3; posterior chain length 344; presentation of pain 338; rare cases 344; running kinematics and 339–40;

running re-education 341–3; shoe selection and shin pain 339; walk-to-run programming 343
biomechanical stress: non-plastic structures, 11–12
biomechanics: bone injury 218, 219; landings 121–9
body composition assessment 40
body cooling: heat and exercise 404–6
body positioning: female athlete 431
bone 212; classification of stress fractures 217; health assessment methods 214; management of stress injuries 220–1; pathopsychology of chronic stress 216; risk factors for injury, 218–20; strength 214; stress injury 215–16; structure of 212–14; supplementation 39
bone mineral density (BMD) 214
brain: pain as output of 223–4; pain neurosignature 225; rehabilitation of body and 229–30
branched chain/essential amino acids (BCAAs/EAAs) 32, 33, 35, 38
bulimia nervosa 433

cardiac MRI 53
cardiac screening 50–1
case studies: back pain in female hockey team 14–15; rehabilitation of ACL injury 17–20; soccer player assessment 72–4
catecholamines: athlete recovery 393, 394
cervical spine injuries (CSI): prevalence 245–6
chop-and-lift techniques: core 166
chronically injured athlete: pain and 228
chronic exertional compartment syndrome (CECS) 337
circulation: nutrition 36–7
citrulline 35, 37, 38, 39
closed chain (CC) rehabilitation: shoulder 264–7
cognitive functional therapy: spine 298–301
cold-water immersion (CWI): athlete recovery 392, 396, 399
competition performance 20
compression garments: athlete recovery 396
concentrated flavonoid extracts 34
conditioning: spine 294, 296, 301
continuous passive motion (CPM) 4
contralateral arm mirroring 262
core 153–4; assessing competency 154–66; global core muscle performance 155, 156, 160–2; half-kneeling chop pass 160–1; keys to stabilization 167; kinetic chain 84–5; local core muscle performance 155–6, 162–6; medicine ball bounce 160, 161; movement pattern screening 155, 156; standing long jump 161–2; Y-balance test 156–9

cortical bone 212–14
cortisol 384; athlete recovery 393, 394
cortisol-modifying agents 40
countermovement jumps (CMJ) 385–6
creatine 35, 38, 40, 397
Crossed Syndromes 276
cryokinetics: foot and ankle 355

deceleration: throwing 141, 143
depth (drop) jump (DJ) 98–9
de Quervain's disease 199, 203, 204
diagnosis: hip and groin 308–10
double-limb landings 122–3, 127
dual energy X-ray absorptiometry (DXA) 214
Dynamic Relocation Test (DRT) 262
Dynamic Rotary Stability Test (DRST) 262

eating disorders: female athlete 432, 433
eccentric bias essential 192
echocardiogram (ECHO) 52; 12-lead (ECG) 51, 52
elbow: biomechanics in sport 274–5; interval golf program 287; interval tennis program 286; interval throwing program 283, 284, 285; isometric strengthening 277, 278; plyometrics 278–83; rehabilitation 275–83, 285–7; Thrower's Ten Program 276; throwing injuries 143–6
electrical stimulation: muscle injury 189–90
elite athletes: landing training program 130–6
Emotional Freedom Technique (EFT) 27
endocrine system: athlete recovery 393, 394
energy balance: nutrition 33
exercise: altitude and 406–10; body cooling 404–6; heat acclimation 404; heat and 401–5; heat gain and loss mechanisms, 402; tendinopathy management 207–8
exercise stress test 53
exit criteria: foot and ankle 353–4; muscle injury 194; neck assessment 255
explosive strength 97
external load 381
extracorporeal shock wave (ECSW) therapy: stress fractures 221
Eye Movement and Desensitisation and Reprocessing (EMDR) 27

fatigue: continuum 381; foot and ankle 360; jet lag 436–7; management 12; marker 383; muscle 79, 185; neuromuscular 385–6; throwing and 147; travelling athlete 436–7
fatty acids 35–6
Federer, Roger 79, 80
female athlete: amenorrhea 432, 433; biomechanical considerations 430–1; body positioning 431; disordered eating 432, 433; female athlete triad 432–4; hormones 431–4;

menstrual cycle 432; osteoporosis 432, 433–4; pregnancy 434; rate of force development (RFD) and power 430; strength and muscle development, 430; strength levels 429–30; training 429–30
fitness marker 383
flexibility training: athletes 169, 176–7; feedback tool 176; kinetic chain 85; periodisation of stretching 171–3; range-of-motion 169; sporting performance 170–1; stretching 169–71, 173–5
follow-through: throwing 141
foot and ankle: acute phase rehabilitation 351–2; agility 363–4; biomechanics 347–8; consequences of injury 348–9; cryokinetics 355; dynamism and ground reaction force 358–9; early afferent input 352–3; exit criteria 353–4; fatigue 360; functional kinematics 354–5; functional performance tests 361–2; impact-free rehabilitation 357–8; injury prevention 367–8; instability training 355–6; lateral and torsional stress 359–60; localized strength 357; mobile adaptor 348; motor control 360; occlusion training 361; positional variation 356; programme construction 350–1; proprioceptive/balance training 355; psychological support 353; rehabilitation 349, 350–67; return to performance 362–3, 365–6; running 347–8, 362–3; sand 359; structure 346–7; taping 366–7; testing limb symmetry 356–7; volume and load consideration 361; walking 347–8; weight-bearing training 360
foot placement: running mechanics 116–19
foot posture: landing 127
force-time graph: landing 125
front foot contact (FFC): throwing 140, 144, 145
functional kinematics: foot and ankle 354–5
Functional Movement Screen 156
Functional Movement Systems (FMS) 155
functional performance: assessments 237–8; foot and ankle 361–2
functional stability threshold (FST) 259, 260
FUNdamental: athlete development 418
fundamental movement screen (FMS) 421

gender: bone injury 218
generic warning index (GWI) 64–5, 72, 73
gingko biloba 32, 37, 39
glenohumeral internal rotation deficiency (GIRD) 89, 148, 203, 263
glenohumeral joint (GHJ) 140, 259, 266
glutamine 35, 38, 40
gluteus maximus 117, 118, 196, 261, 313, 315
gluteus medius 85, 109, 315

gluteus minimus 313, 315
glycine 32, 33, 35, 39
golf: interval program 287
gravitational forces (Gz): neck injuries 245, 247, 249
green tea 32, 33, 34, 39
groin see hip and groin
Groth, Samuel 86, 87
ground reaction force (GRF): bone 218–19; foot and ankle 346–7, 349, 358, 362; kinetic chain 83; knee 323–5, 328–9; landing 122–5, 127; maximal power 97; running 106, 108, 115; shin pain 338, 342
growth hormone (GH): athlete recovery 393, 394

hamstring: rehabilitation 17–20, 190, 191; running 112–13
healing process: anti-catabolic agents 38; meals supporting 33
heart rate: internal load measure 381–2
heart rate recovery (HRR) 383
heart rate variability (HRV) 383–4, 389
heat: acclimation 404; body cooling 404–6; exercise and 401–5; gain and loss mechanisms 402; illness, injury and performance risks 403–7
heel-off running 107, 108, 116–18
hip and groin: anatomical diagnosis 308–10; biomechanical assessment of 310–12; differential diagnosis 308; level 1 performance 312, 313–16; level 2 performance 312, 316–18; level 3 performance 312, 318–19; level 4 performance 312, 319–20; magnetic resonance imaging (MRI) 309–10; presenting problem 307–8; rehabilitation 312–20; return to competition 320
hips: landing technique 125–6; range of motion 313–14; running 118–19
hockey players: back pain in female 14–15
Holter test, 24-hour 53
holy basil 40
hop and stop: core 155, 156, 161–2
hormones: female athlete 431–4
hot-water immersion (HWI): athlete recovery 392, 396, 399
hydration: travelling athlete 438, 440–1
hypothalamic-pituitary-adrenal (HPA) axis, feedback system 23

ice: muscle injury 187
iliopsoas 89, 110–14, 118, 203, 308–9, 314–15
imaging 49: muscle injury 186; tendinopathy 204
imbalances: kinetic chain 88, 90, 91
immune action: support and stimulation 37, 38
immune system: athlete recovery 393, 394

impact-free rehabilitation: foot and ankle 357–8

inflammation: eating to support and regulate 34; fatty acids 35–6; immune system reaction 36; step-by-step guide 34

injured athlete: reducing anxiety in 25–6

injury: kinetic chain 79–80

injury performance: landing training 129

injury prevention 11–12, 28; assessing susceptibility 68–9; foot and ankle 367–8; muscle re-injury 195–6; neck 256; throwing 143–6

injury risk model 13–14; factors 13; training interventions 14

injury risk profiling 62–3; assessments 68–70, 73–4; case study 72–4; developing a screening tool 64–71; disrupting injury equation 63–4; generic warning index (GWI) 64–5, 72, 73; risk factors 67; screening frequency 71–2; specific warning index (SWI) 66, 73

in-season training 373; balancing training and recovery 374–6; strength and power strategies, 376–7

instability training: foot and ankle 355–6

insurance: travelling athlete 443

internal impingement: throwing 142–3

internal load: heart rate 381–2

jet lag: travelling athlete 436–7

joint position sense (JPS) 260, 264, 266

joint stress: kinetic chain 80

jump and hop assessment 98–9

kinetic chain 77, 91; assessing 80; asymmetries 88–90, 91; biomechanical analysis 82; developing 83; flexibility training 85; hip and groin 316–17; imbalances 88, 90, 91; injury 79–80; knee 323–4; musculoskeletal screening 82, 83; neck as part of 250; performance 78–9, 81–2; plyometric training 84; sport-specific training 83–4; technical correction 85, 88; tests of 81; training movements 83–4; training the core 84–5; types and variations of athletic 77–8; weightlifting 84

knee: force-absorber and force-generator 322–3; kinetic chain 323–4; landing technique, 125–6; load-compromised athlete 334–5

knee rehabilitation: capacity to decelerate 330–1; phases of 324–34; protection and healing 325–7; reactivation of muscles 326–7; removing effusions 325–6; return to contact training 332–4; return to function 328–31; return to performance 331–4; sand-based training 331–2; strength and motion 327–8; trampoline drills 332

landings: athlete training for injury prevention 129; biomechanics of 121–9; considerations for good technique 125–9; developing ability 133–6; mobility development 133; monitoring load 136; training program design for elite athletes 130–6; wrong 129

lateral and torsional stress: foot and ankle 359–60

lifting see Olympic lifting

light exposure: travelling athlete 437, 439

limb symmetry: foot and ankle 356–7

load compromised athlete (LCA) 5–6; knee injury 334–5

load transfer: hip and groin 317

localized strength: foot and ankle 357

long-term athlete development (LTAD): aerobic endurance 420–1; athletic development 424, 425; athletic foundation 422–3; FUNdamental 418; models of 417–19, 422–7; motor skill development 419; optimal sports performance 415–16; performance actualisation 425, 426, 427; performance development 424–5, 426; physical literacy 419; rationale for 416–17; skilled performance 421; speed 420; strength 420; trainability of youth 419–21; training to compete 419; training to train 418; training to win 419; windows of opportunity 419–21

low back pain (LBP) 91, 289, 291–4, 296–7, 302

lower-limb, throwing 148–9

lysine 40

magnetic resonance imaging (MRI): hip and groin 309–10; muscle injury 186; tendinopathy 204

maximal power 97–8

maximal strength 96

medial tibial stress syndrome (MTSS) 337, 338, 342–3

medical examination: health screening 49; imaging studies 49; neurological screening 48–9; respiratory disease screening 48; travelling athlete 441–3

medical history, 47–8, 51–2; form, 54–9

medications: muscle injury 188

medicine ball throws: core 155, 160, 161

melatonin 437, 440

menstrual cycle: female athlete 432

mobile adaptor: foot and ankle 348

mobility development: landing technique 133

monitoring training load: biochemical markers 384; cortisol 384; countermovement jumps (CMJ) 385–6; data analysis 387–8; day-to-day application 388, 389; dose-response relationship 380–1; fatigue 381, 383; fitness

383; heart rate 381–2; heart rate recovery (HRR) 383; heart rate variability (HRV) 383–4; interpreting data 386–7; muscle damage 384; neuromuscular fatigue 385–6; physiological markers 383; quantifying 381; rating of perceived exertion (RPE) 382, 387, 389; salivary *vs.* blood markers 385; testosterone 384; testosterone/cortisol ratio 385; wellness inventories 383

motor control: foot and ankle 360; spine 292–3

movement pattern screening: core 155, 156

movement proficiency: assessment 69–70, 74

movement training: spine 299–300

multidimensional speed and agility (MDSA) 9–10

multidirectional performance: hip and groin 318–19

muscle 183–4; architecture 183; damage 384; fibre type 183; function 181–2; injury process 184–5; pathophysiology 185; plasticity of 184; structure 183

muscle injury: acute phase 187–90; dynamic correspondence 192; eccentric bias essential 192; electrical stimulation and occlusion training 189–90; exit criteria 194; grading 186–7; hamstring rehabilitation 191; ice 187; loading 188; managing 187–95; preventing re-injury 195–6; progressive loading 190–4; reconditioning 193; repair 185; return to running 192; return to training and performance 194–5; role of imaging in 186; specific testing 194–5

muscle slack 112

muscle tendon junction (MTJ) 183–4

muscle tendon unit (MTU): as force amplifier 182; imaging 186; as shock absorber 182

musculoskeletal screening: kinetic chain 82, 83

musculoskeletal system: role of tendons 199–200

neck: assessment 248–9; characteristics of healthy 247–50; exit criteria 255; injury prevention 256; managing injuries 250–5; pain in athletes 246–7; part of kinetic chain 250; prevalence of injuries in sport 245–6; return to performance 255

neurological screening 48–9

neuromatrix 224–6; sports 226–7

neuromuscular control: landing 127–8

neuromuscular fatigue 385–6, 389

neuromuscular system: athlete recovery 392

neurosignatures: pain 224–6

nutrition: acid/base balance 34; altitude training 409; athlete recovery 396–7; deficiencies 34; energy balance 33; fatty acids 35–6; injury-specific supplementation 39;

rebuilding the athlete 36–9; regeneration 37; return to competition 39–40; stabilising the athlete 32–6; strategies 31, 32; travelling athlete 438, 440–1

obliques 154, 276, 315

occlusion training: foot and ankle 361; muscle injury 189–90

Olympic lifting: landing training program 130–3

one-repetition maximum (1RM) 96, 97

optimal sports performance 415–16

ornithine alpha ketoglutarate (OAKG) 35, 37, 38

osteoporosis: female athlete 432, 433–4

over-stretching: muscle 185

over-striding: running danger 115

overtraining syndrome 381

oxytocin 23–4

pain: challenge of 223; chronically injured athlete 228; neuromatrix and neurosignatures 224–6; output of brain 223–4; personal experiences 227; sporting performance 227–8; tendon 206–7

pain neuromatrix 224–6

patellar tendon 83, 121, 126, 199, 202–4, 206, 208–10, 323, 330

pathophysiology: chronic bone stress 216; muscle injury 185

peel back phenomenon: throwing, 143

pelvis: injury-free running, 110–11; throwing, 144

performance: jet lag, 437; kinetic chain, 78–9, 81–2

performance actualisation: long-term athlete development (LTAD) 425, 426, 427

performance development: LTAD 424–5, 426

performance model 8

peripheral quantitative computed tomography (pQCT) 214, 215

physical examination 51–2

placebo effect 24, 25, 396

plantar fascia 199, 203, 347

plyometrics: elbow 278–83; kinetic chain 84; knees 328, 334; shoulder 267–70

positional variation: foot and ankle 356

positive psychology interventions (PPIs) 25–6, 28

positive running model 108–9

post-traumatic stress disorder (PTSD) 26–7

posture: hip and groin 313

power training, 376–7

pregnancy: female athlete 434

pre-habilitation needs 50

pre-participation screening (PPS) 45, 46; cardiac MRI 53; cardiac screening 50–1;

consequences of process 49–50;
echocardiogram 52; elite 46; exercise stress
test 53; Holter test 53; medical examination
48–9; medical history 51–2, 54–9; physical
examination 51–2; process 46–8
pre-season training 373; balancing training
and recovery 374–6
Profile of Mood State Questionnaire 382
proprioception: foot and ankle 355
protein synthesis: regeneration 37
psychology 22; ABCDE method 26;
application of theory in practice 25–6;
identifying psychological ill health 26–7;
injury prevention 28; motivation 26;
psychological health, 28–9; reducing anxiety
in injured athlete 25–6; returning to sport
27–8; support for foot and ankle 353;
theoretical basis of rehabilitation 22–4;
thoughts and beliefs in rehabilitation, 24
psychoneuroimmunology (PNI) 22, 25
pycogenol 37

quadratus lumborum 67, 89, 162

rapid eccentric/active lengthening contraction:
muscle 184
rate of force development (RFD) 96–7; female
athlete 429, 430
rating of perceived exertion (RPE) 20, 382,
387, 389
reactive agility test (RAT) 101–2, 364
reconditioning: 4; model 5, 6
recovery strategies: athletes 394–5
red blood cell analysis 34, 35
regeneration: nutrition 37
registration: travelling athlete 443
rehabilitation 3, 229; brain and body 229–30;
closed chain 264–7; competition
performance 20; criteria-driven approach
16; elbow 275–83, 285–7; end-stage 235,
236; foot and ankle 350–67; hip and groin
312–20; integrated scapulothoracic 271–2;
knee 324–34; model of 233; neck injuries
250–5; philosophy 349; psychology 22–4;
quantifying process 236–7; restoration of
sensorimotor system 264; restoration of
shoulder functional range of motion 263,
264; return to throwing 149; running 114;
scapula 270–2; shoulder 262, 263; strength
and conditioning 15–16, 20; success of 240–1;
tendinopathy 208; thoughts and beliefs in
24; throwing 149, 152
rehabilitation needs 50
rehab shakes 35
resistance exercise: athlete recovery 392–3

respiratory disease screening 48
return to competition: hip and groin 320
Return to Competition (RtC), 3, 4; model of
transition from injury, 233; nutrition, 39–40;
phases, 7–8
return to contact training: knees 332–4
return-to-performance (RTP): criteria 95–6,
103; end-stage rehabilitation 235, 236; foot
and ankle 365–6; knees 331–4; neck 255;
rehabilitation programme 234–5
return to play: spine pain 302
Return to Play (RTP) 7–8; monitoring
returning athlete 240; role of coach 239–40;
sport- and position-specific testing 238, 239;
strength and conditioning (S&C) 232;
success of rehabilitation 240–1; training vs.
fitness test 239
Return to Running Program 9, 10, 192, 328
return to sport: tendon pain recovery 209–10
Reuleaux, Franz 77
rhodioloa rosea 40
risk see injury risk profiling
risk factors: bone injury 218–20; injury risk
model 13; lower back pain 14; sporting
injuries 67
rotator cuff: importance of 261
rugby tackle: functional joint instability 260
rugby training: exit criteria 194; field testing
238, 239
runners: tibial stress fracture 338
running: accelerated program 193; foot and
ankle 347–8; hip and groin 318; kinematics,
339–40; re-education 341–3; return to 192,
362–3; technique philosophies 339; walk-to-
run programming 343
running-based anaerobic spring test
(RAST) 102
running mechanics: foot placement 116–19;
full contact 115–16; hamstring loading
phase 112, 113; heel-off 116–17; heel-off
to toe-off 118–19; importance of pelvis
110–11; injury 112–19; muscle slack 112;
over-striding danger 115; positive running
model 108–9; running cycle 106–8;
scissors motion 114–16; toe-off posture
109–10, 112; transverse plane movements
117–18

salivary vs. blood markers 385
sand-based training: foot and ankle 359; knees
331–2
scapula: importance of 261; rehabilitation of,
270–2
schizandra 40
scissors motion: running 114–16

screening: assessment frequency 71–2; benefits of 46; cardiac 50–1; principles of 45–6; *see also* pre-participation screening (PPS)
secretagogues 37, 40
shin pain: biomechanical overload syndrome 337–8; biomechanical overload syndrome (BOS) 337, 344; shoe selection 339
shoulder: assessment of integrated function 261–2; closed chain rehabilitation 264–7; dynamic defence of 260–1; functional stability threshold 259, 260; integrated scapulothoracic rehabilitation 271–2; plyometrics 267–70; range of motion 148; rehabilitation 262, 263; rehabilitation of scapula 270–2; restoration of functional range of motion 263, 264; rotator cuff importance 261; restoration of sensorimotor system 264; scapula importance 261; strength 148
shoulder abduction: throwing 144, 146
shoulder injuries: throwing 139, 142–3
side-lying external rotation (SLER) 194, 266, 268
single-limb landings 122, 126–7
sleep: travelling athlete 440
soft-tissue injuries: supplementation 39
soft tissue therapies: athlete recovery 395–6
specific warning index 66, 73
speed: athlete development 420
spine pain: assessment and monitoring tools 302; assessment framework for athletes 290; characteristics 291–2; cognitive functional therapy 298–301; diagnosis 291; extrinsic factors 292; injury mechanism 289, 291; intrinsic factors 292–7; management planning 297–8; managing acute 297–8; prevention 302; psychological factors 296–7; return to play 302; team approach 302–3
sports: applying neuromatrix paradigm in 226–7; conditioning hip and groin 317–18; elbow biomechanics 274–5; field testing 238, 239; massage for athlete recovery 395–6; pain and performance 227–8; stretching after 174–5; stretching before 173–4
sport-specific training: hip and groin 319–20; kinetic chain 83–4
sprained ankle: brain response to 224
sprinting speed 100
standing long jump: core, 155, 161–2
strength: athlete development 420; athletic 96; female athlete 429–30; landing training program 130–3
strength and conditioning (S&C) 11, 232; case studies 14–15, 17–20; coach 20, 232;

end-stage rehabilitation 236; foot and ankle 352–3, 357–8, 360, 365–6; injury prevention 11–12; injury risk model 13–15; rehabilitation 15–16, 20; return to competition model 233
strength training 376–7
stress injuries: bone 215–16; classification of fractures 217
stress-strain index (SSI) 214
stretching 169–71; after exercise 174–5; athlete recovery 395; avoiding 176; before exercise 173–4; periodisation of 171–3; pre-exercise programme design 174, 175; training program 173–5
stride: throwing 140, 143
striding out: landing 126–7
sudden cardiac arrest (SCA) 50–1
sudden cardiac death (SCD) 50–1
supplementation: injury-specific 39

taping: foot and ankle 366–7
team approach: spine pain 302–3
technical correction: kinetic chain 85, 88
tendinopathy: Achilles 208; diagnosing 204; imaging 204; management of 199; mobility and weakness 203; patellar 208; principles of exercise prescription 207–8; progression to 201–4; rehabilitation 208; risk factors 201–2; staging 205–6
tendon: in-season load management 209; pain 205; pain management 206–7; returning to sports 209–10; role of tenocyte in function 200–1; role within musculoskeletal system 199–200
tennis: interval program 286
testosterone 384; athlete recovery 393, 394
testosterone/cortisol ratio 385
Thrower's Ten Program 276
throwing: golf 287; interval program 284, 285; tennis 286
throwing mechanics: analysis of biomechanics 140–2; arm pain 139–40; assessment of 146, 149, 152; elbow injuries 143–6; fatigue 147; lower-limb 148–9; physical adaptations in throwers 148; rehabilitation 149, 152; shoulder injuries 142–3; trunk function 148–9; whole body motions 139, 149–50; workloads 146–7
time under tension (TUT): training 261, 340, 373, 376–7
toe-off: running, 107, 108–12, 114, 117–19
trabecular bone 212–14
training: around injury 4–5; athlete development 418–19; balancing recovery and 374–6; de-training timescales 373–4;

developmental 375; developmental stimuli 373–4; maintenance 376; stretching in program 173–5; *see also* in-season training; monitoring training load; pre-season training
training load 136
training movement: kinetic chain 83–4
trampoline: gravitational forces 254; knee-injured athlete 331, 332
transverse plane movements: running 117–18
travelling athlete: fatigue 436–7; hydration 440–1; jetlag 436–7; medical considerations 441–3; melatonin 440; nutrition 438, 440–1; planning travel 437–9; registration and insurance 443; sleep hygiene 440; vaccination 442
TRIMP (Training Impulse) concept 382
trophy position 85, 86
trunk flexion: throwing 144
trunk function: throwing 148–9
trunk motion: landing 128–9
trunk rotation: throwing 144
turmeric 33, 38

ultrasound (US): muscle injury 186
ultraviolet B (UVB) radiation: bone injury 218
upper body propulsion: hip and groin 319

vaccinations: travelling athlete 442
vasodilation: nutrition 36–7
vitamin C 32, 39, 40
vitamin D: bone injury 218
volume/load training: foot and ankle 361

walking: foot and ankle 347–8
warning index 64–5, 72, 73
weight-bearing training: foot and ankle 360
weightlifting: kinetic chain 84
wellness 383, 389
workloads: throwing 146–7
World Anti-Doping Agency (WADA) 37, 39, 440

Y-balance test: core 156–9
youth: athlete development 419–21